Advance praise for *The Bad Doctor*

'This unputdownable graphic novel, like all great literature, makes you feel slightly less alone. Ian Williams gently points out what's under our noses but what we might not yet have managed to articulate. It shows us – through good observation and by being funny – how the ordinary is extraordinary.'
—Philippa Perry

'Skilfully told, relentlessly honest, often funny and painfully true… this is courageous work. It undercuts the accepted nonsense that doctors are – or should be expected to be – seraphic beings, exalted above the rest of humanity. It should be read by every student and practising professional out there, and in the larger world as well. Ian Williams is my hero and I wish he were my doctor, too!'
—David Small

'Amazing… crafted with a consistent wit in which the cartoon narrator spares himself no less than his patients. This profoundly honest doctor pursues his humanitarian mission while exorcising personal demons. Williams gives us a dose of insight and laughter that is germane not only to the comics medium, but also to medicine itself.'
—Justin Green

'A helpful, insightful adventure into the dynamic of the doctor/patient relationship. *The Bad Doctor*'s elegant renderings illuminate the mind and explore the relationships that don't always have a happy ending. A very original and honest view of a highly personal examination of the human psyche.'
—Ron Turner, Last Gasp Comics

The BAD DOCTOR

IAN WILLIAMS

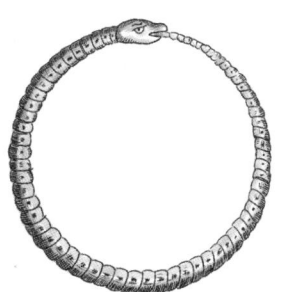

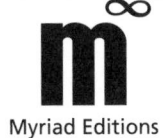

Myriad Editions

First published in 2014 by

Myriad Editions
59 Lansdowne Place
Brighton BN3 1FL, UK

www.myriadeditions.com

1 3 5 7 9 10 8 6 4 2

A CIP catalogue record for this book is available from
the British Library.

ISBN: 978-1-908434-28-9

Printed in Lithuania on paper sourced from sustainable forests.

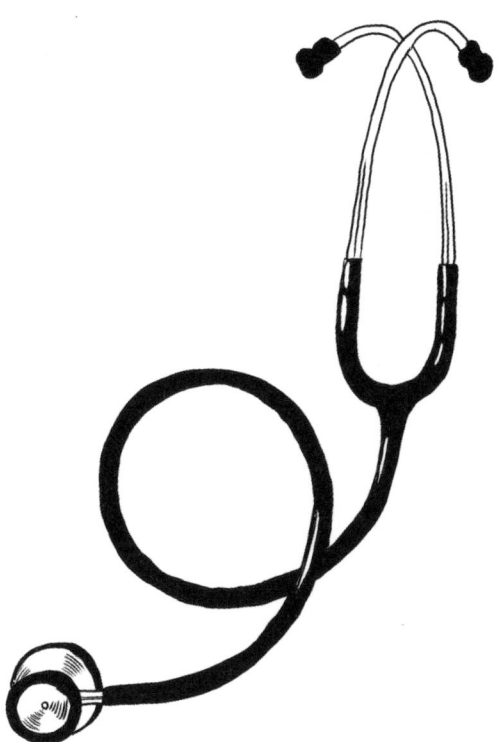

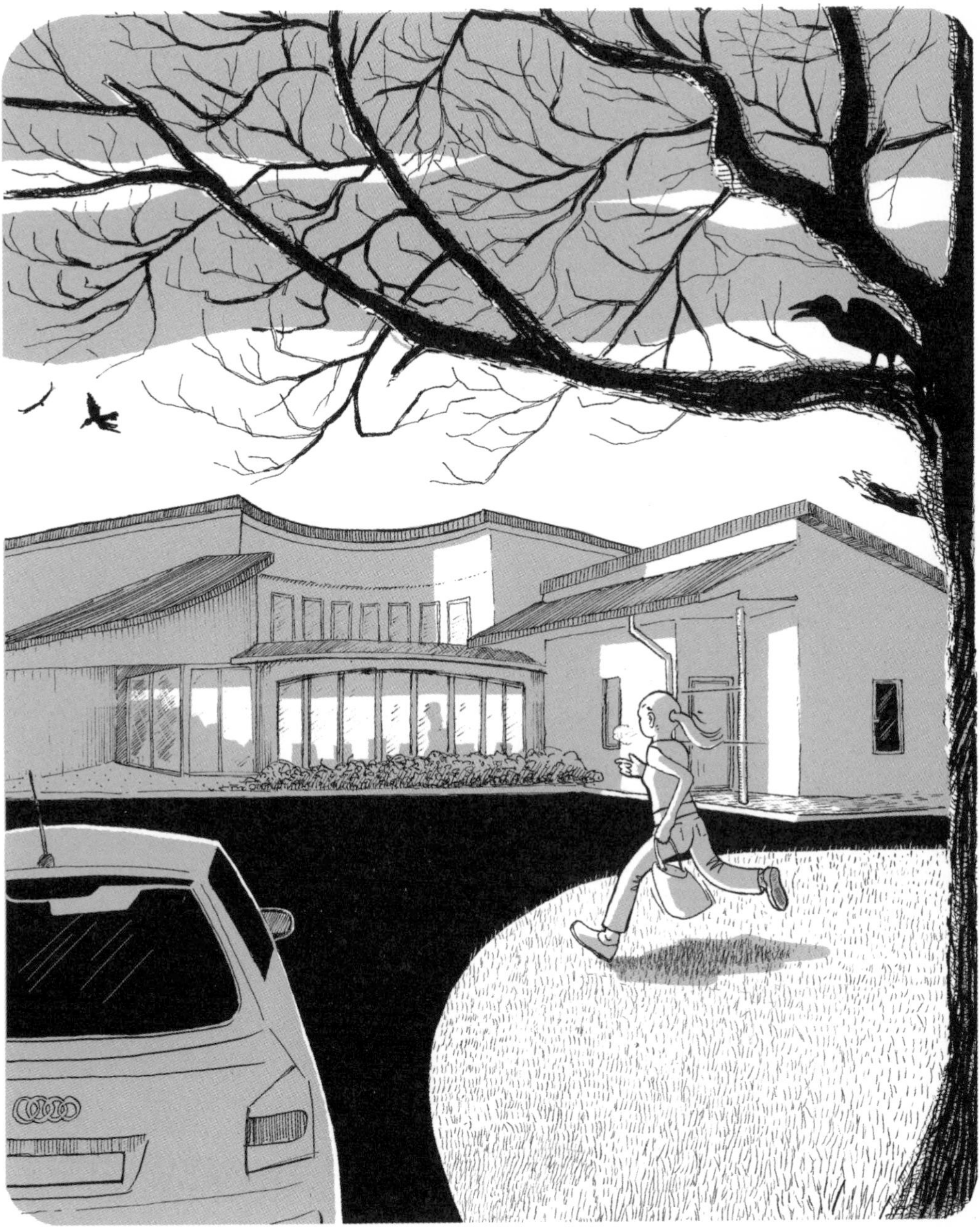

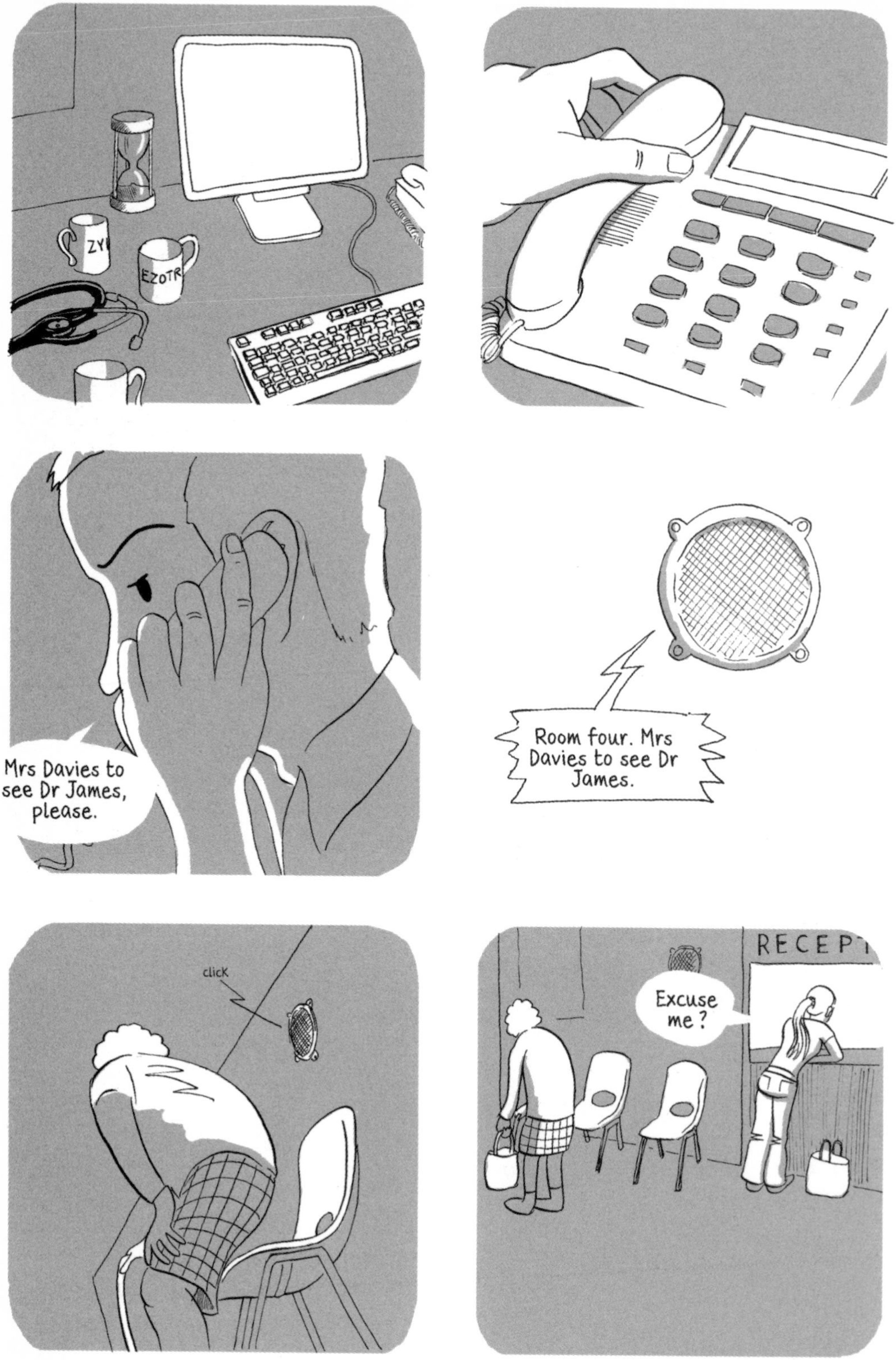
Mrs Davies to see Dr James, please.
Room four. Mrs Davies to see Dr James.
click
RECEPT
Excuse me?

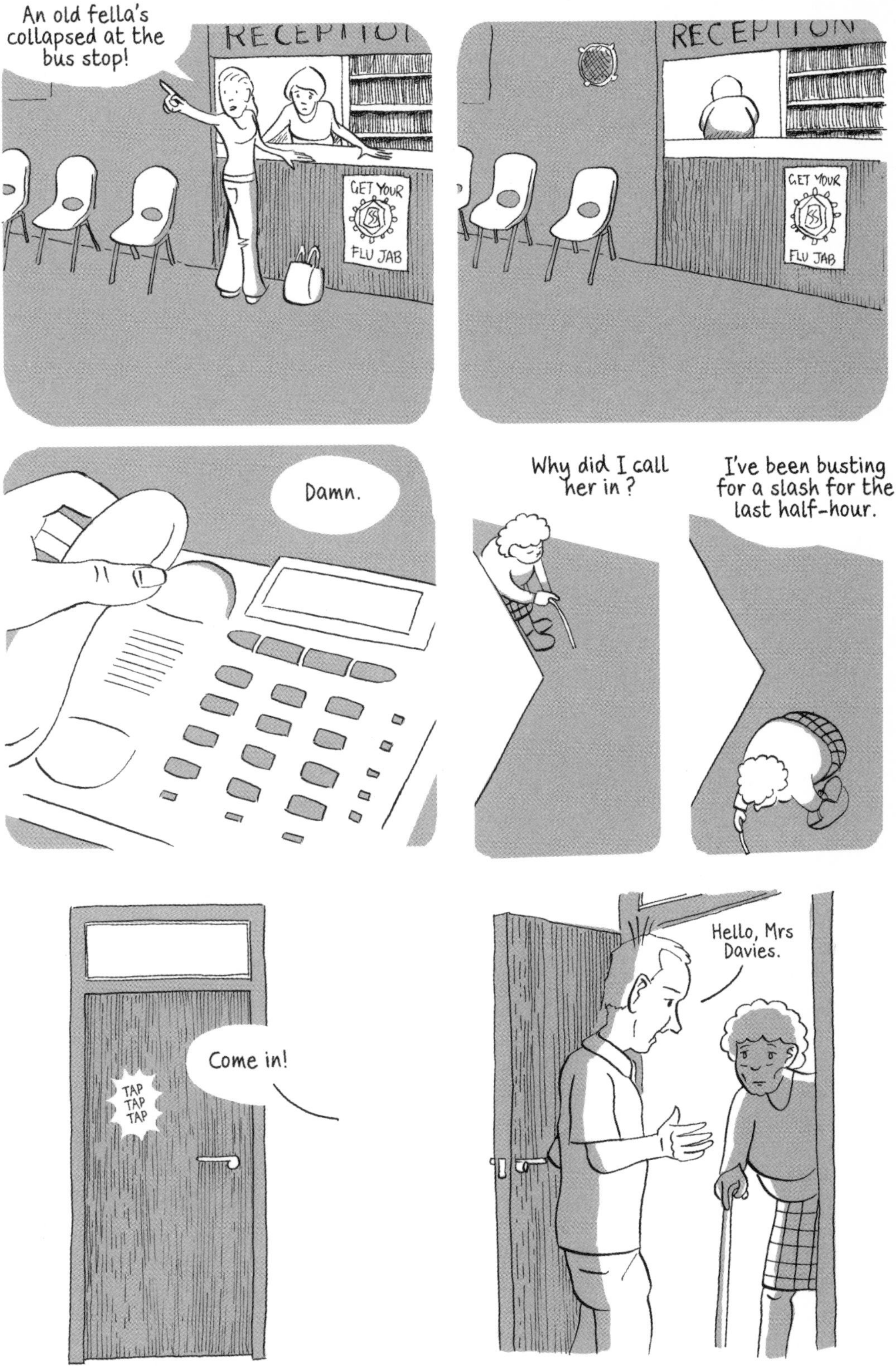
An old fella's collapsed at the bus stop!
RECEPTION
GET YOUR FLU JAB
RECEPTION
GET YOUR FLU JAB
Damn.
Why did I call her in?
I've been busting for a slash for the last half-hour.
TAP TAP TAP
Come in!
Hello, Mrs Davies.

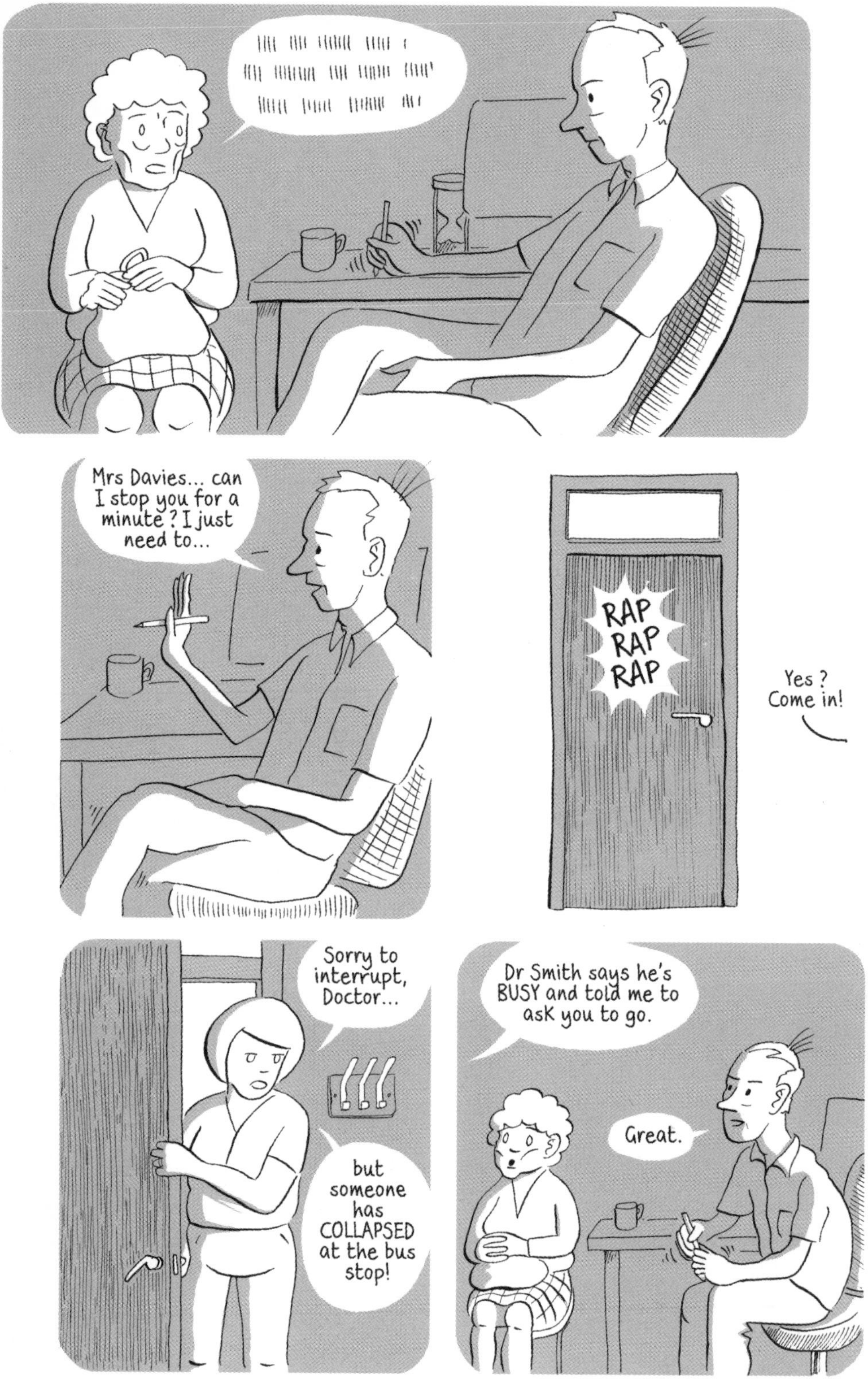

Mrs Davies... can I stop you for a minute? I just need to...
RAP RAP RAP
Yes? Come in!
Sorry to interrupt, Doctor...
but someone has COLLAPSED at the bus stop!
Dr Smith says he's BUSY and told me to ask you to go.
Great.

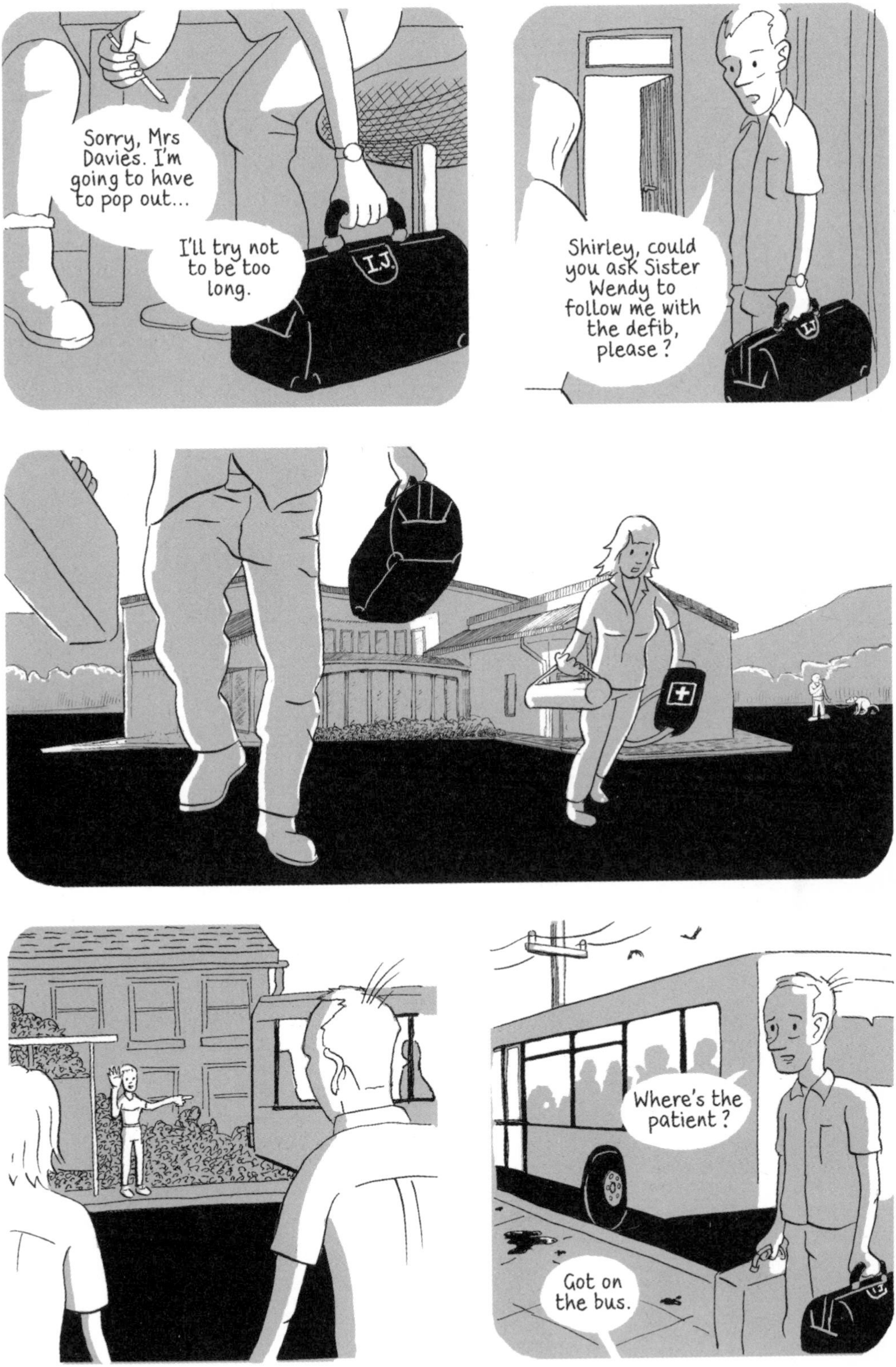
Sorry, Mrs Davies. I'm going to have to pop out...
I'll try not to be too long.
I.J.
Shirley, could you ask Sister Wendy to follow me with the defib, please?
Where's the patient?
Got on the bus.

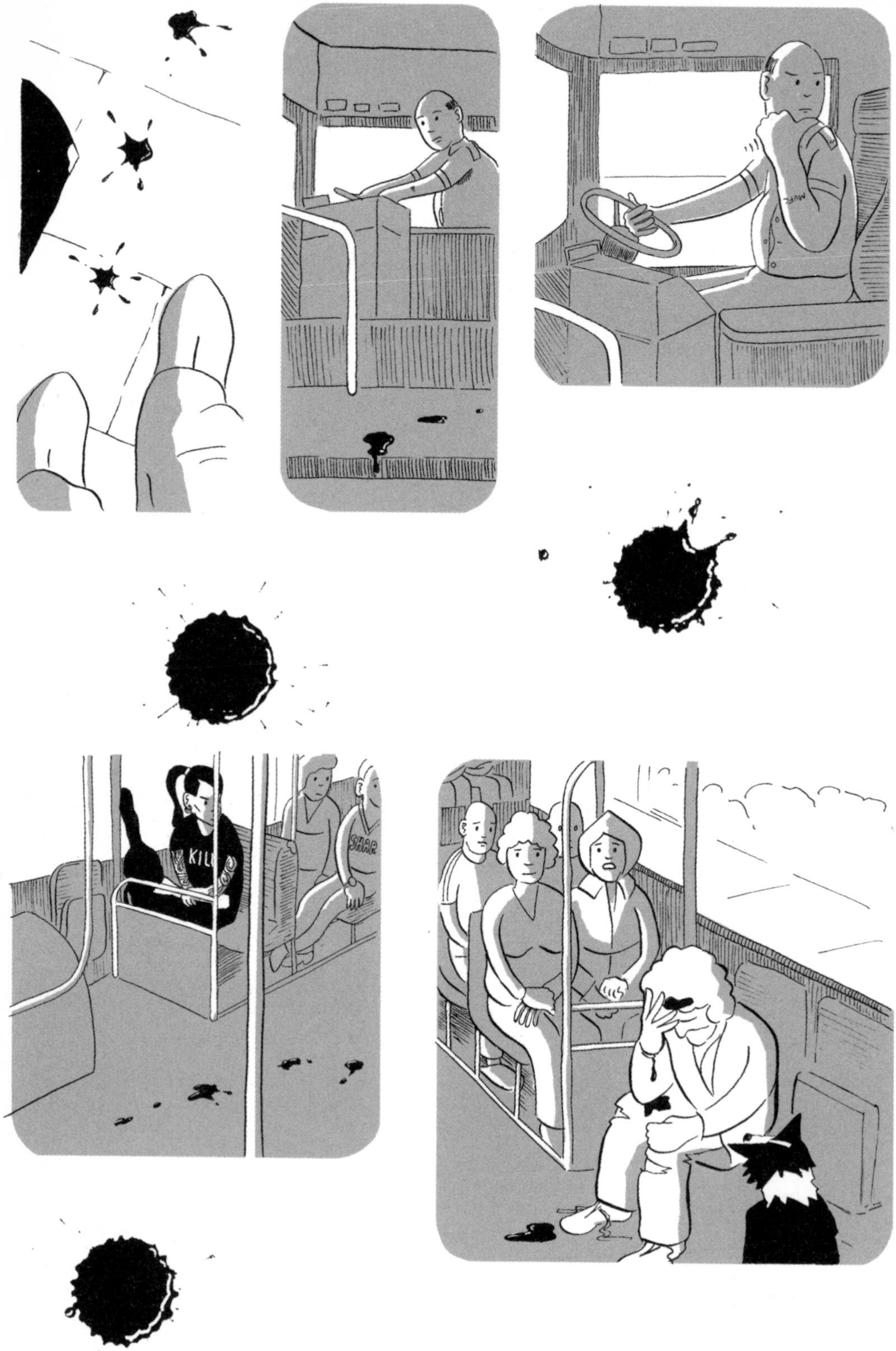

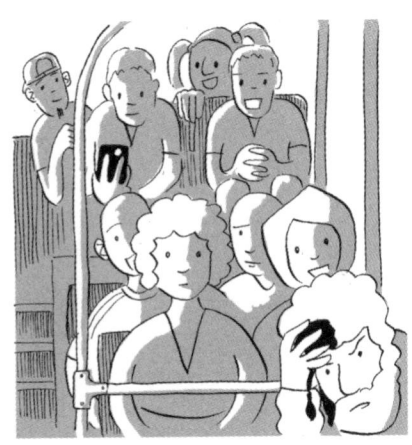

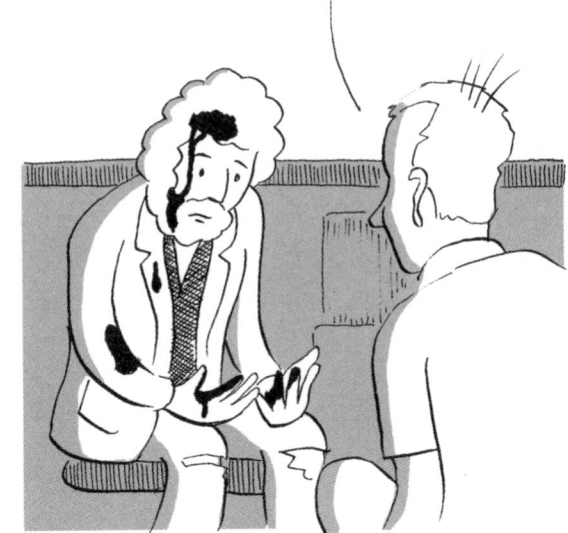

Hello, sir, I'm Dr James.

What happened?

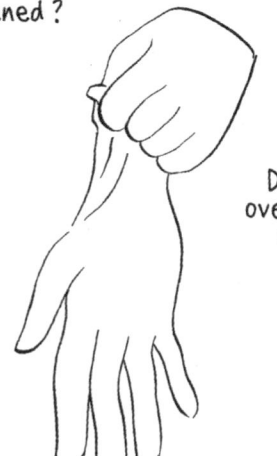

Did you trip over or did you collapse?

Can I have a look?

Iwan...

You gettin' this shit, bud?

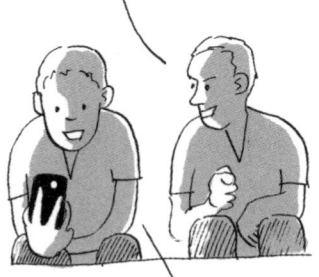

Yeah! Heheheh.

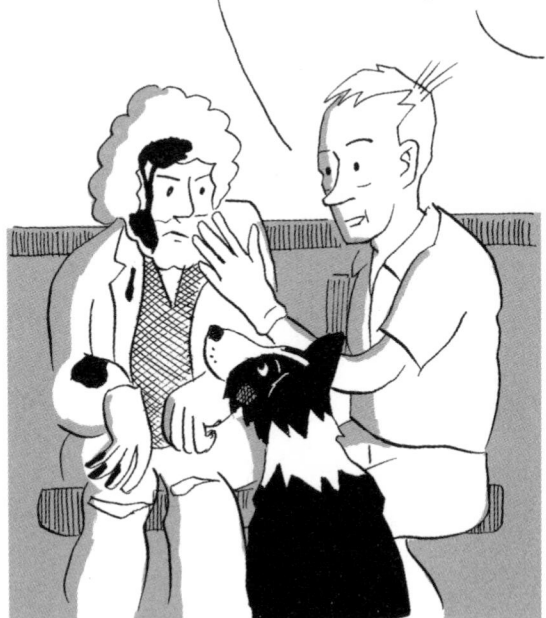

GERROFFF!

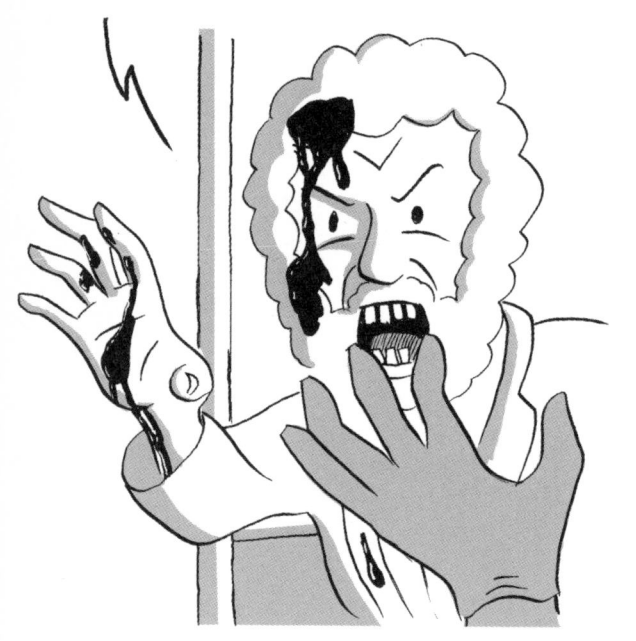

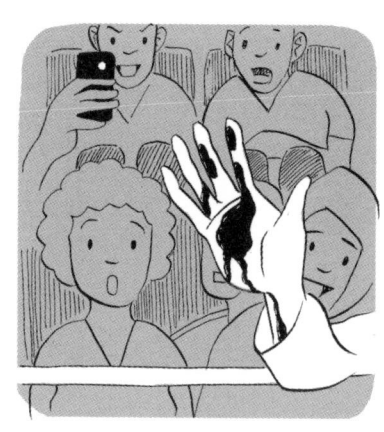

OK... how about coming back to the surgery so we can...

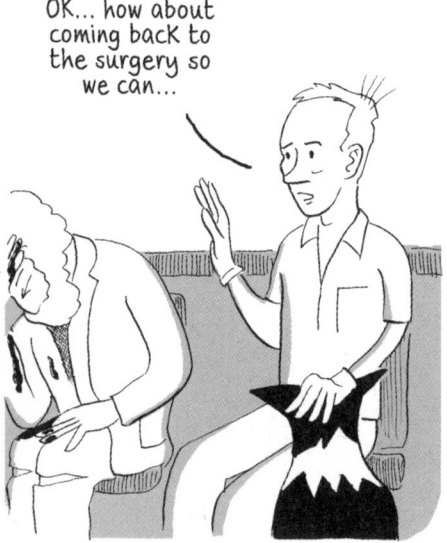

DON'T TOUCH THE DOG!

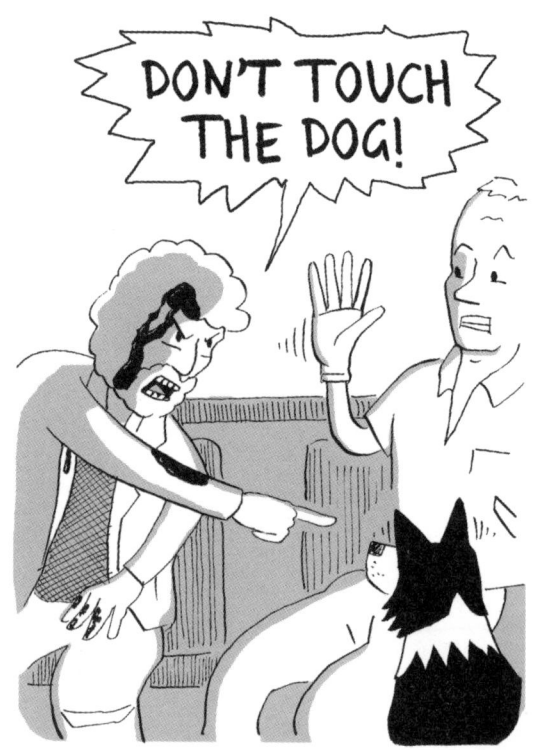

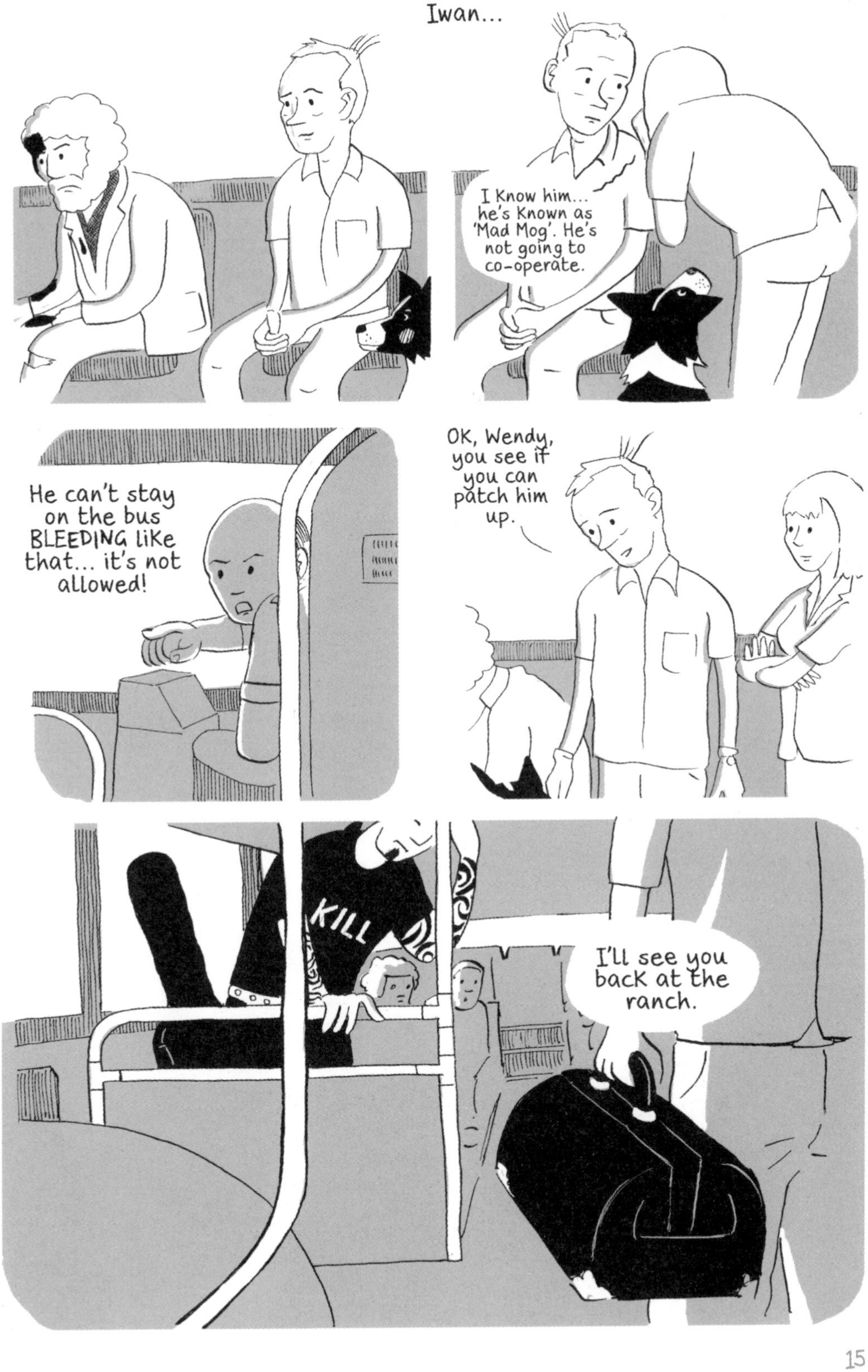

Iwan...
I know him... he's known as 'Mad Mog'. He's not going to co-operate.
He can't stay on the bus BLEEDING like that... it's not allowed!
OK, Wendy, you see if you can patch him up.
KILL
I'll see you back at the ranch.

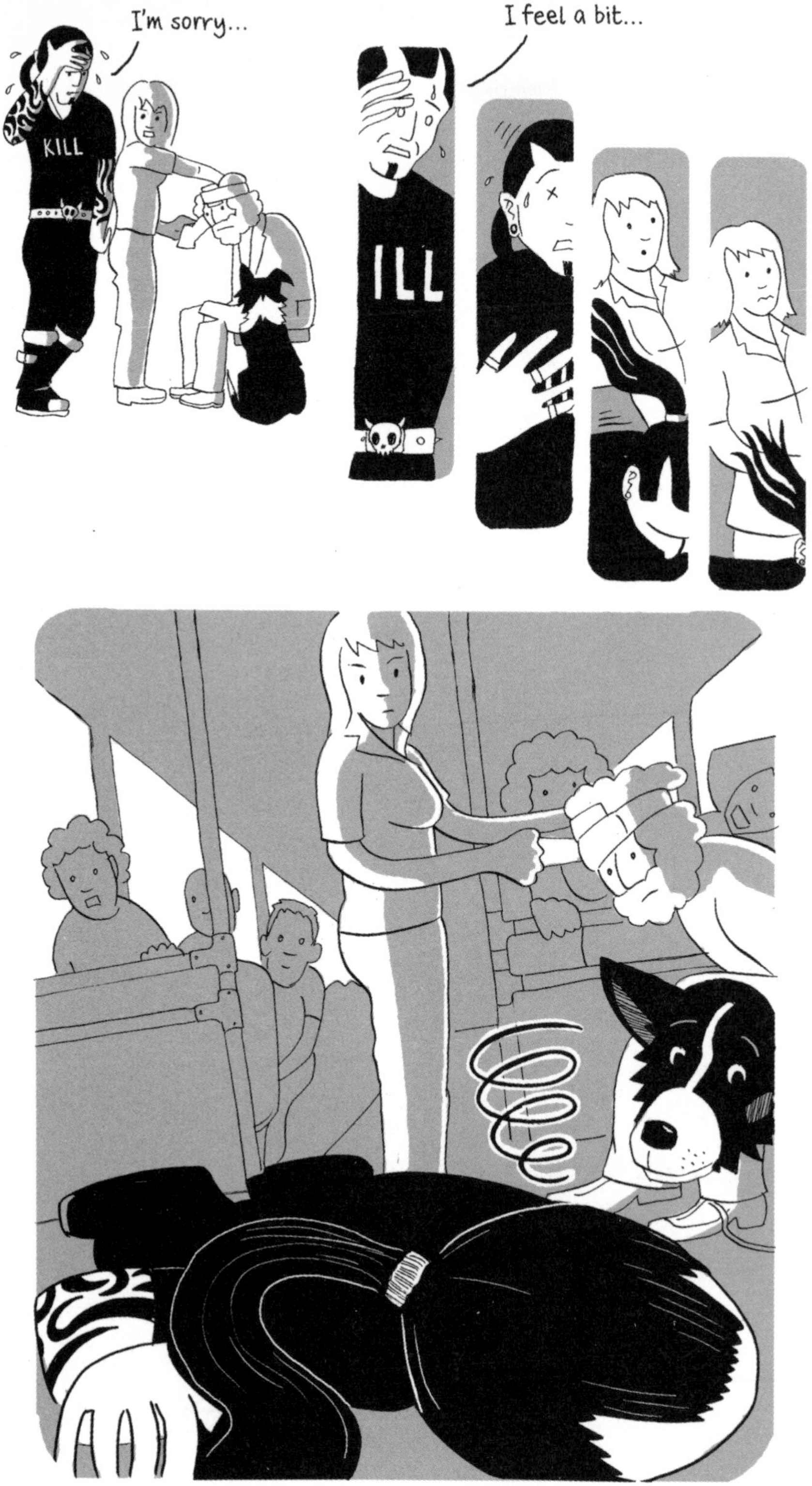
I'm sorry...
KILL
I feel a bit...
ILL

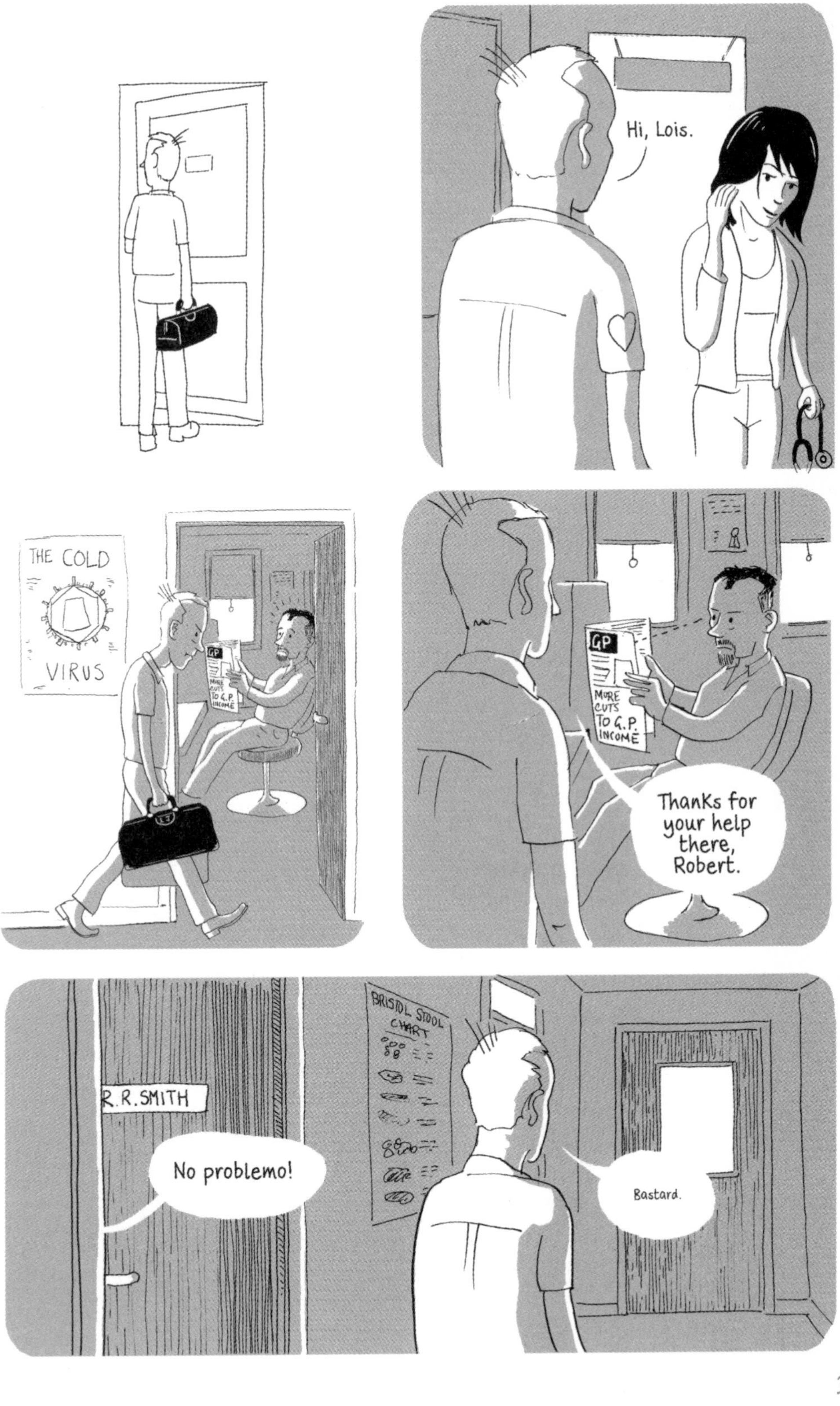
Hi, Lois.
THE COLD VIRUS
GP
MORE CUTS TO G.P. INCOME
GP
MORE CUTS TO G.P. INCOME
Thanks for your help there, Robert.
BRISTOL STOOL CHART
R.R.SMITH
No problemo!
Bastard.

STAFF TOILE
SIGH.
OK, I'm back!
DR I. JAMES
Sorry to keep you waiting, Mrs Dav...
I.J
Thank FUCK she's gone!

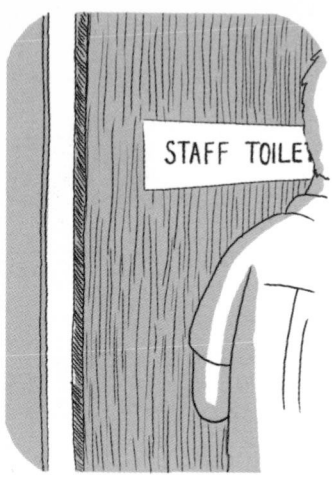

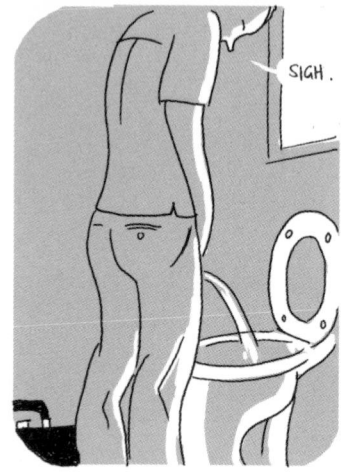

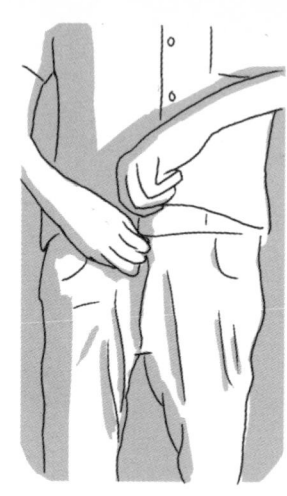

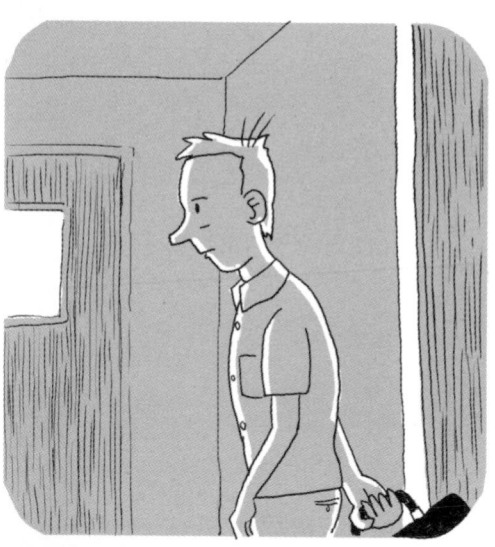

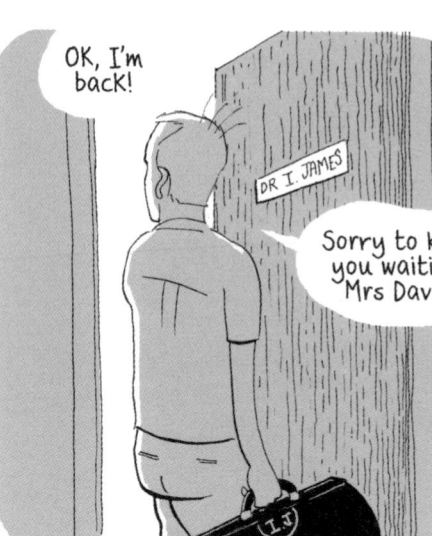

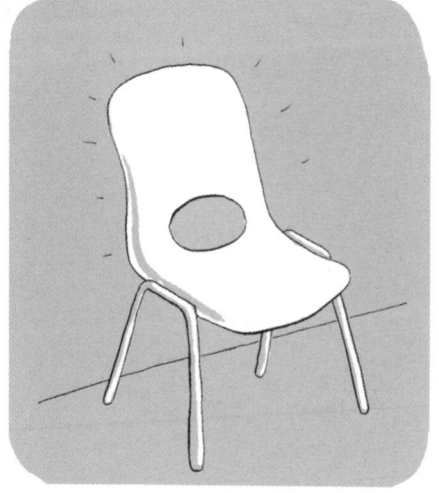

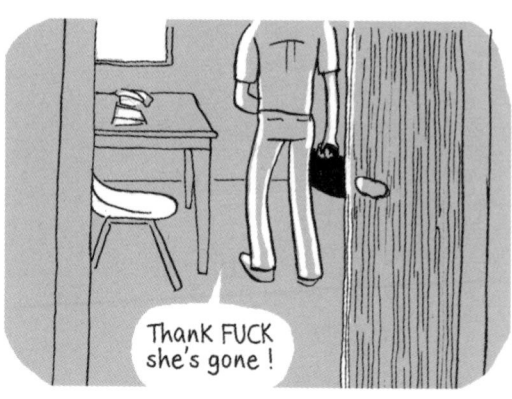

(SIGH)
Who's next then ?

Lovely photographs, Doctor!

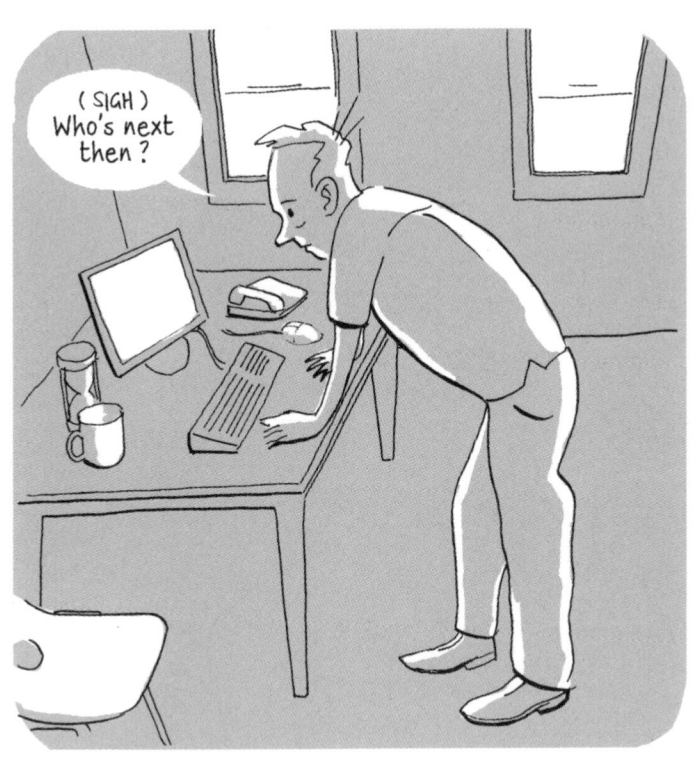

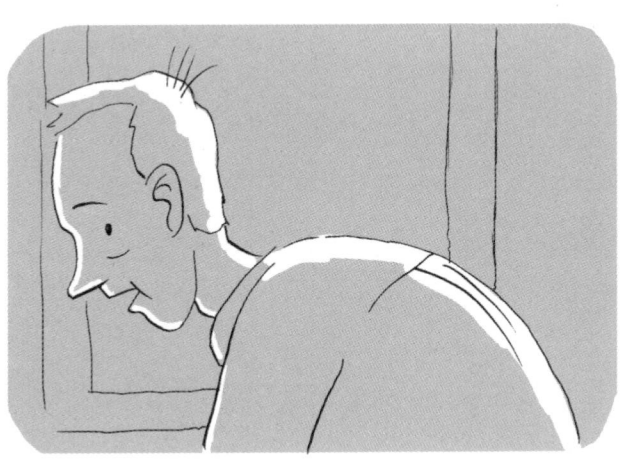

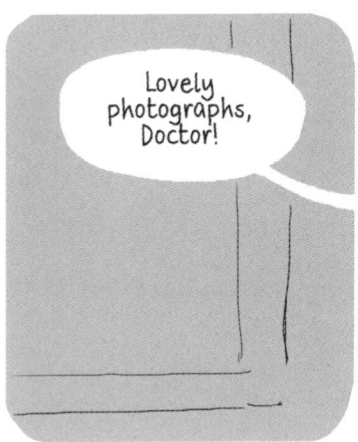

Did you take them ?

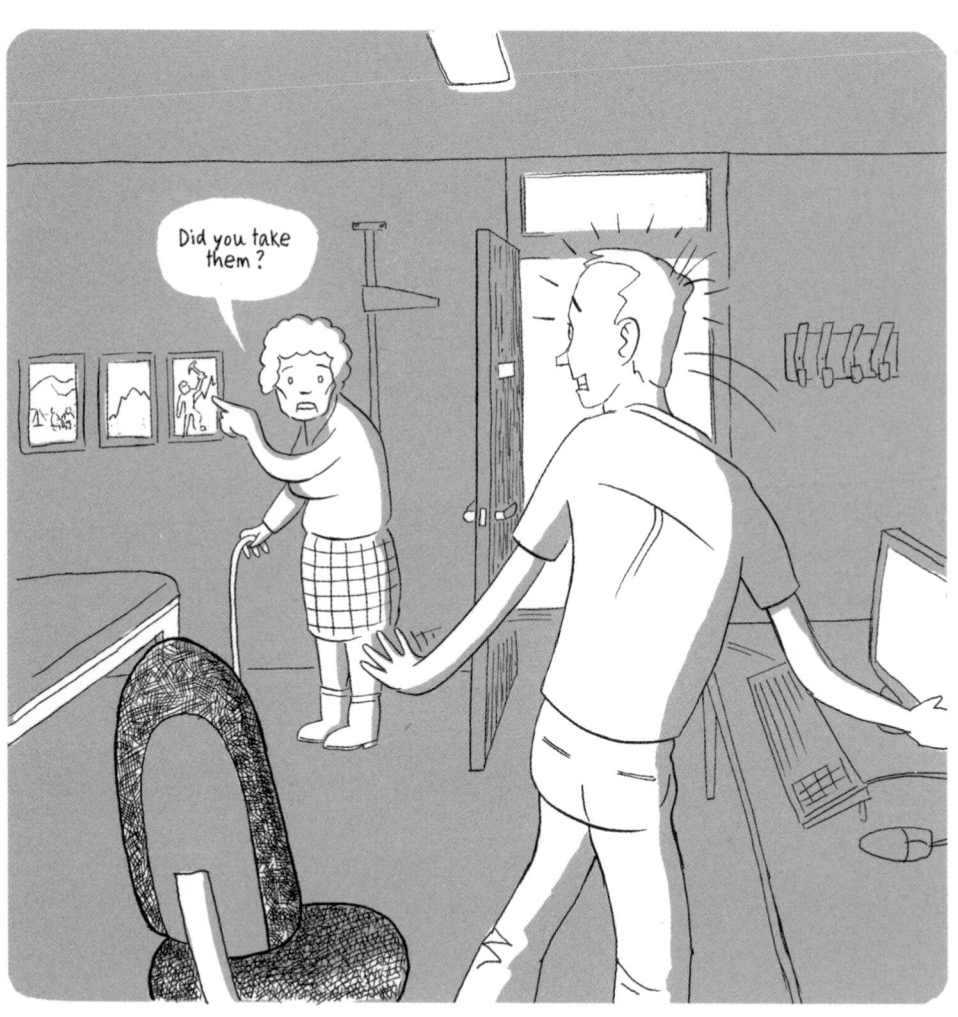

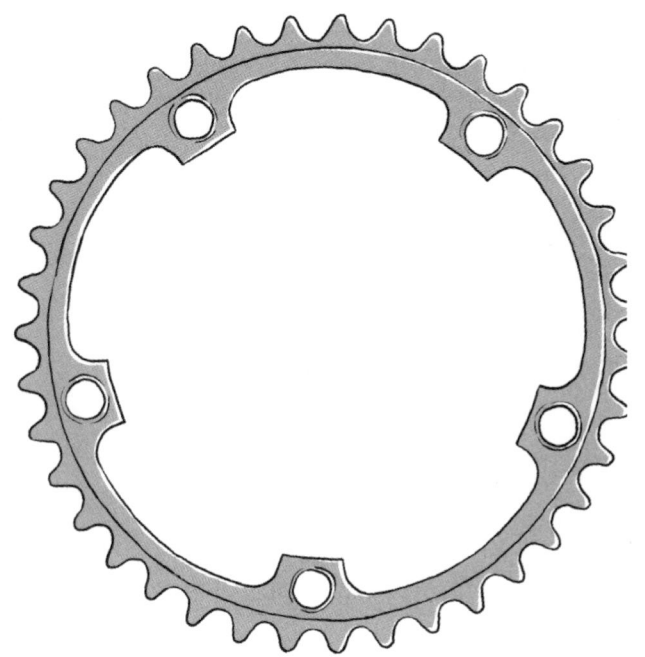

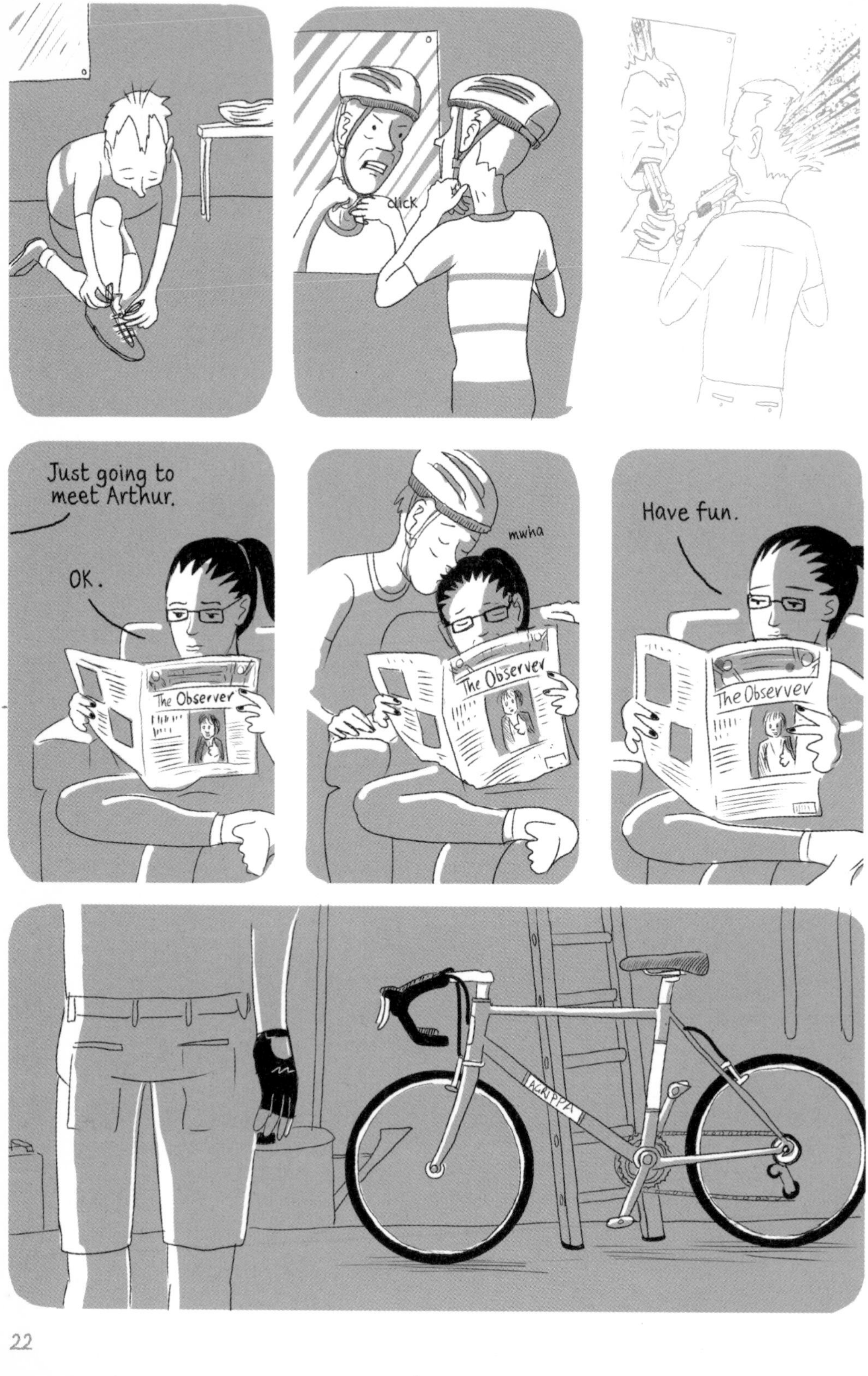
click
Just going to meet Arthur.
OK.
The Observer
mwha
The Observer
Have fun.
The Observer
AGRIPPA

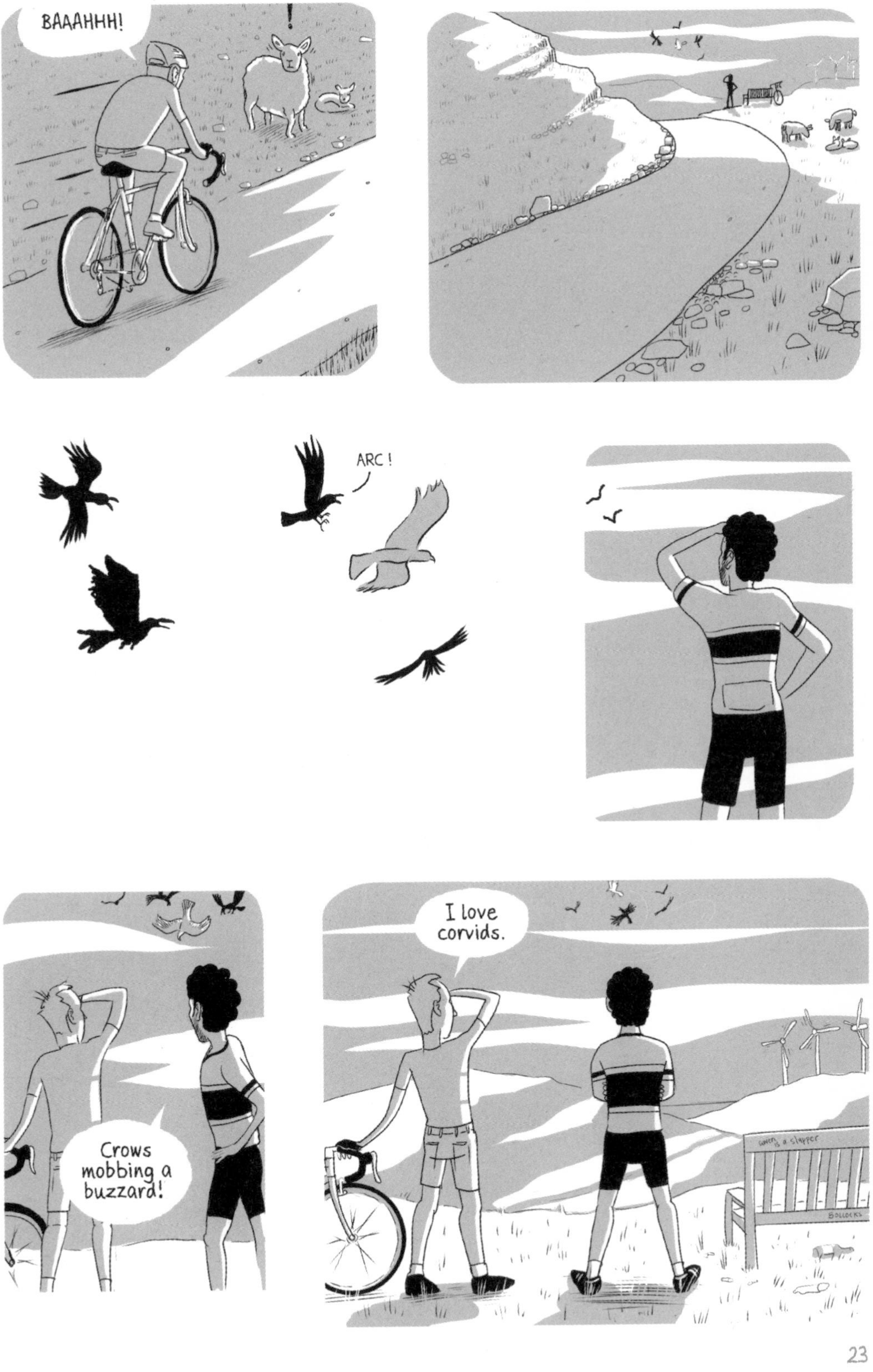
BAAAHHH!
!
ARC!
Crows mobbing a buzzard!
I love corvids.
Gwen is a slapper
BOLLOCKS

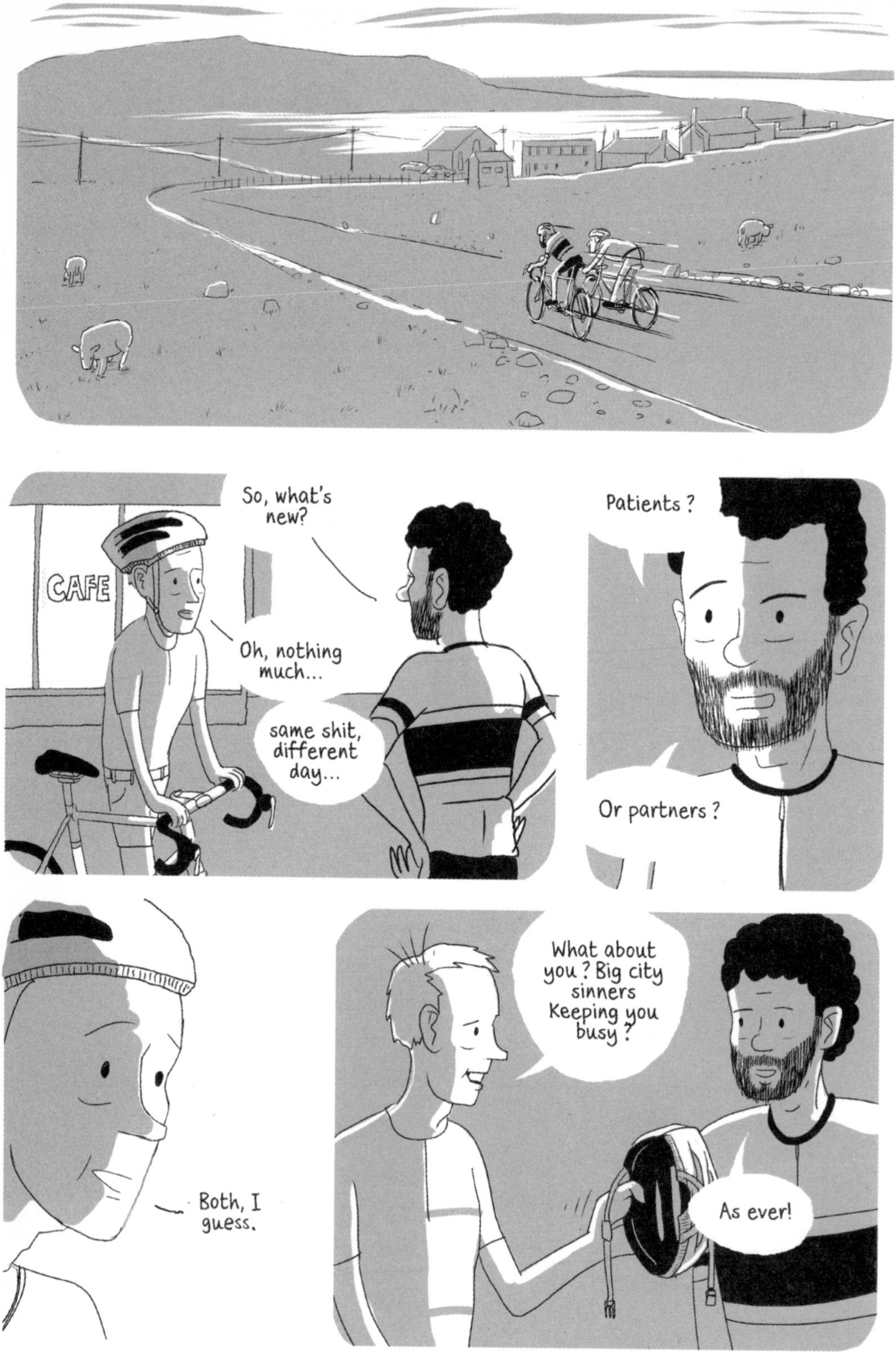
So, what's new?
Oh, nothing much...
same shit, different day...
Patients ?
Or partners ?
Both, I guess.
What about you ? Big city sinners Keeping you busy ?
As ever!

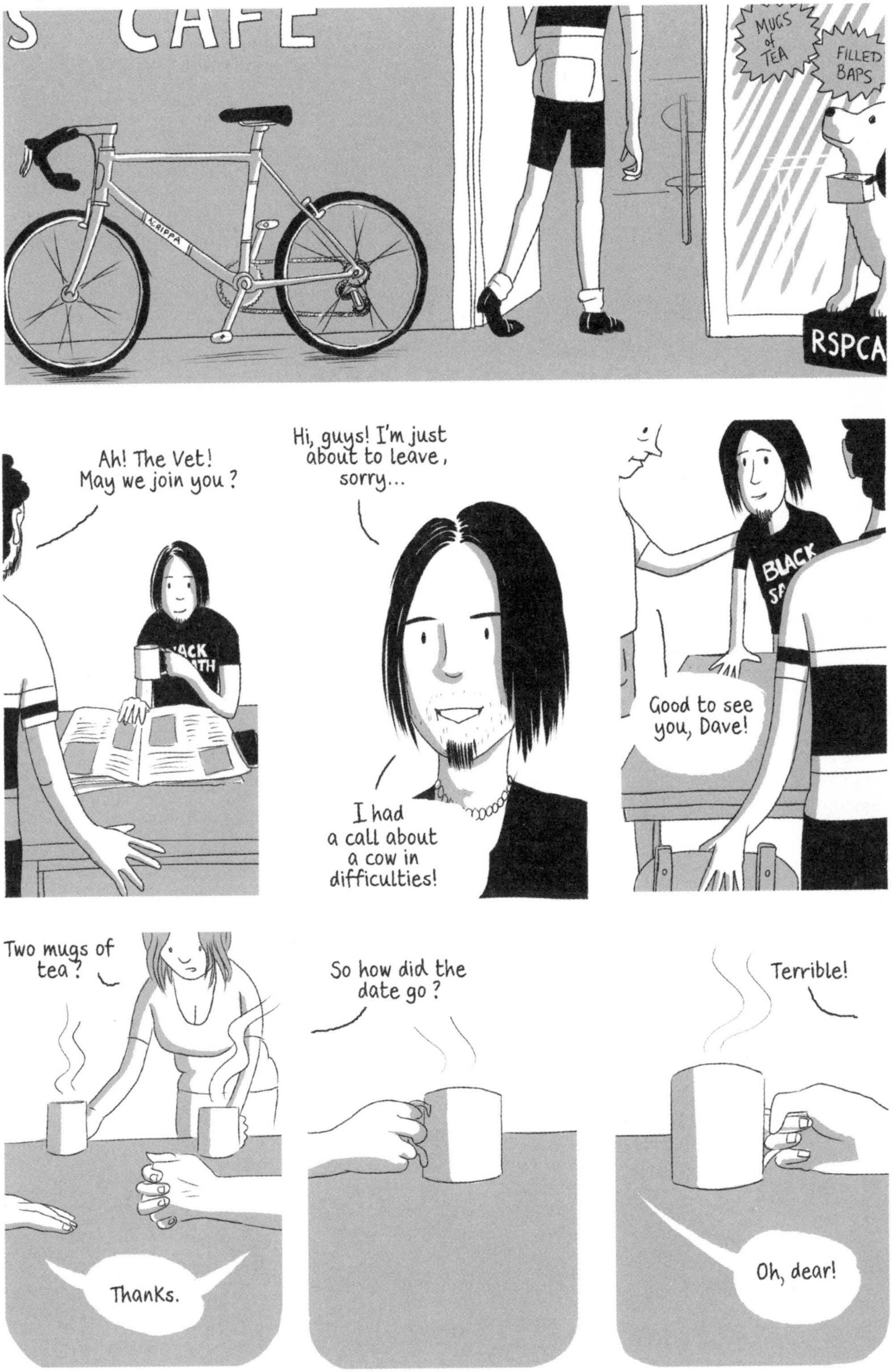
S CAFE
MUGS of TEA
FILLED BAPS
RSPCA
Ah! The Vet! May we join you?
Hi, guys! I'm just about to leave, sorry...
I had a call about a cow in difficulties!
Good to see you, Dave!
Two mugs of tea?
Thanks.
So how did the date go?
Terrible!
Oh, dear!

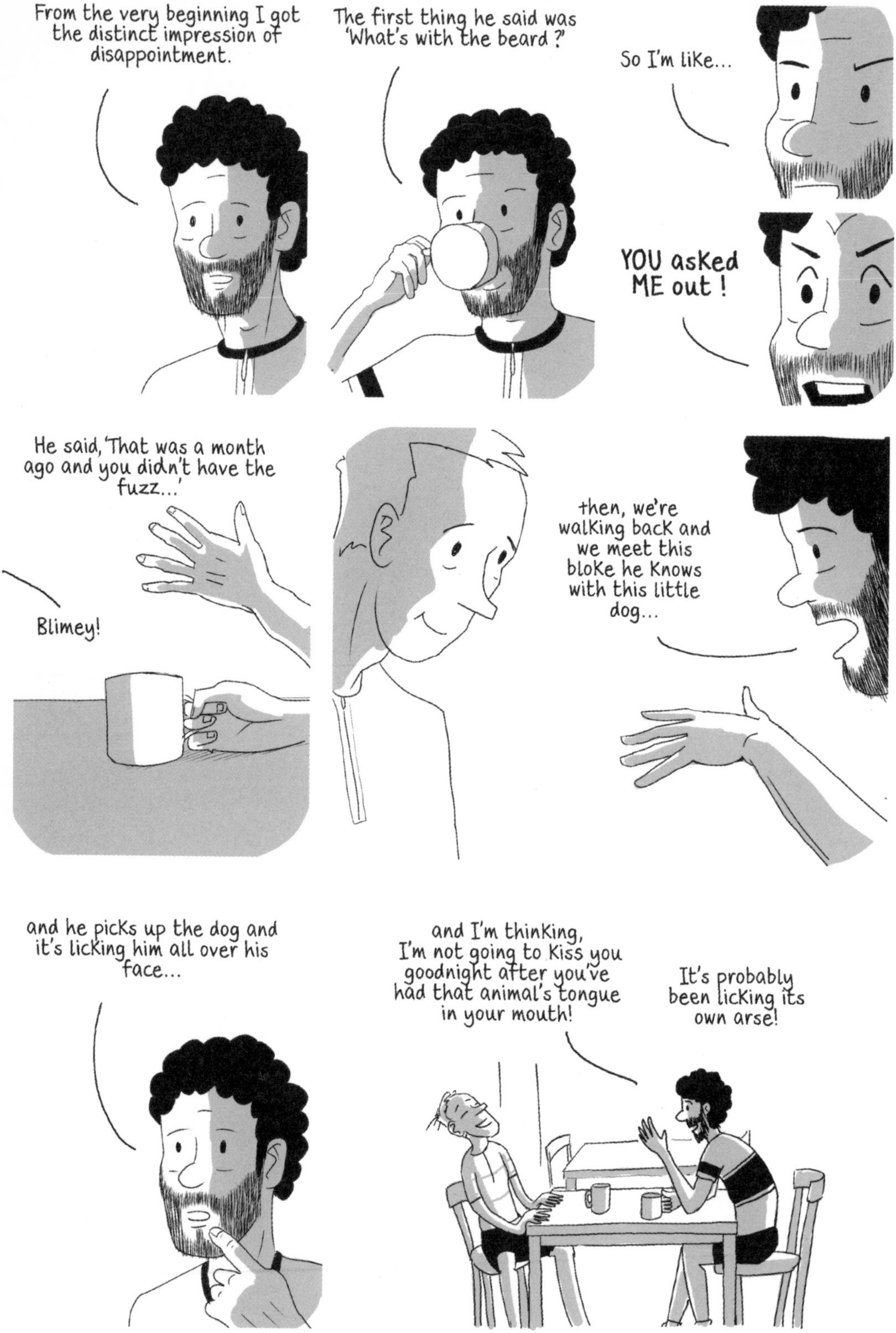
From the very beginning I got the distinct impression of disappointment.
The first thing he said was 'What's with the beard?'
So I'm like...
YOU asked ME out!
He said, 'That was a month ago and you didn't have the fuzz...'
Blimey!
then, we're walking back and we meet this bloke he knows with this little dog...
and he picks up the dog and it's licking him all over his face...
and I'm thinking, I'm not going to kiss you goodnight after you've had that animal's tongue in your mouth!
It's probably been licking its own arse!

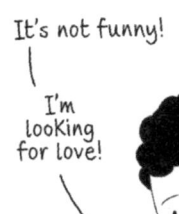

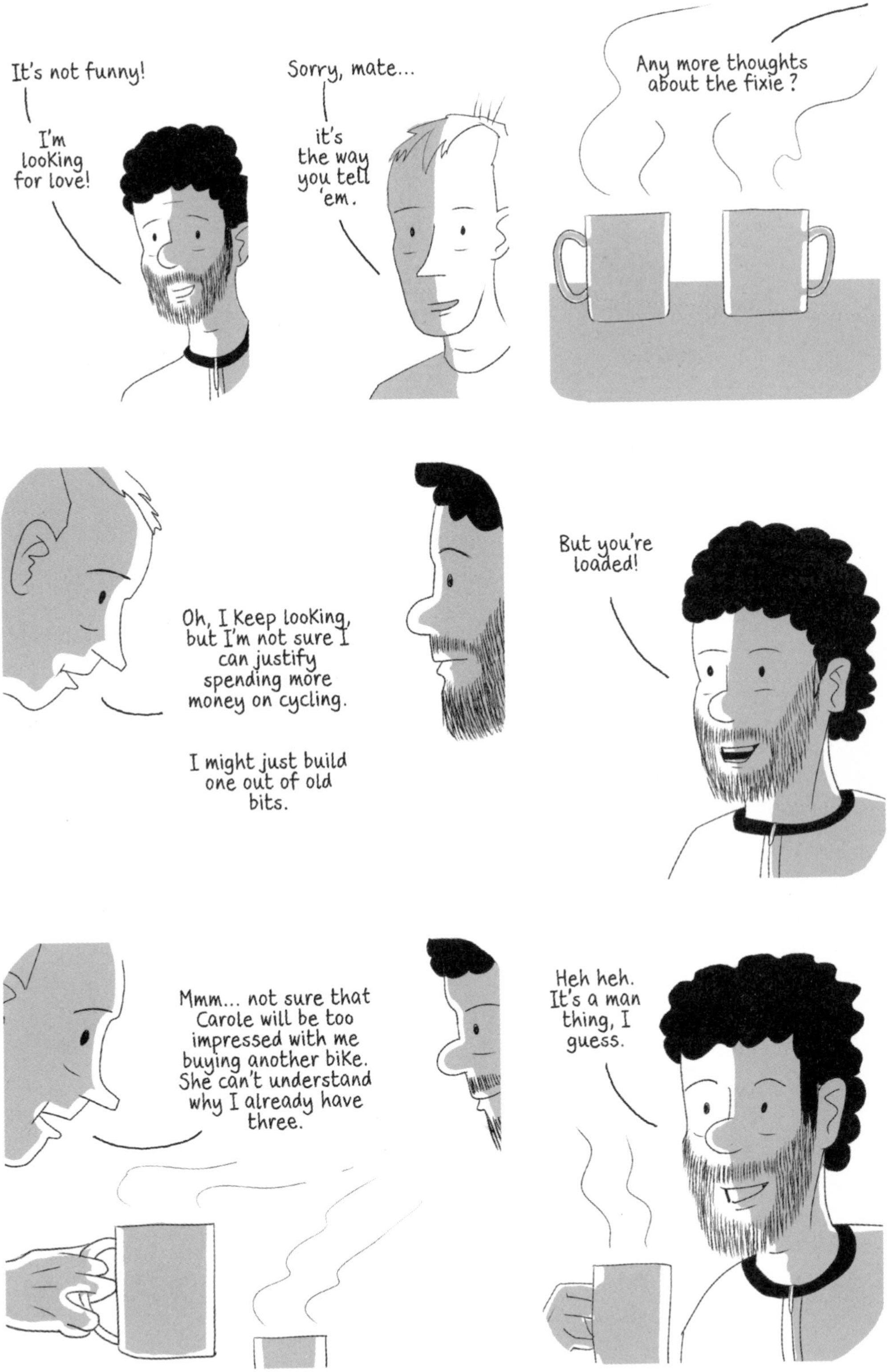

It's not funny!

I'm looking for love!

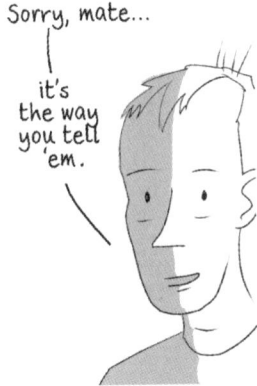

Sorry, mate...

it's the way you tell 'em.

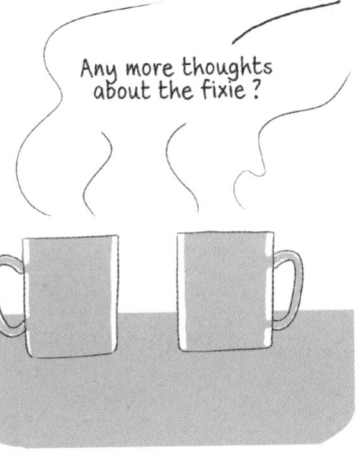

Any more thoughts about the fixie?

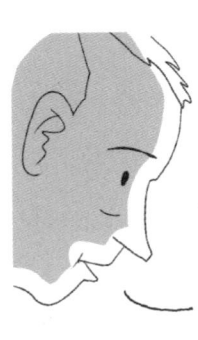

Oh, I keep looking, but I'm not sure I can justify spending more money on cycling.

I might just build one out of old bits.

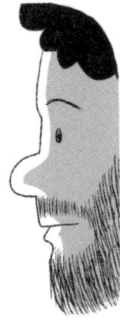

But you're loaded!

Oh, I keep looking, but I'm not sure I can justify spending more money on cycling.

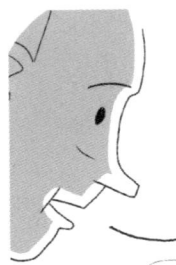

Mmm... not sure that Carole will be too impressed with me buying another bike. She can't understand why I already have three.

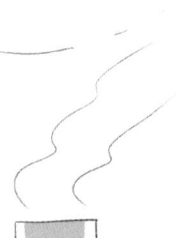

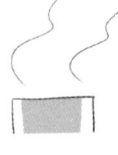

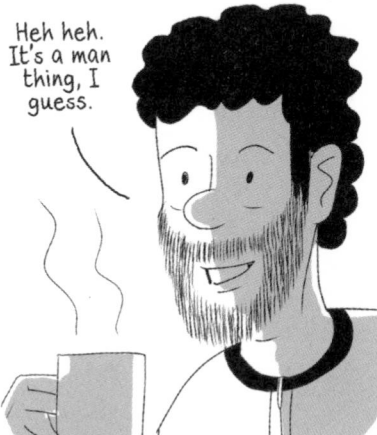

Heh heh. It's a man thing, I guess.

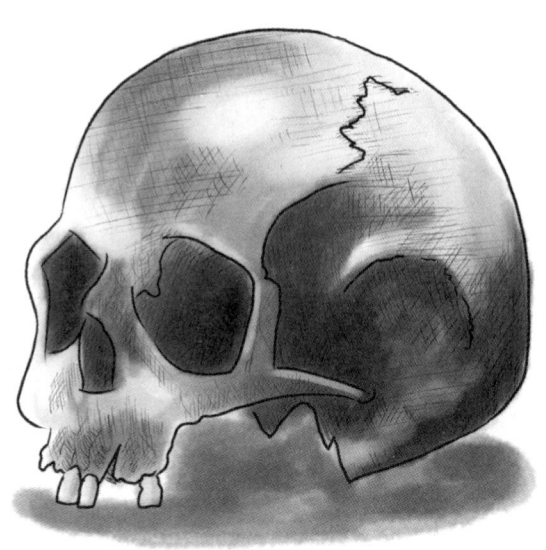

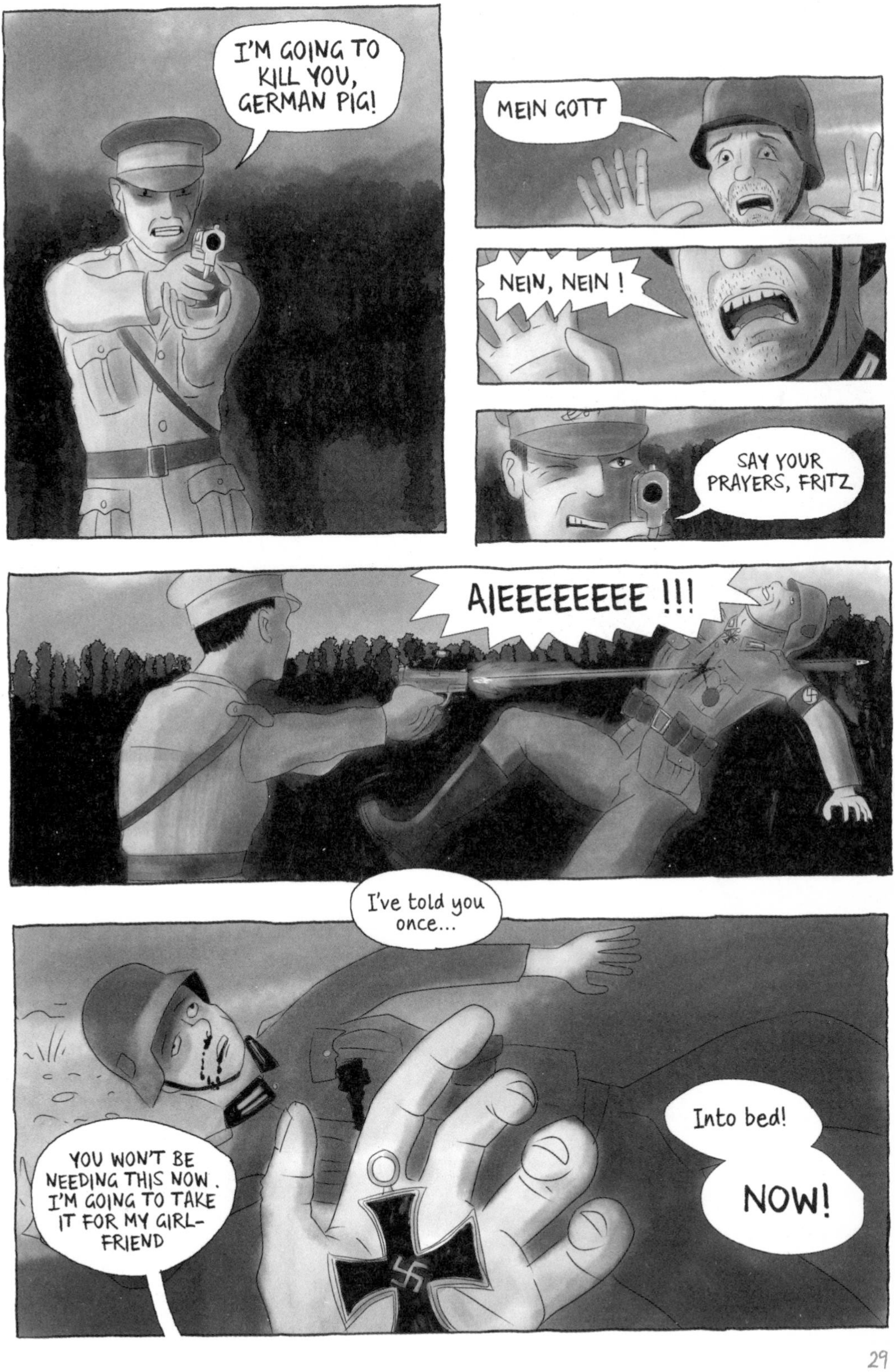
I'M GOING TO KILL YOU, GERMAN PIG!
MEIN GOTT
NEIN, NEIN !
SAY YOUR PRAYERS, FRITZ
AIEEEEEEEE !!!
I've told you once...
YOU WON'T BE NEEDING THIS NOW. I'M GOING TO TAKE IT FOR MY GIRL-FRIEND
Into bed!
NOW!

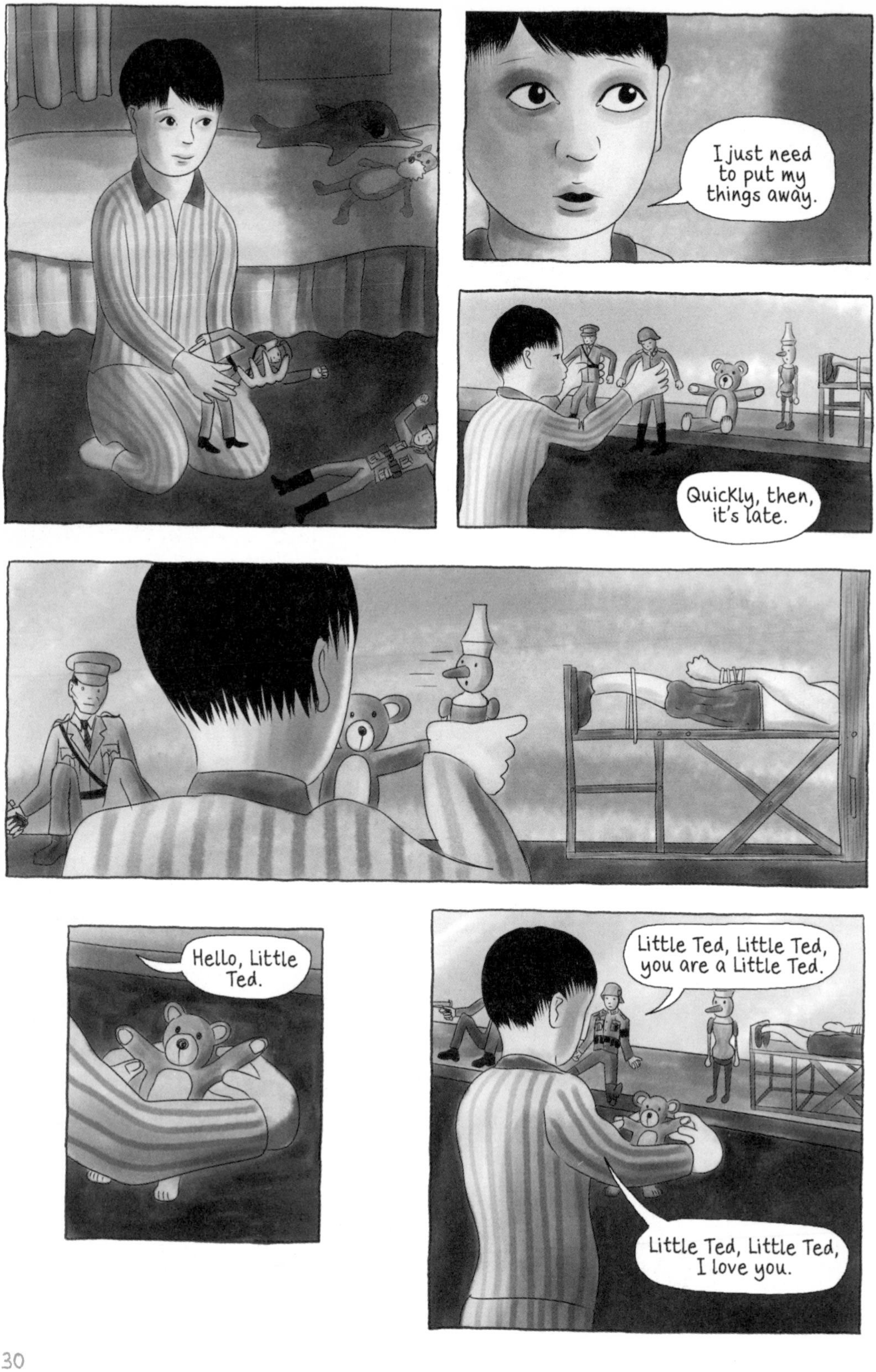
I just need to put my things away.
Quickly, then, it's late.
Hello, Little Ted.
Little Ted, Little Ted, you are a Little Ted.
Little Ted, Little Ted, I love you.

PAT
Goodnight, Dolphin.
Goodnight, Pyjama Dog.
PAT
PAT
Goodnight, Frog.
PAT PAT
Goodnight, Dolphin.
PAT PAT
Goodnight, Pyjama Dog.
PAT PAT
Goodnight, Frog.
PAT PAT PAT
Goodnight, Dolphin.
Goodnight, Pyjama Dog.
PAT PAT PAT

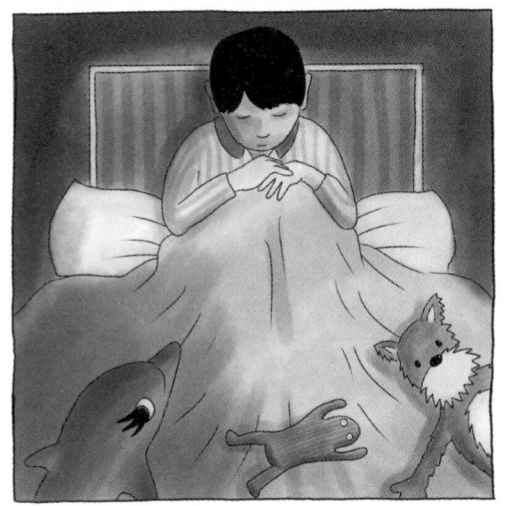

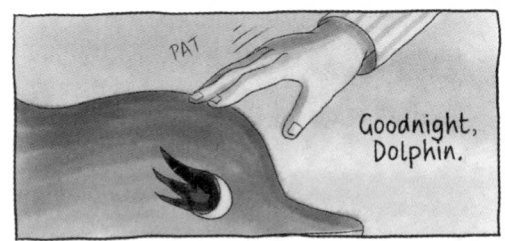

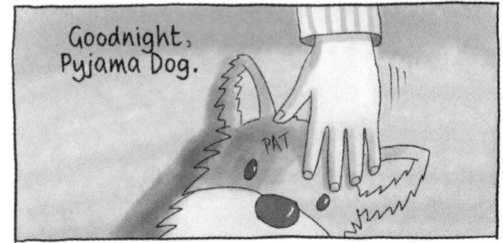

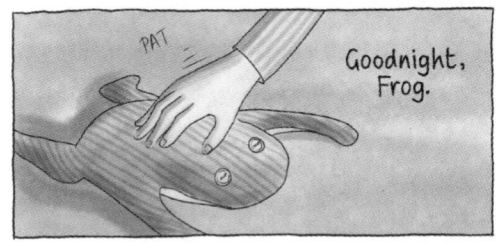

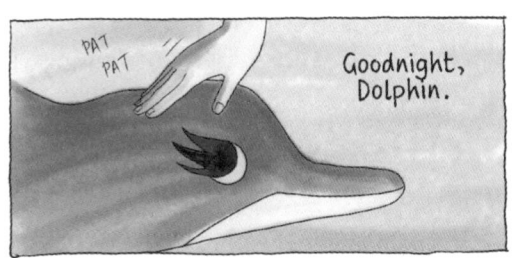

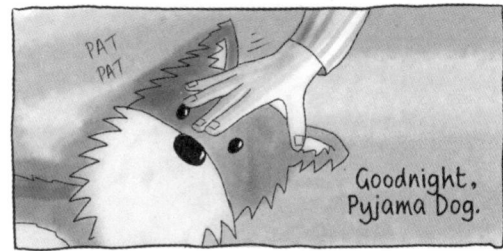

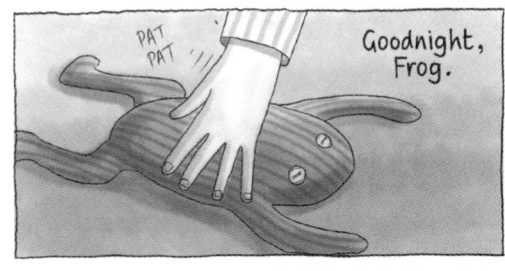

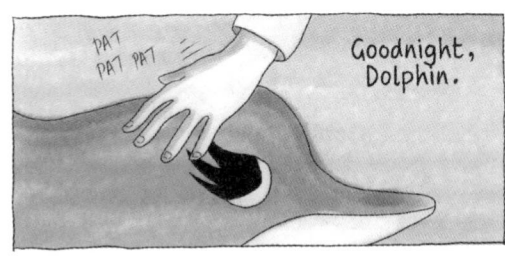

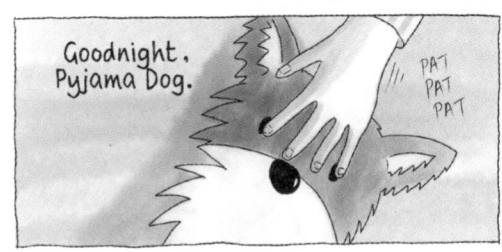

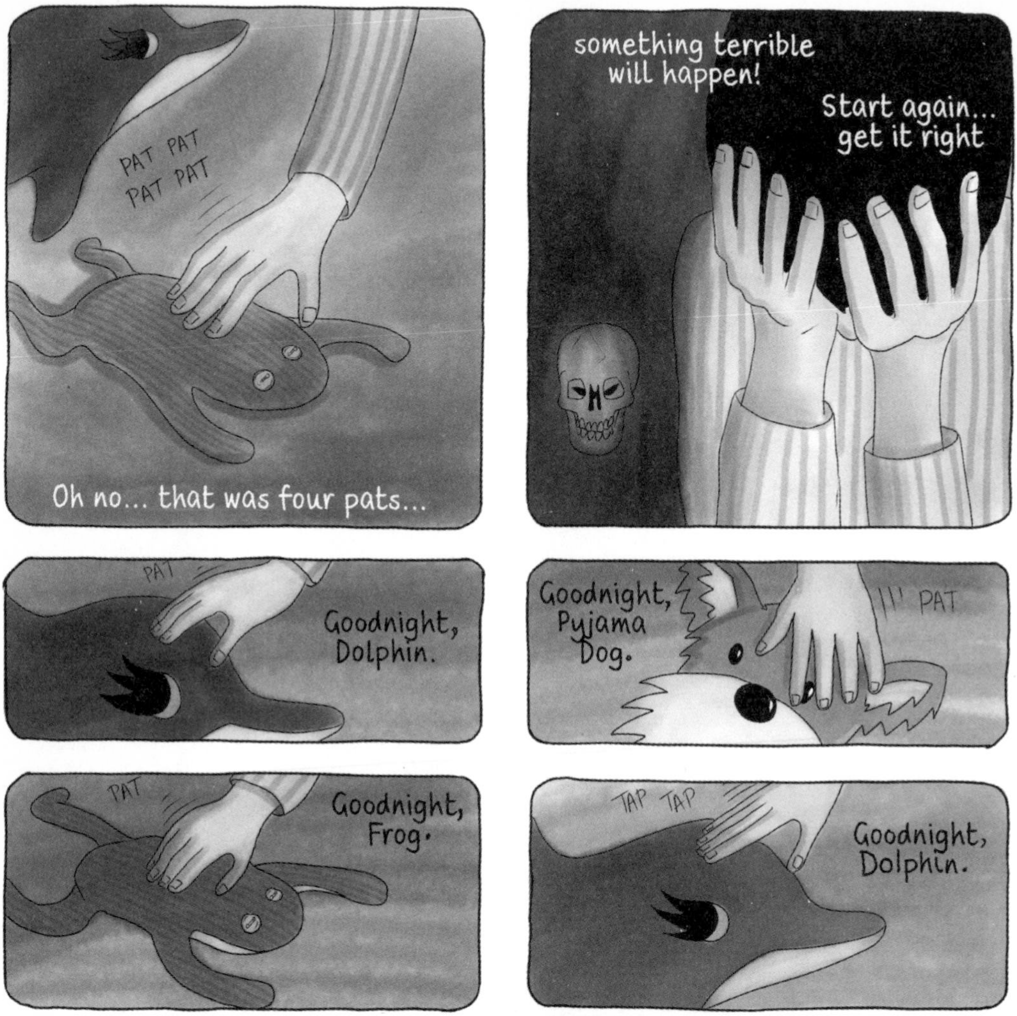
PAT PAT
PAT PAT
Oh no... that was four pats...
something terrible
will happen!
Start again...
get it right
PAT
Goodnight,
Dolphin.
PAT
Goodnight,
Pyjama
Dog.
PAT
Goodnight,
Frog.
TAP TAP
Goodnight,
Dolphin.

AND SO ON, UNTIL...

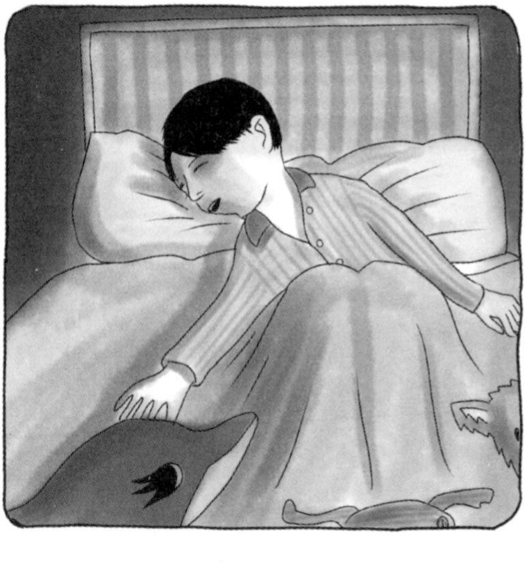

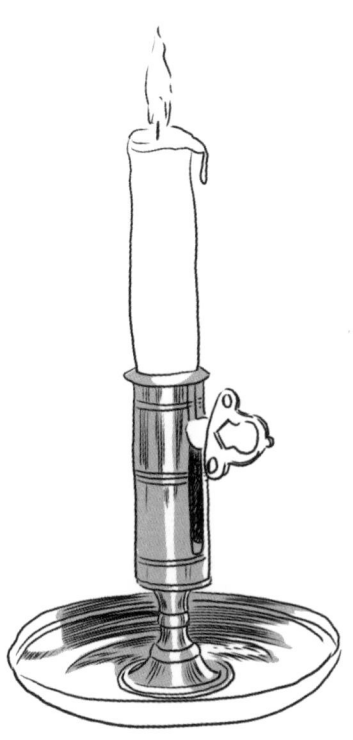

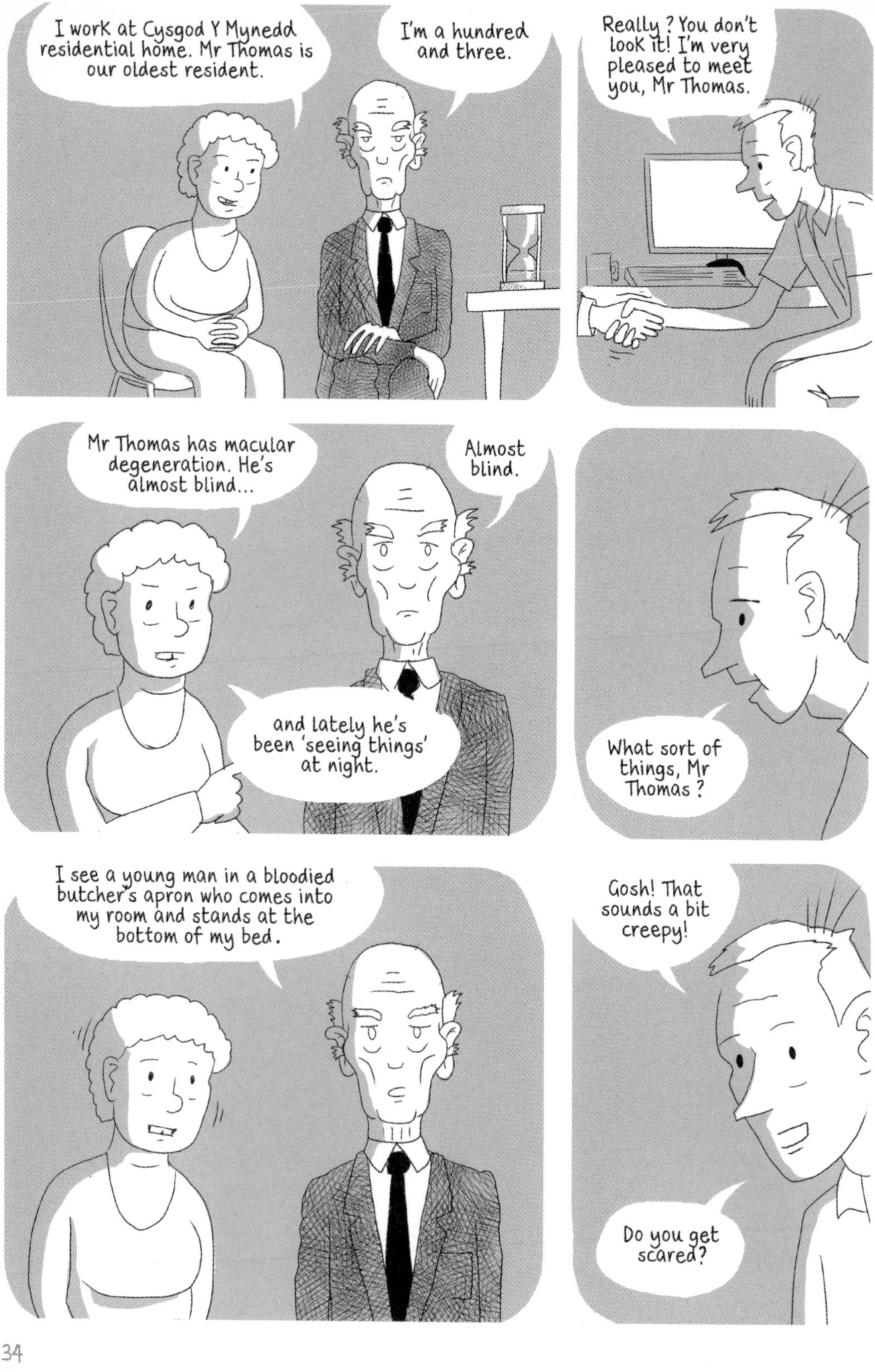
I work at Cysgod Y Mynedd residential home. Mr Thomas is our oldest resident.
I'm a hundred and three.
Really? You don't look it! I'm very pleased to meet you, Mr Thomas.
Mr Thomas has macular degeneration. He's almost blind...
Almost blind.
and lately he's been 'seeing things' at night.
What sort of things, Mr Thomas?
I see a young man in a bloodied butcher's apron who comes into my room and stands at the bottom of my bed.
Gosh! That sounds a bit creepy!
Do you get scared?

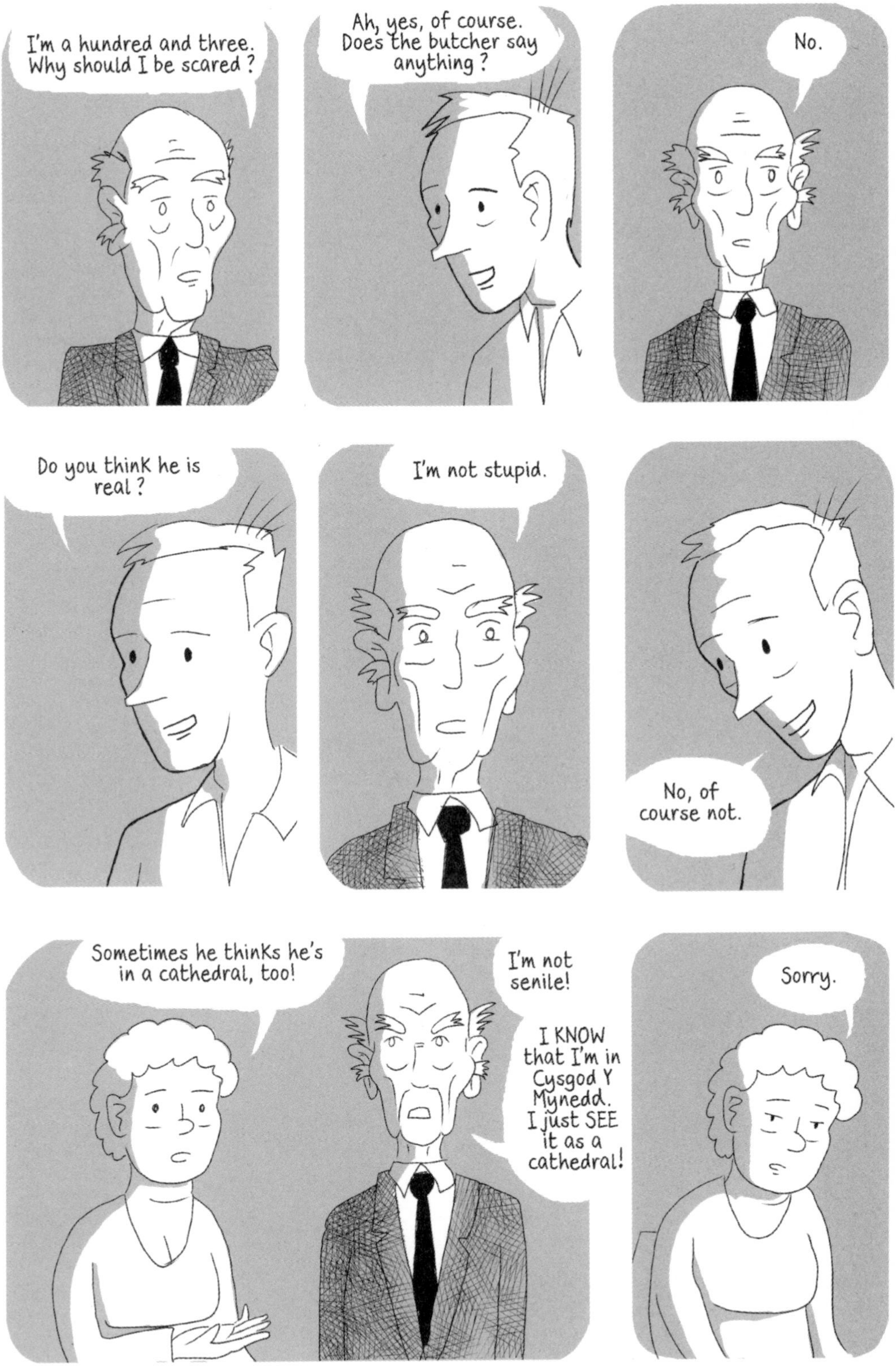
I'm a hundred and three. Why should I be scared?
Ah, yes, of course. Does the butcher say anything?
No.
Do you think he is real?
I'm not stupid.
No, of course not.
Sometimes he thinks he's in a cathedral, too!
I'm not senile!
I KNOW that I'm in Cysgod Y Mynedd. I just SEE it as a cathedral!
Sorry.

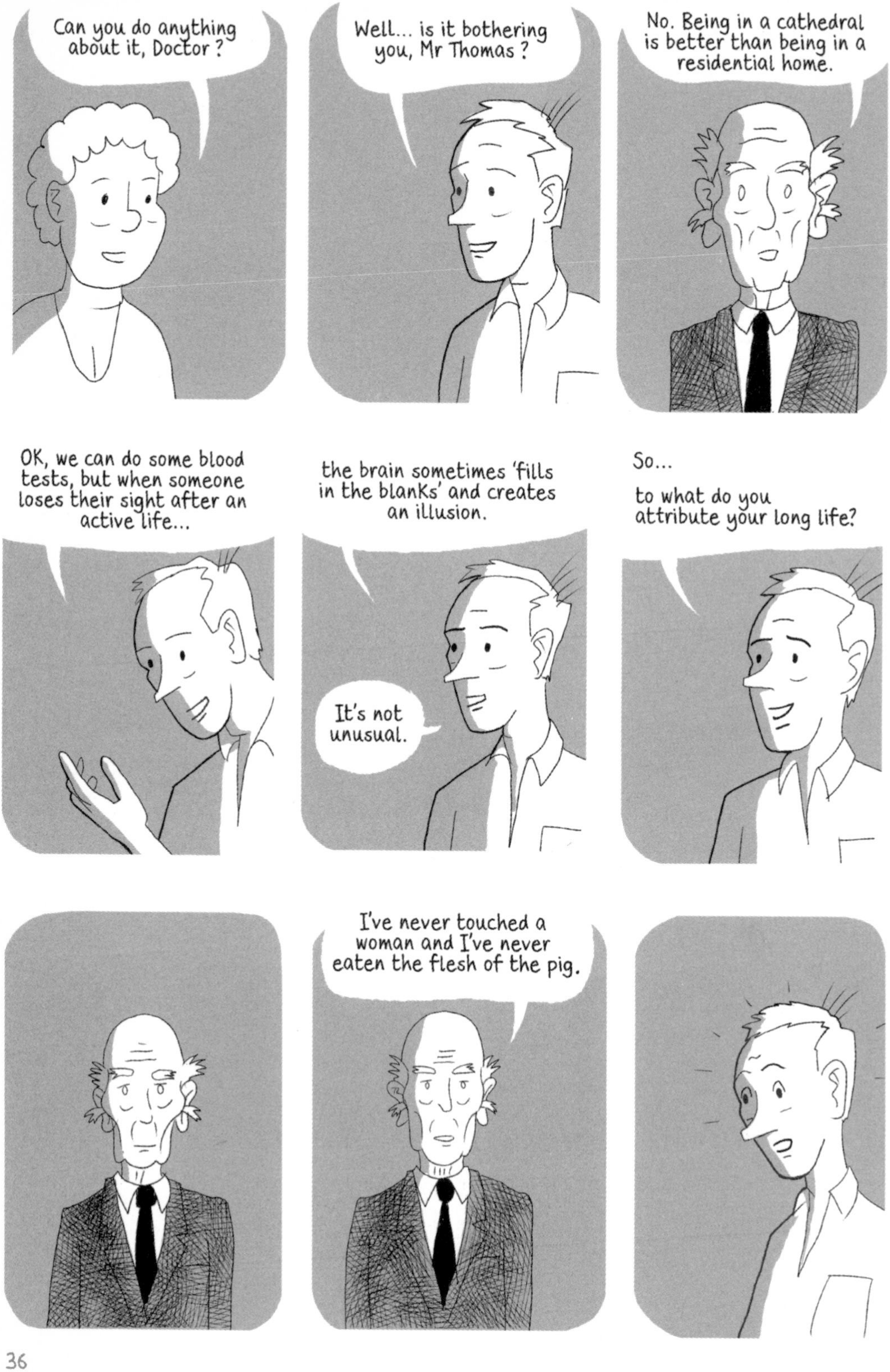
Can you do anything about it, Doctor ?
Well... is it bothering you, Mr Thomas ?
No. Being in a cathedral is better than being in a residential home.
OK, we can do some blood tests, but when someone loses their sight after an active life...
the brain sometimes 'fills in the blanks' and creates an illusion.
It's not unusual.
So...
to what do you attribute your long life?
I've never touched a woman and I've never eaten the flesh of the pig.

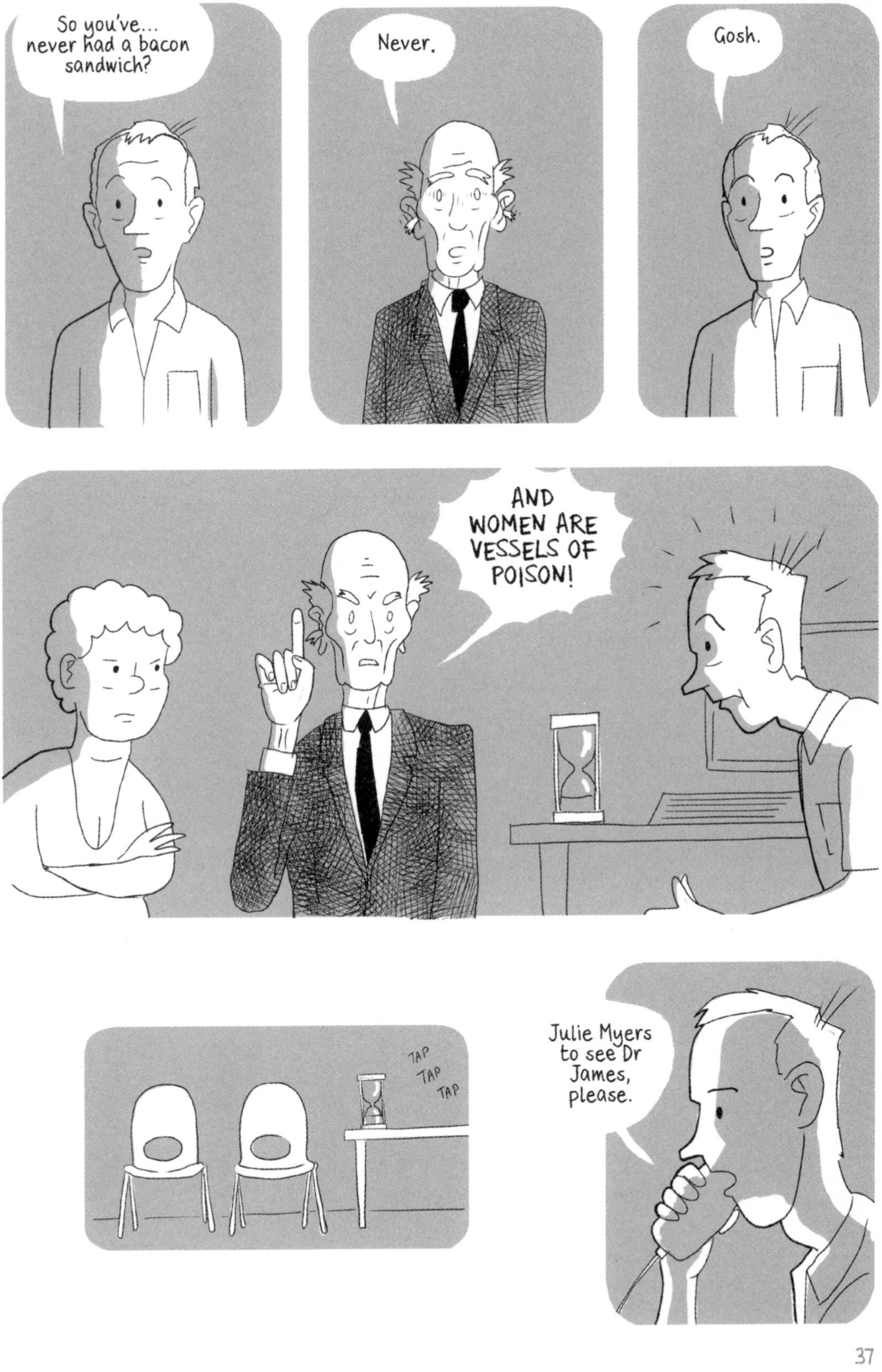
So you've... never had a bacon sandwich?
Never.
Gosh.
AND WOMEN ARE VESSELS OF POISON!
TAP TAP TAP
Julie Myers to see Dr James, please.

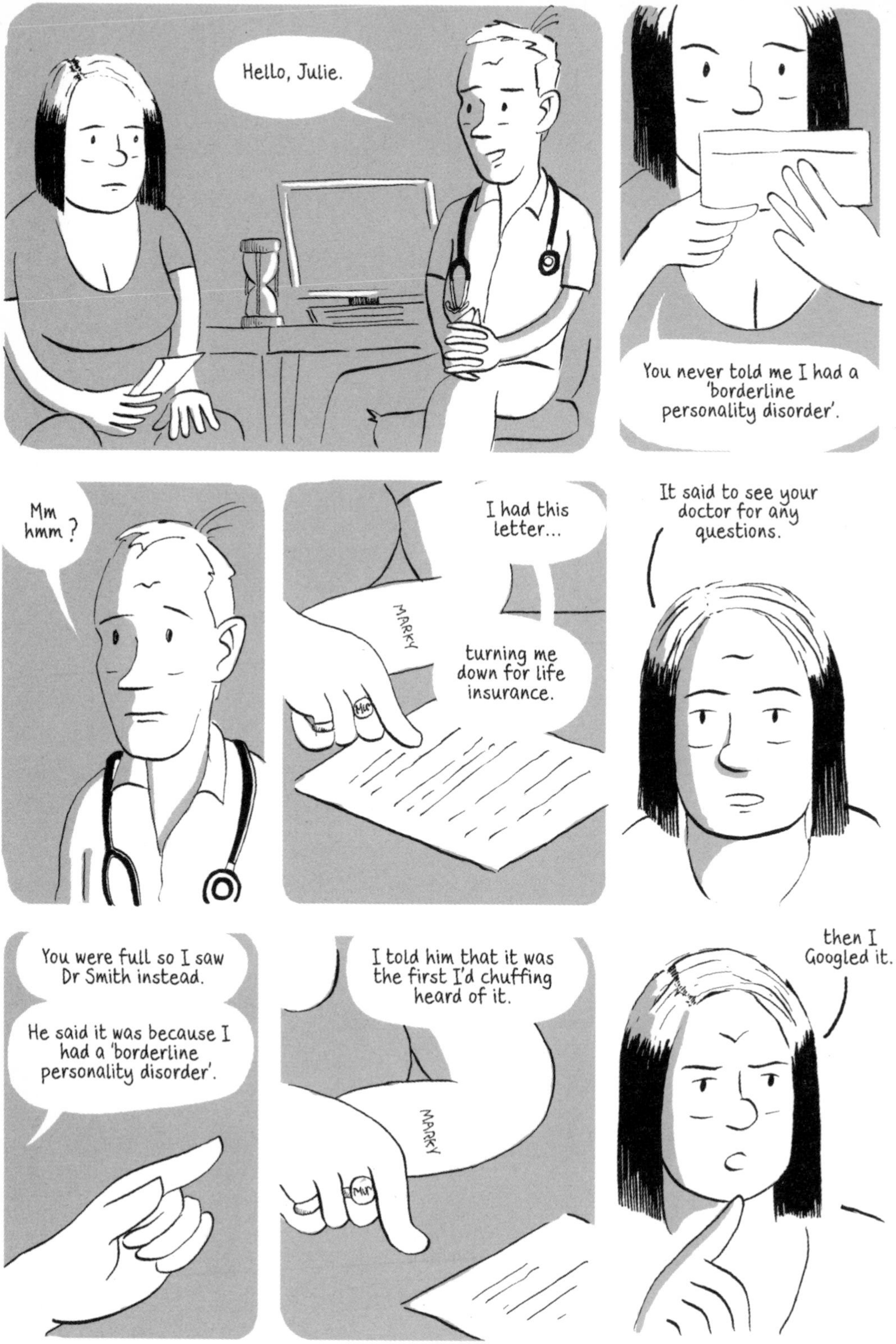
Hello, Julie.
You never told me I had a 'borderline personality disorder'.
Mm hmm?
I had this letter...
turning me down for life insurance.
MARKY
It said to see your doctor for any questions.
You were full so I saw Dr Smith instead.
He said it was because I had a 'borderline personality disorder'.
I told him that it was the first I'd chuffing heard of it.
MARKY
then I Googled it.

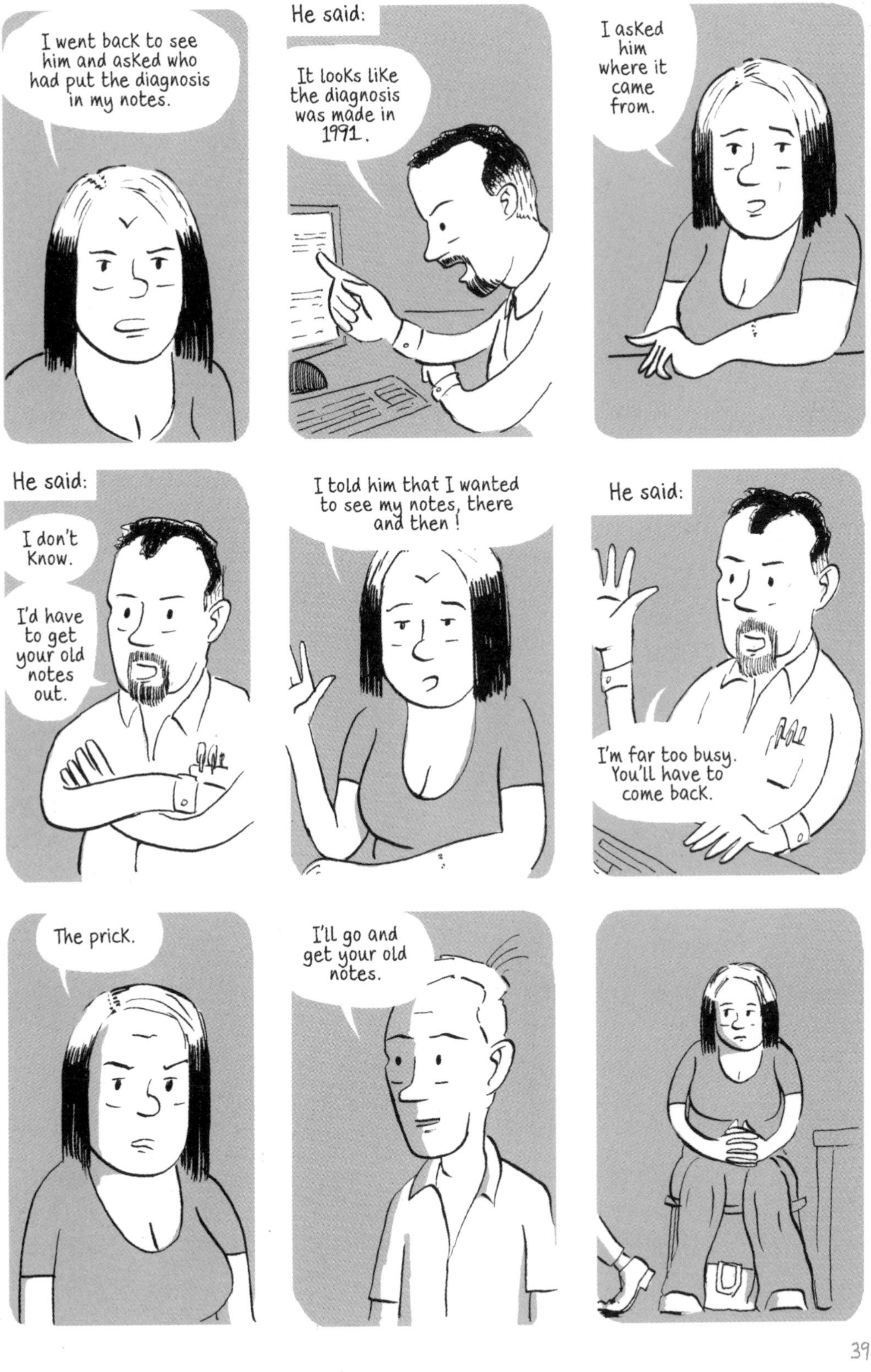
I went back to see him and asked who had put the diagnosis in my notes.
He said:
It looks like the diagnosis was made in 1991.
I asked him where it came from.
He said:
I don't know.
I'd have to get your old notes out.
I told him that I wanted to see my notes, there and then!
He said:
I'm far too busy. You'll have to come back.
The prick.
I'll go and get your old notes.

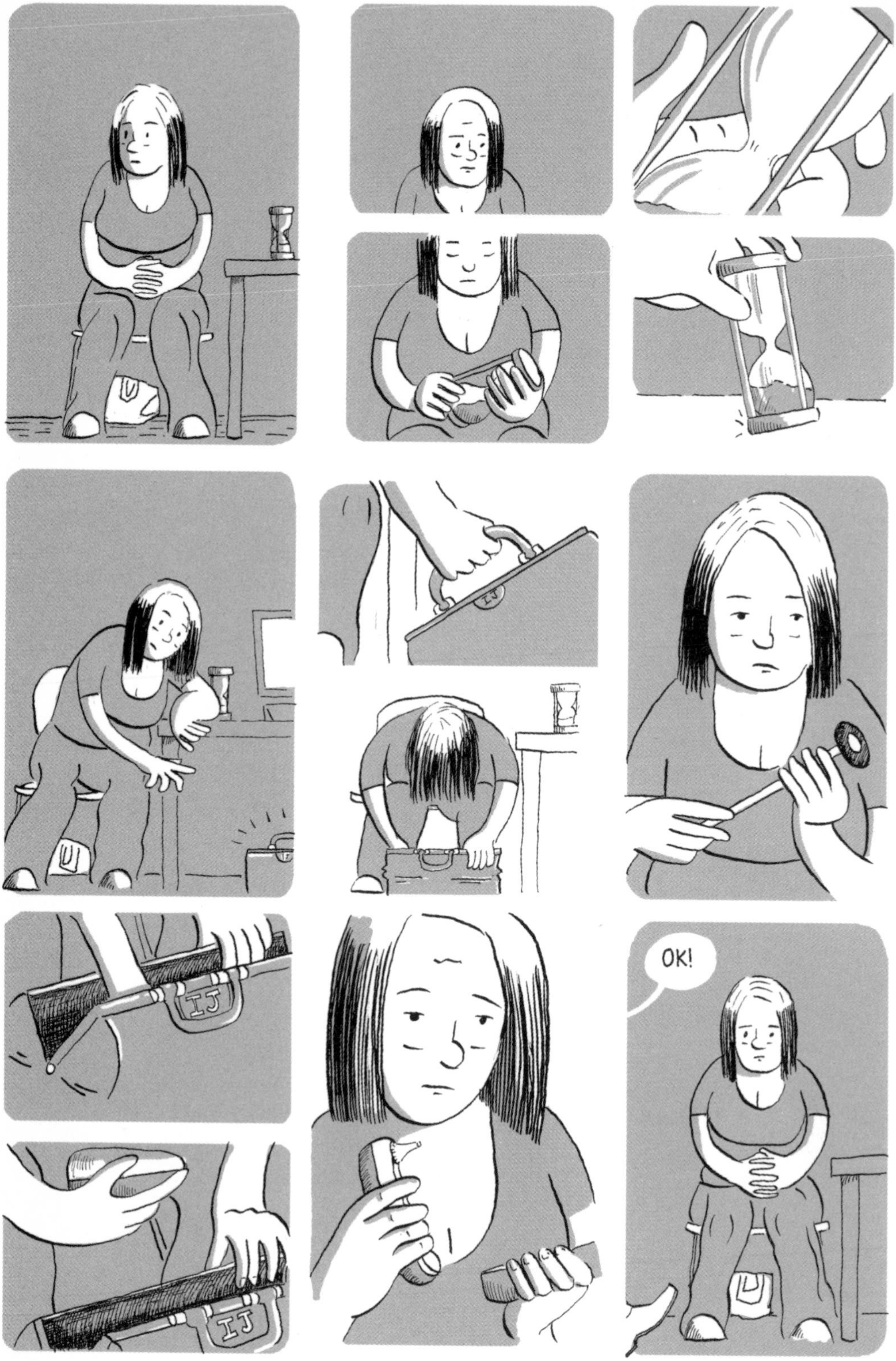

OK!

Let's have a look.
Looks like you saw a psychiatrist in 1991.
ONCE! I was having a really shitty time.
I'd just found Barry in bed with my friend.
I went a bit nuts...
MUM
MUM
I did some things I'm not proud of...
There's a note from the psychiatrist. He remarks that you 'might have a borderline personality disorder'.
Then someone underlined it.
Julie, could you leave this with me for a day or two?

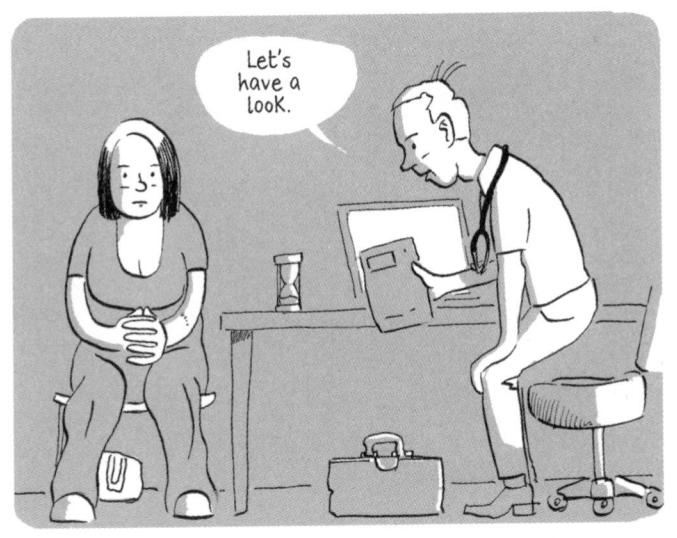

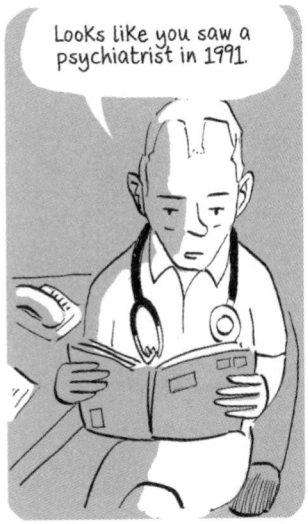

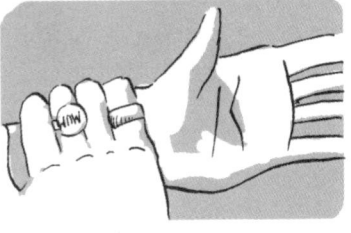

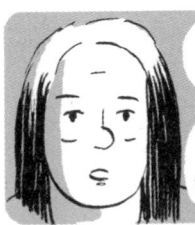

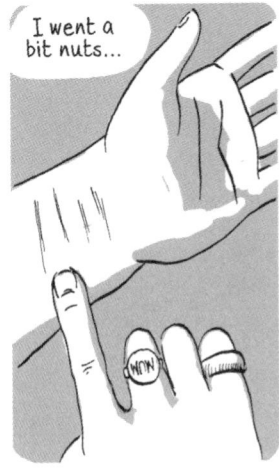

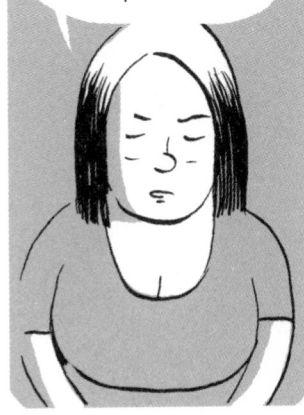

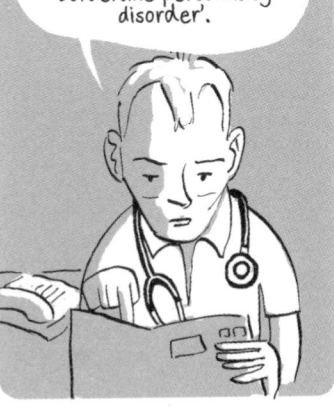

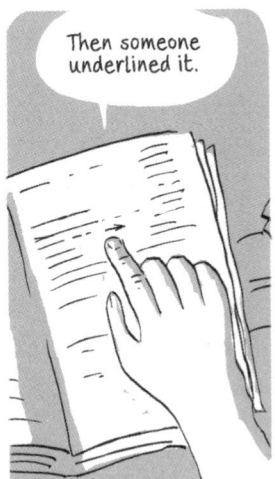

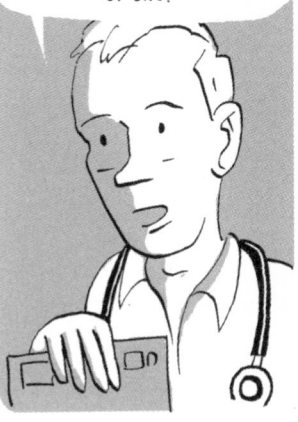

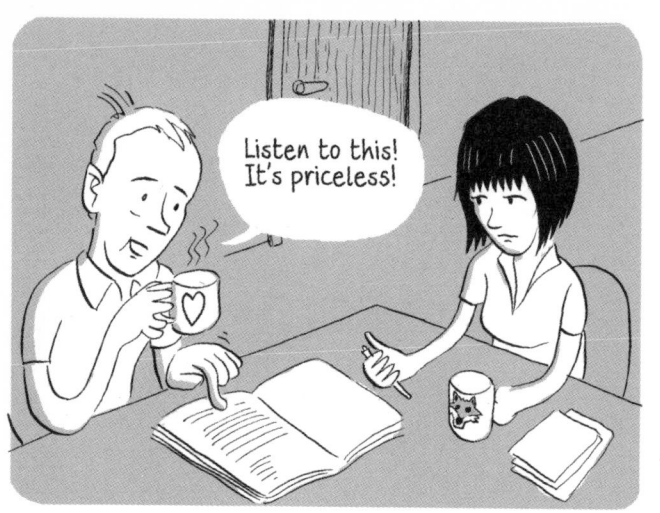

Listen to this! It's priceless!

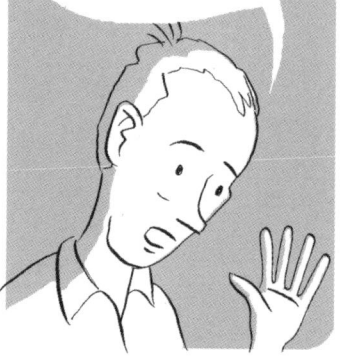

'She is a rather difficult and unpleasant woman who may, I suspect, have a borderline personality disorder.'

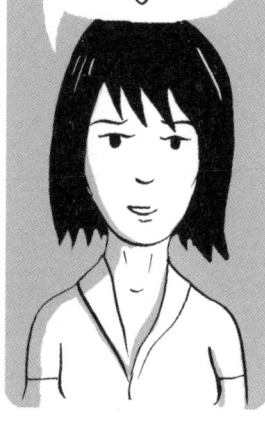

Consultants don't write letters like that any more!

Too right!

Somewhere along the line that comment got turned into a diagnosis.

Probably when her notes were summarised.

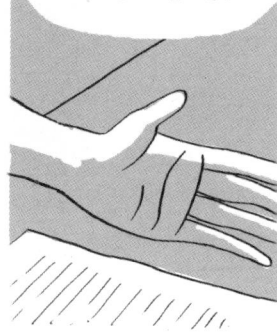

Then it got Read Coded and put on her electronic record and hey presto, she's branded a B.P.D.

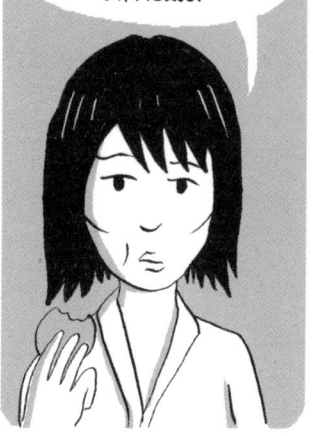

She is pretty weird and difficult.

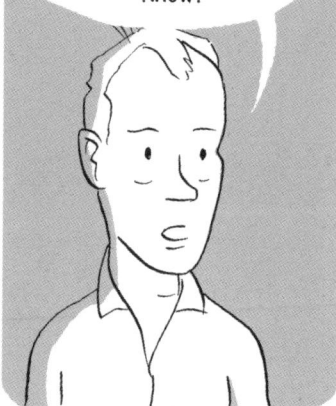

Well, yes, but no more so than a lot of people we know.

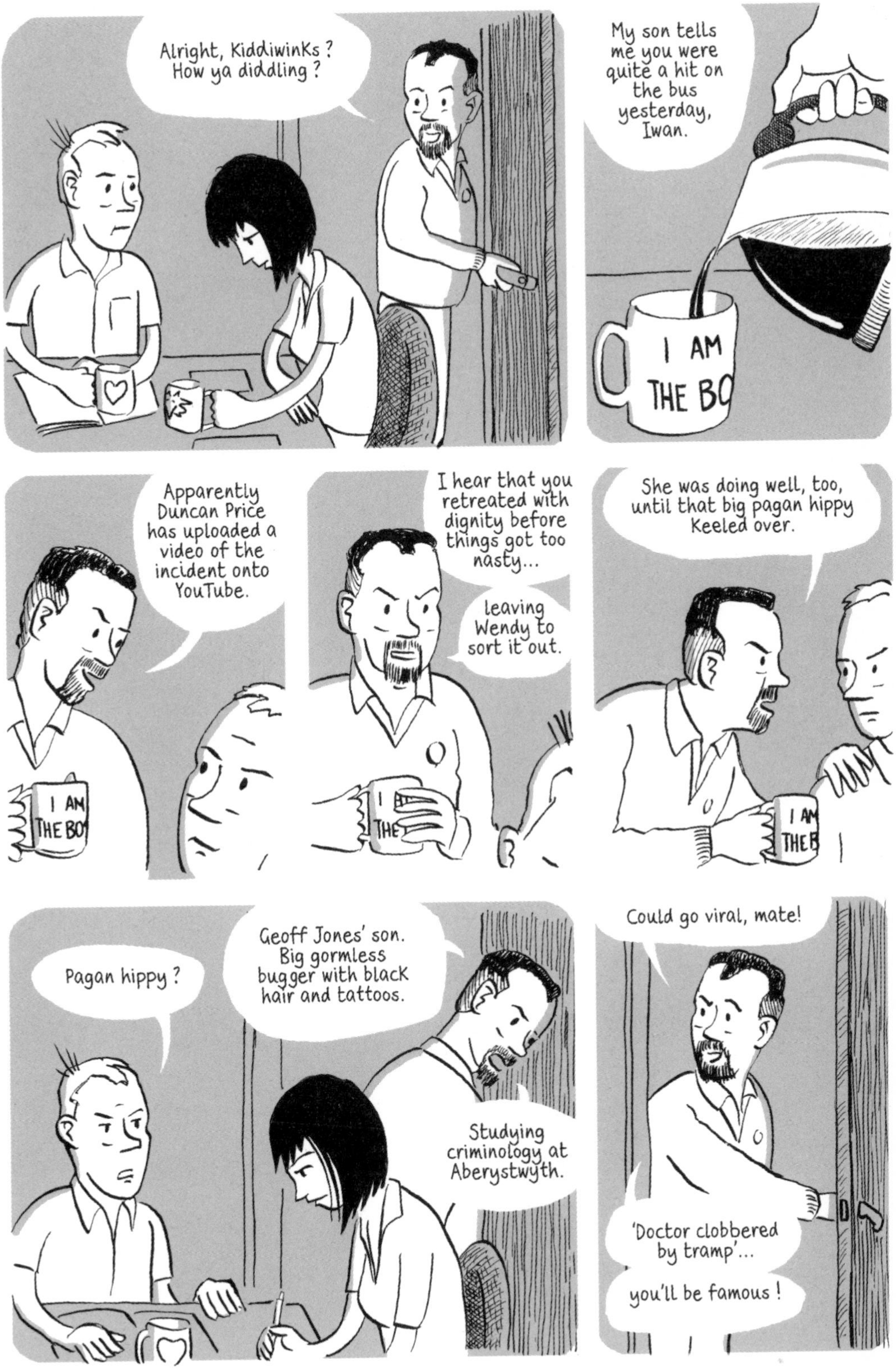

Alright, Kiddiwinks ? How ya diddling ?
My son tells me you were quite a hit on the bus yesterday, Iwan.
I AM THE BO
Apparently Duncan Price has uploaded a video of the incident onto YouTube.
I AM THE BO
I hear that you retreated with dignity before things got too nasty...
leaving Wendy to sort it out.
She was doing well, too, until that big pagan hippy Keeled over.
Pagan hippy ?
Geoff Jones' son. Big gormless bugger with black hair and tattoos.
Studying criminology at Aberystwyth.
Could go viral, mate!
'Doctor clobbered by tramp'...
you'll be famous !

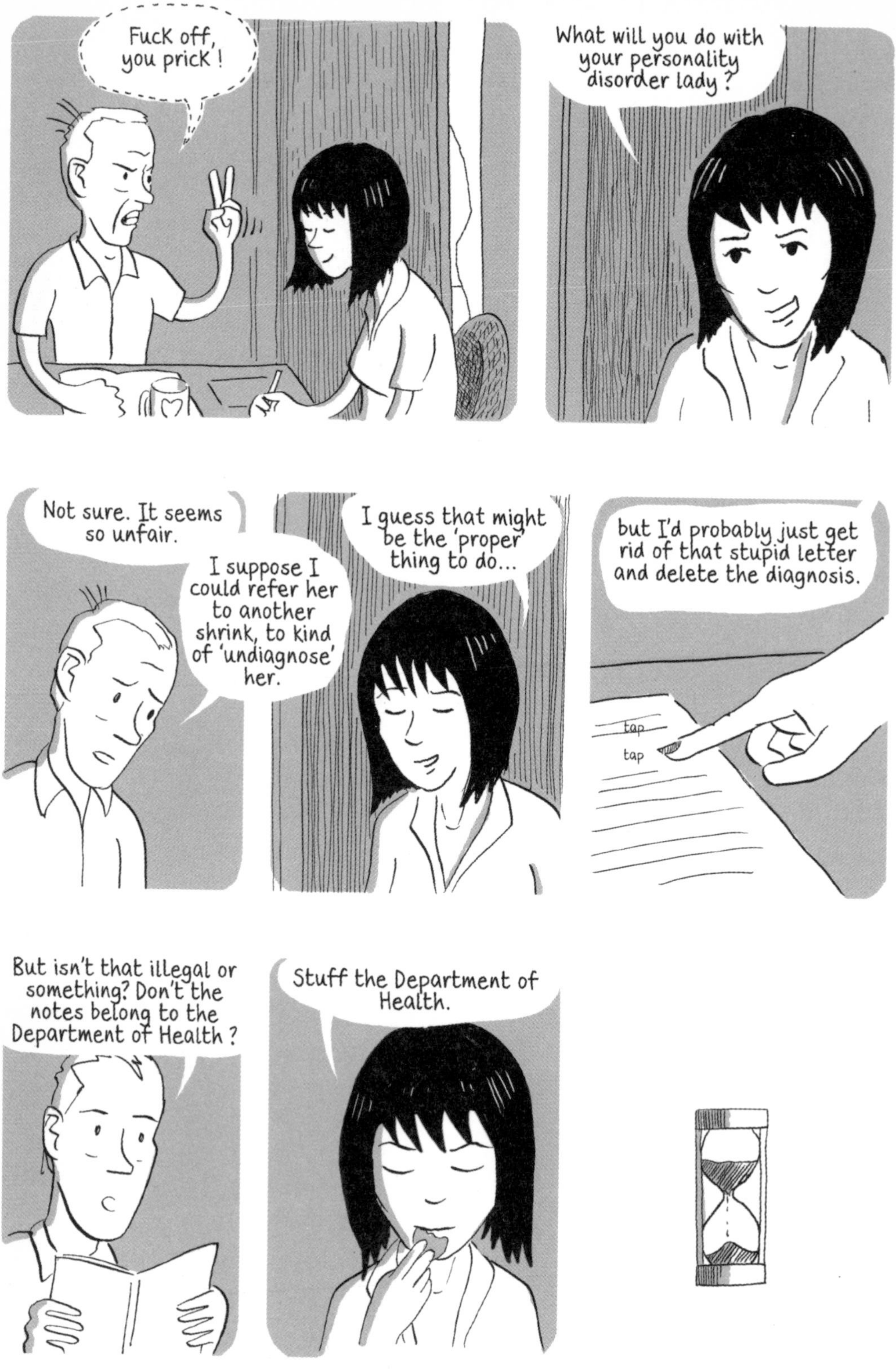
Fuck off, you prick!
What will you do with your personality disorder lady?
Not sure. It seems so unfair.
I suppose I could refer her to another shrink, to kind of 'undiagnose' her.
I guess that might be the 'proper' thing to do...
but I'd probably just get rid of that stupid letter and delete the diagnosis.
tap
tap
But isn't that illegal or something? Don't the notes belong to the Department of Health?
Stuff the Department of Health.

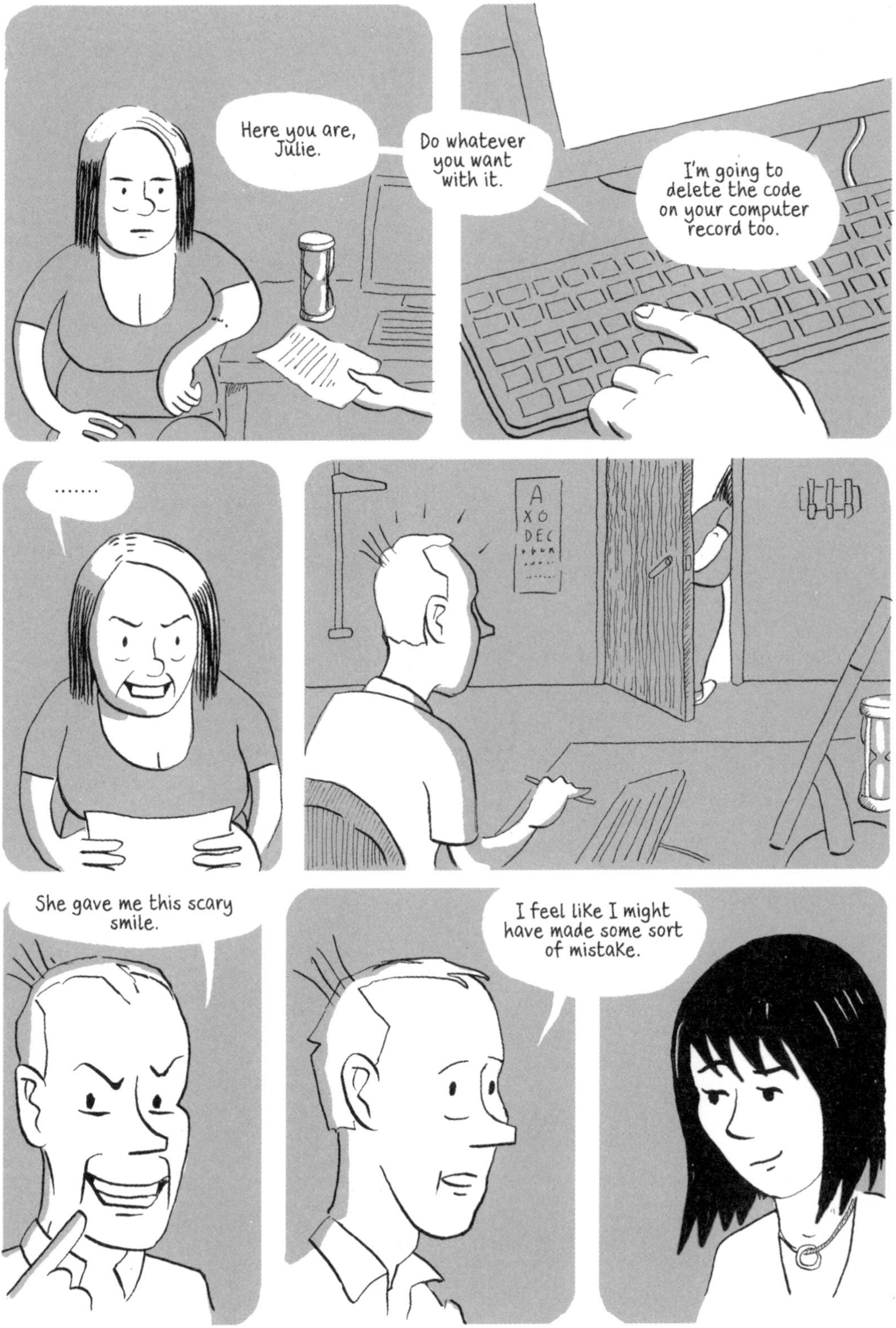
Here you are, Julie.
Do whatever you want with it.
I'm going to delete the code on your computer record too.
....
She gave me this scary smile.
I feel like I might have made some sort of mistake.

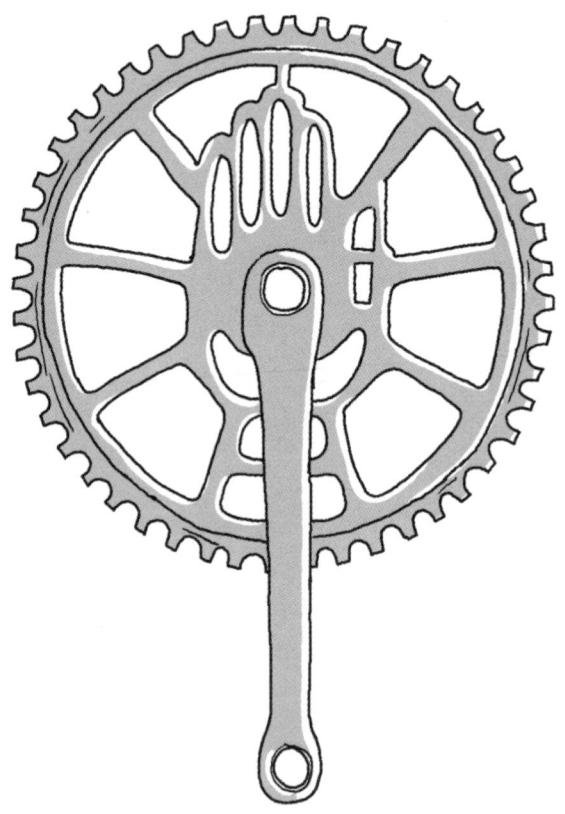

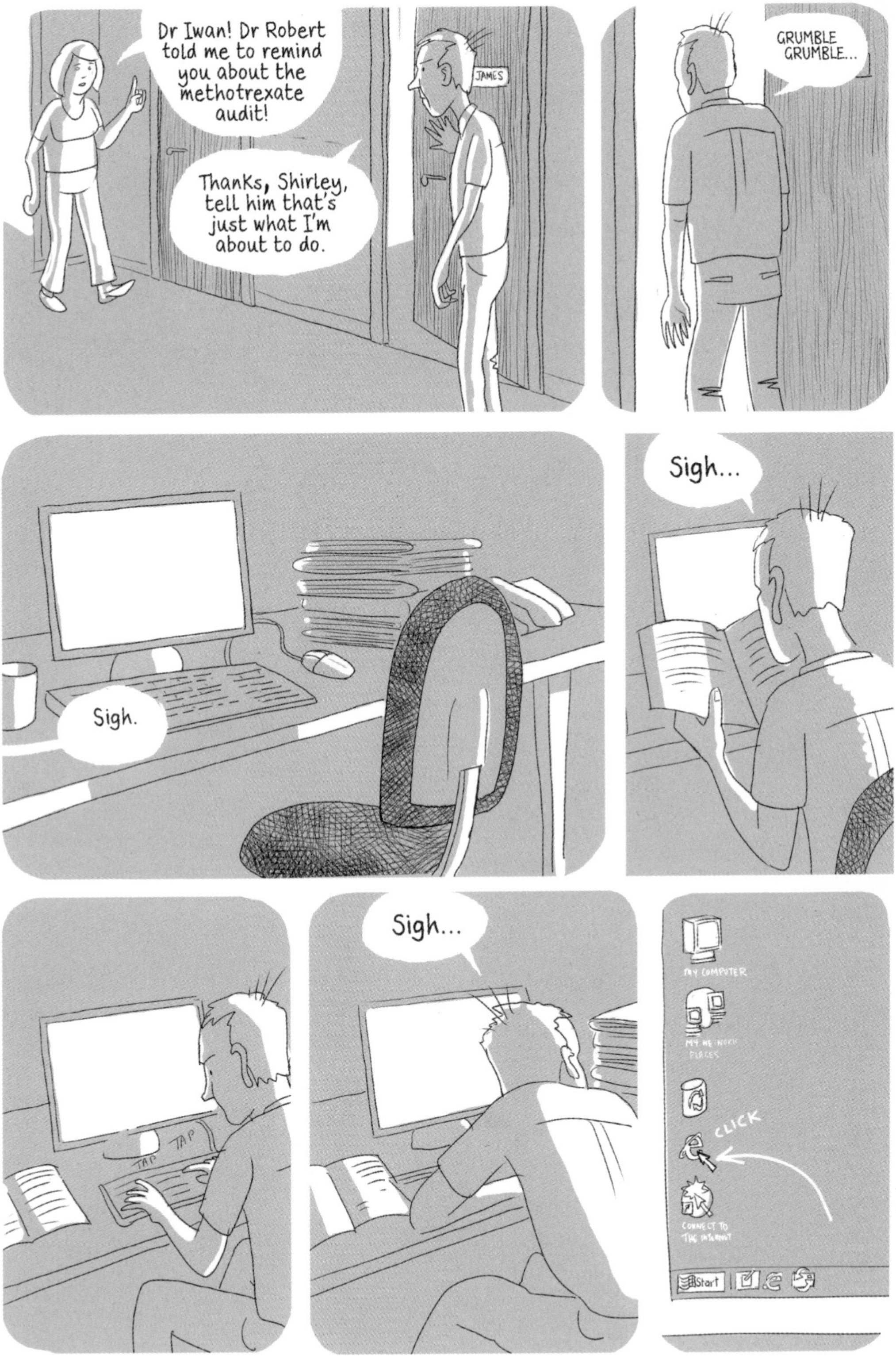
Dr Iwan! Dr Robert told me to remind you about the methotrexate audit!
JAMES
Thanks, Shirley, tell him that's just what I'm about to do.
GRUMBLE GRUMBLE...
Sigh.
Sigh...
TAP
TAP
Sigh...
MY COMPUTER
CLICK
CONNECT TO THE INTERNET
Start

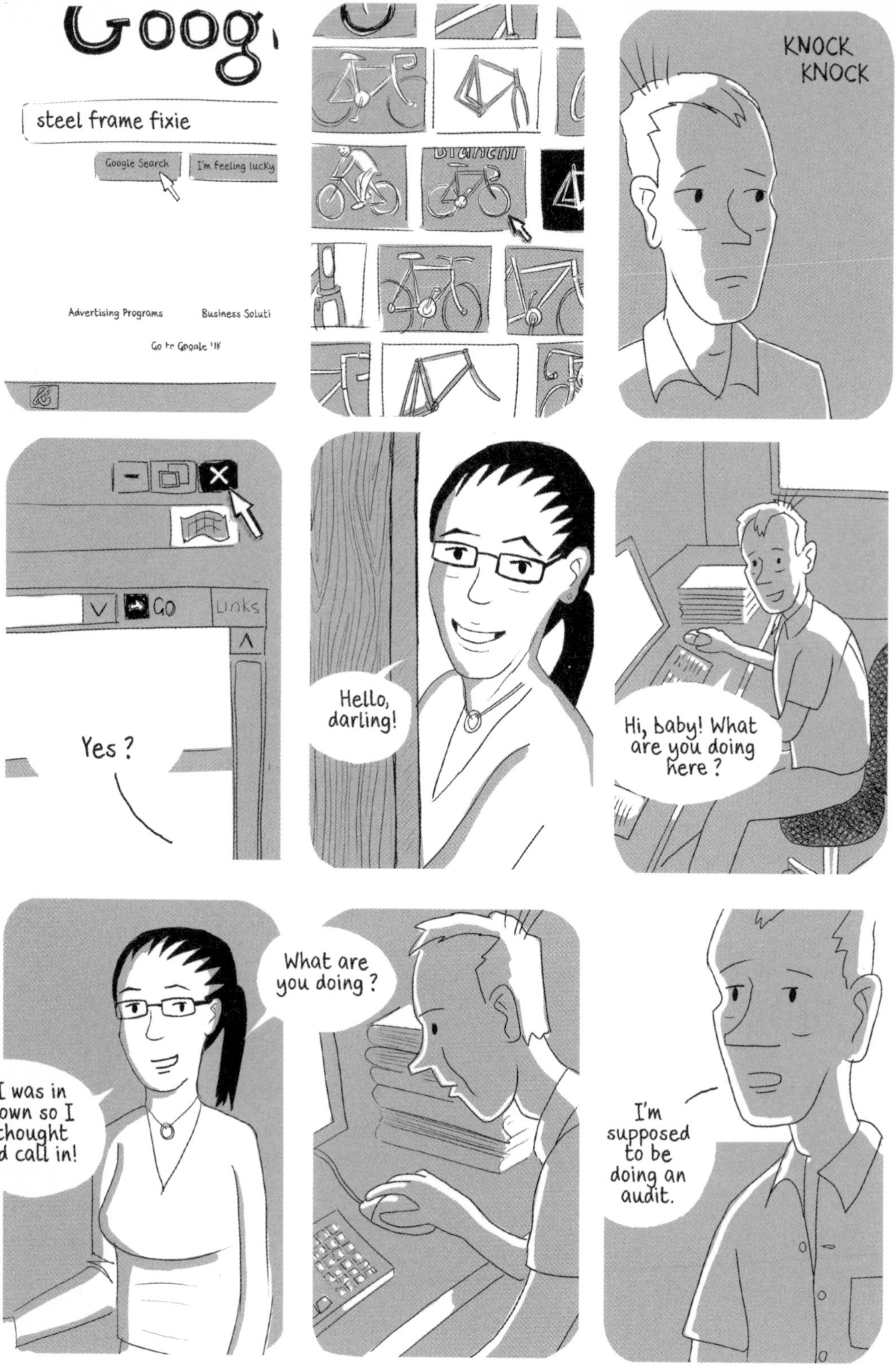
Goog
steel frame fixie
Google Search
I'm feeling lucky
Advertising Programs
Business Soluti
Bianchi
KNOCK KNOCK
GO
Links
Yes ?
Hello, darling!
Hi, baby! What are you doing here ?
I was in town so I thought I'd call in!
What are you doing ?
I'm supposed to be doing an audit.

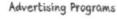

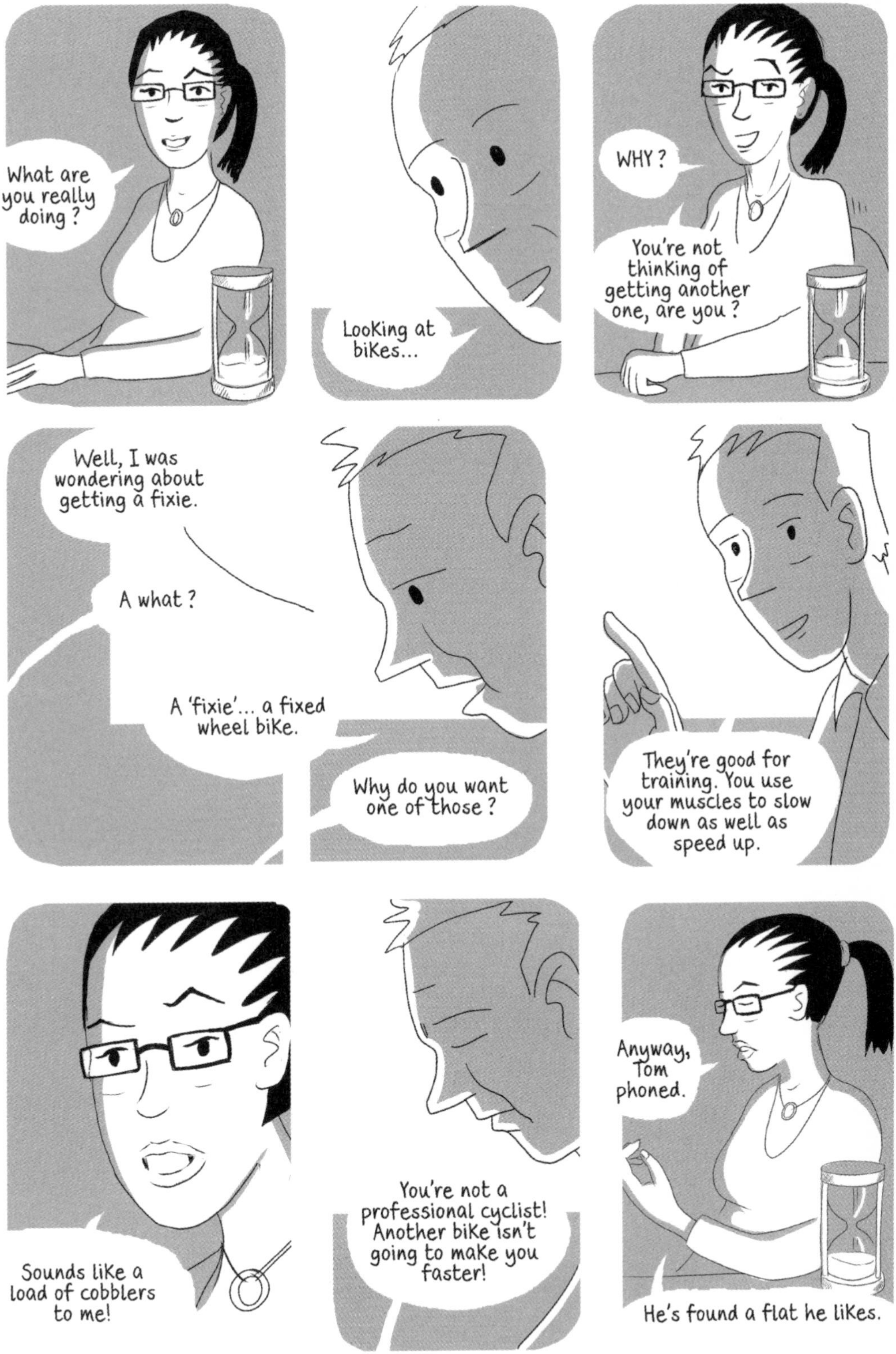
What are you really doing?
Looking at bikes...
WHY?
You're not thinking of getting another one, are you?
Well, I was wondering about getting a fixie.
A what?
A 'fixie'... a fixed wheel bike.
Why do you want one of those?
They're good for training. You use your muscles to slow down as well as speed up.
Sounds like a load of cobblers to me!
You're not a professional cyclist! Another bike isn't going to make you faster!
Anyway, Tom phoned.
He's found a flat he likes.

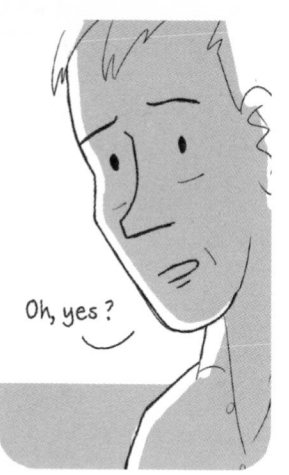

Oh, yes?

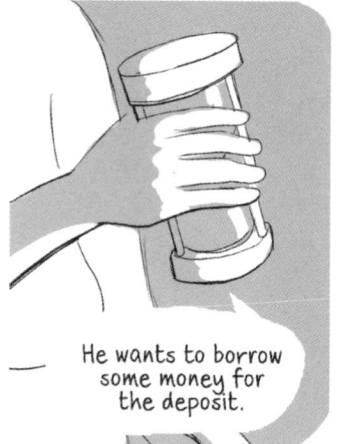

He wants to borrow some money for the deposit.

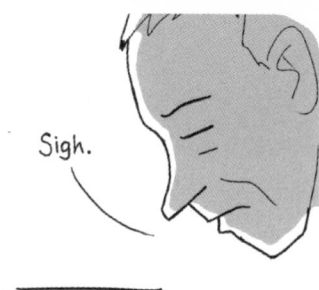

Sigh.

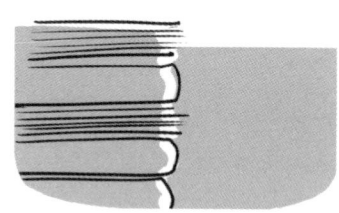

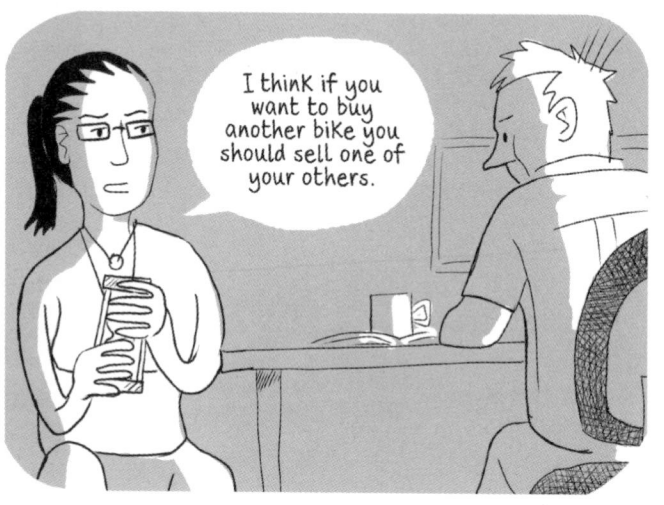

I think if you want to buy another bike you should sell one of your others.

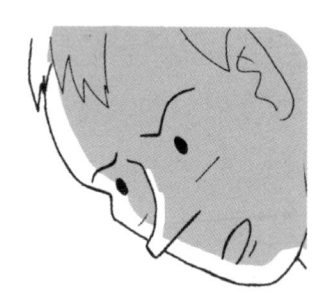

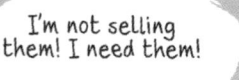

I'm not selling them! I need them!

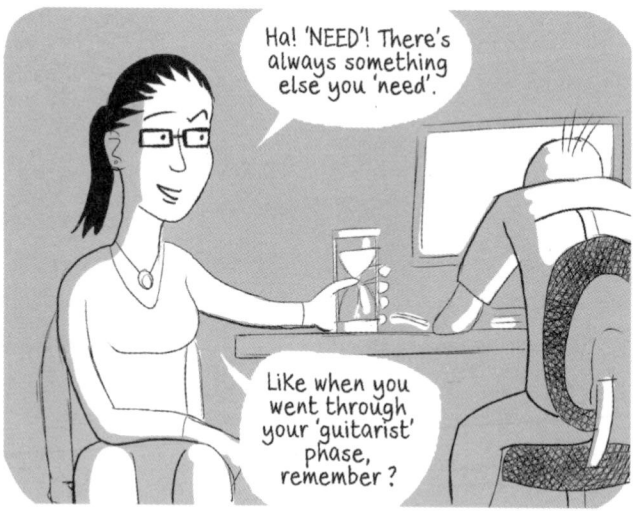

Ha! 'NEED'! There's always something else you 'need'.

Like when you went through your 'guitarist' phase, remember?

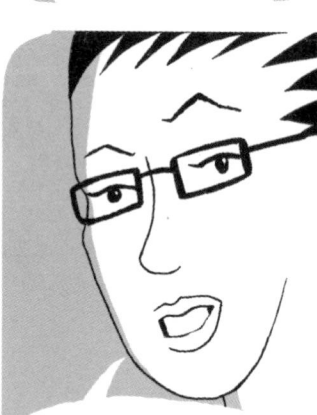

Hmmm... when you start obsessing about gear, it's usually a sign you're not happy...

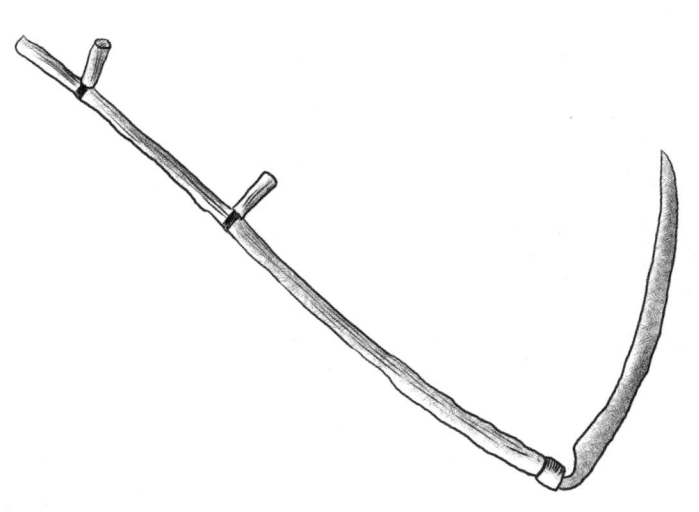

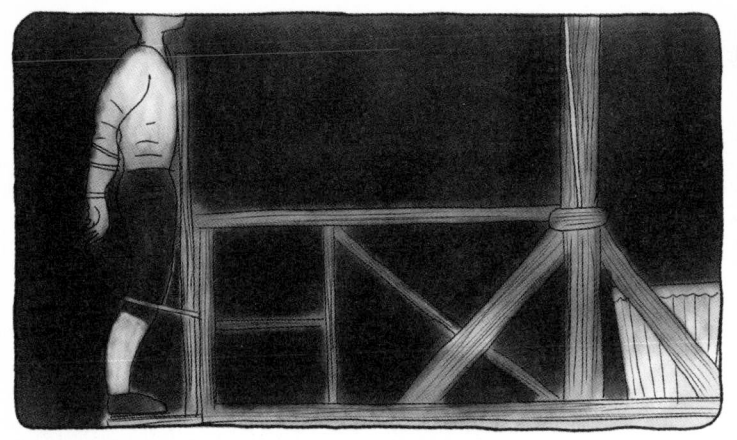
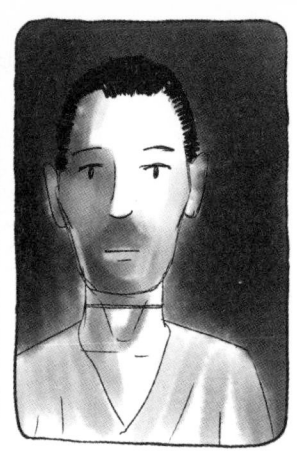
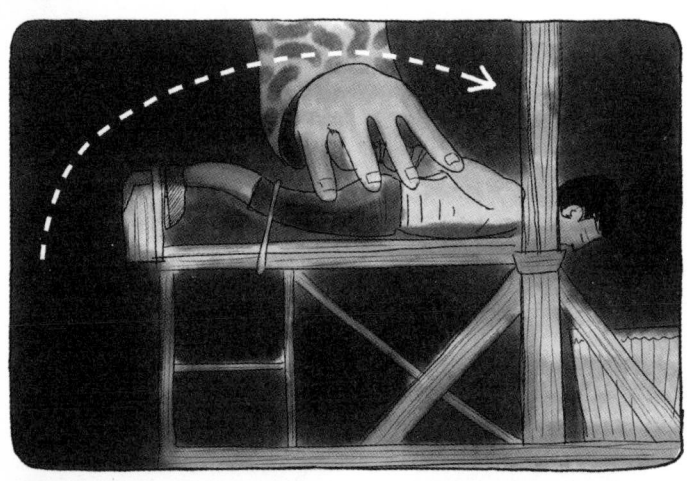
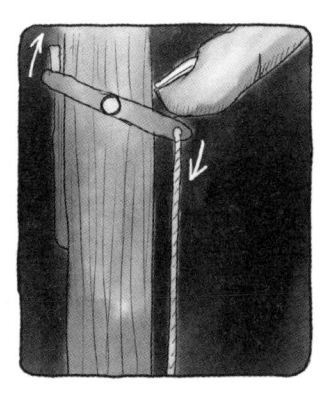
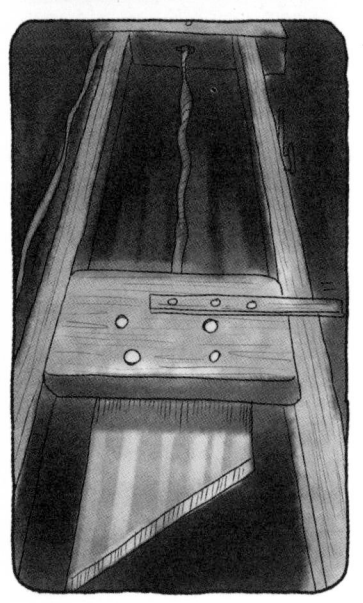
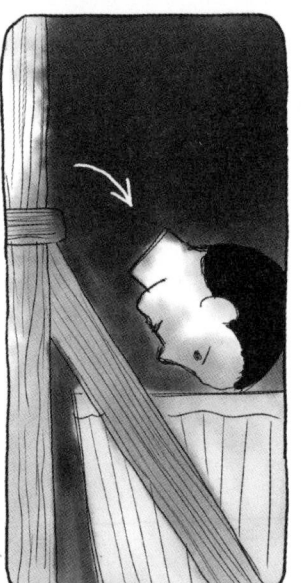
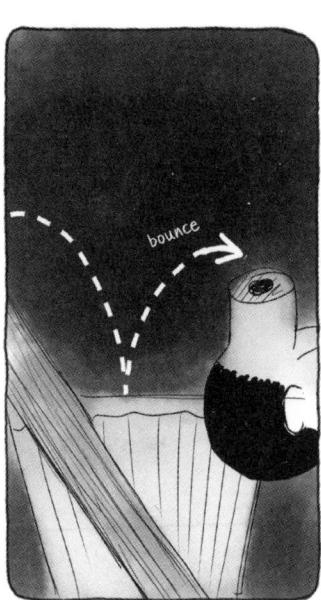

bounce

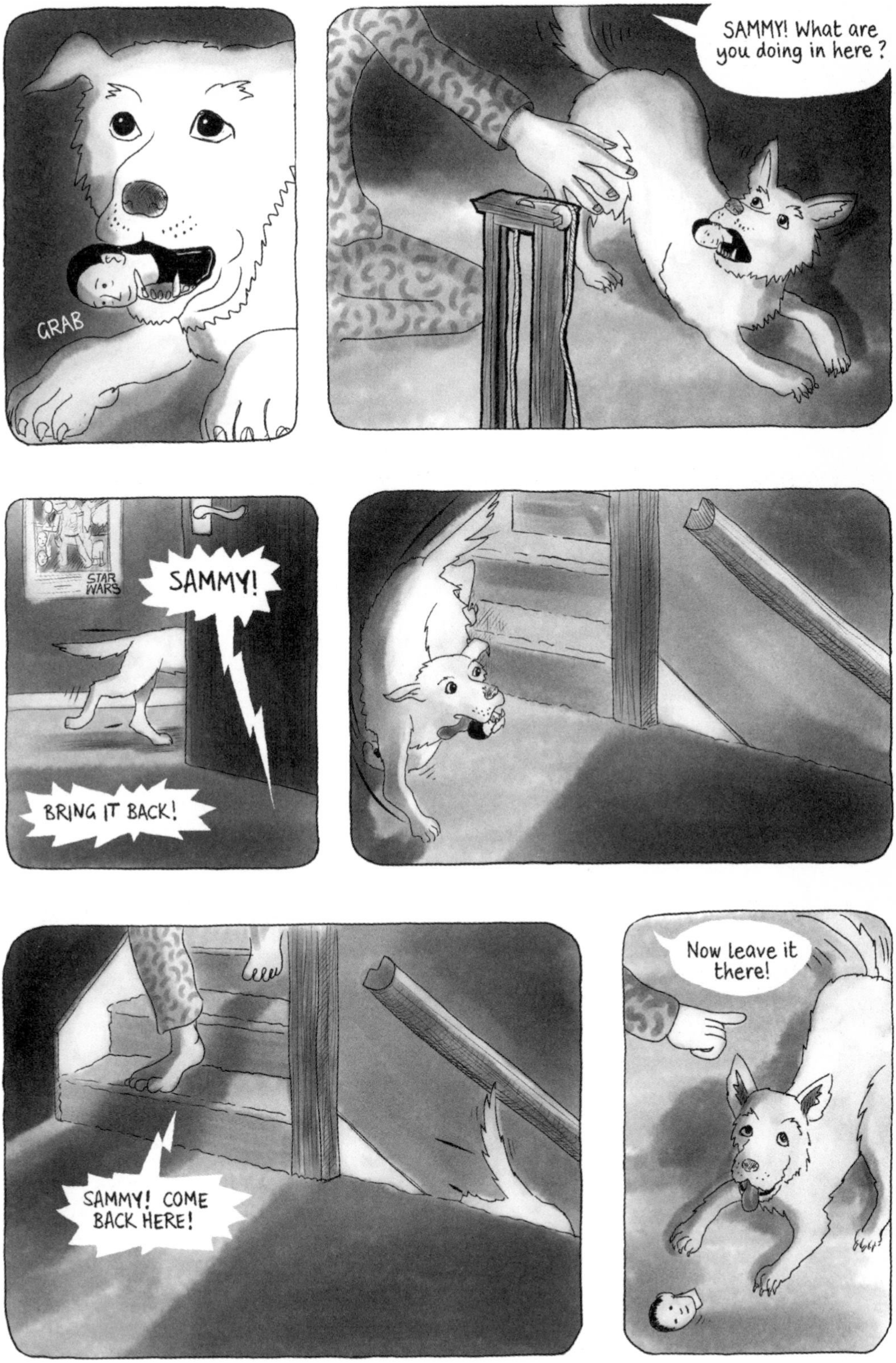
GRAB
SAMMY! What are you doing in here?
STAR WARS
SAMMY!
BRING IT BACK!
SAMMY! COME BACK HERE!
Now leave it there!

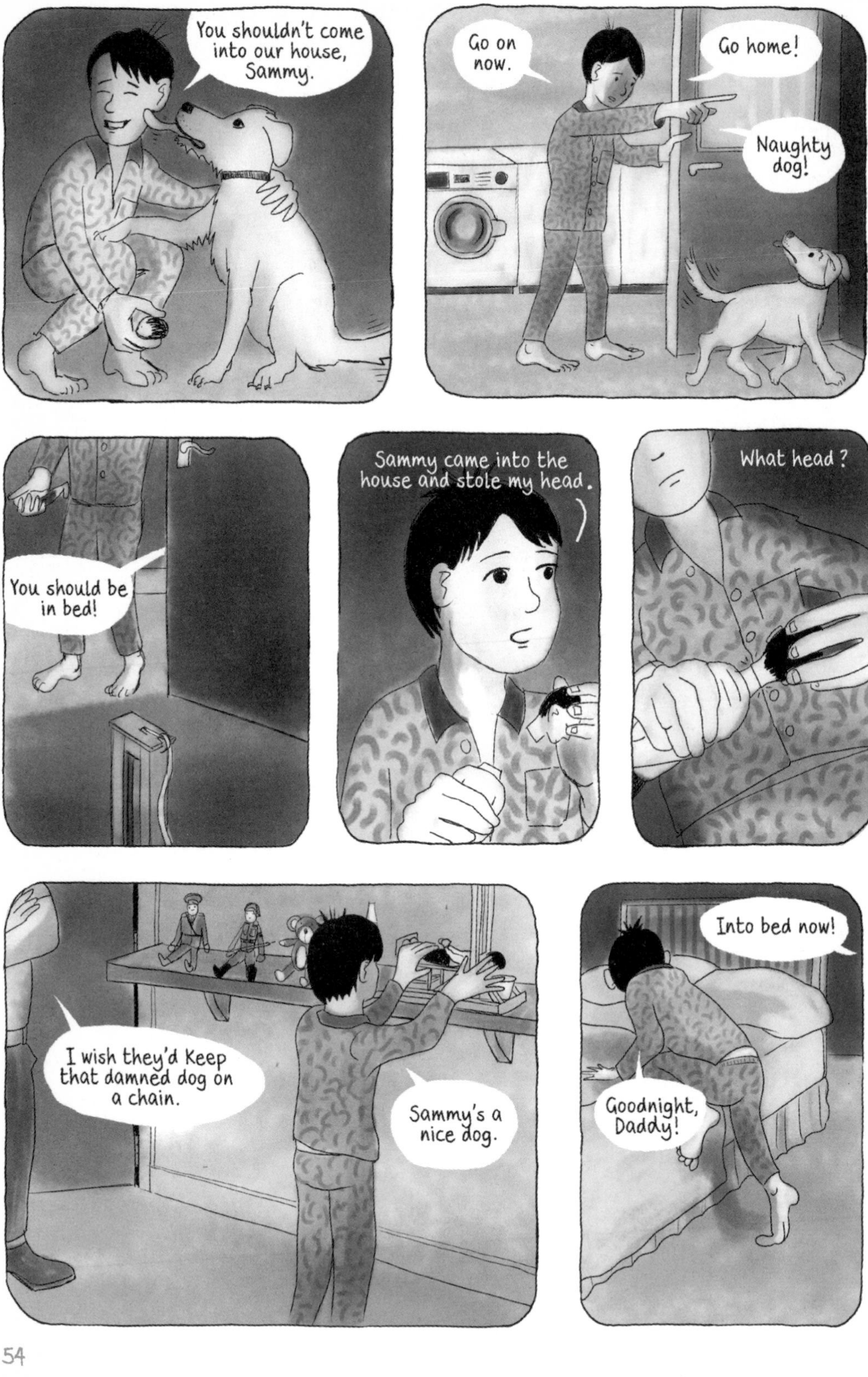
You shouldn't come into our house, Sammy.
Go on now.
Go home!
Naughty dog!
You should be in bed!
Sammy came into the house and stole my head.
What head?
I wish they'd Keep that damned dog on a chain.
Sammy's a nice dog.
Into bed now!
Goodnight, Daddy!

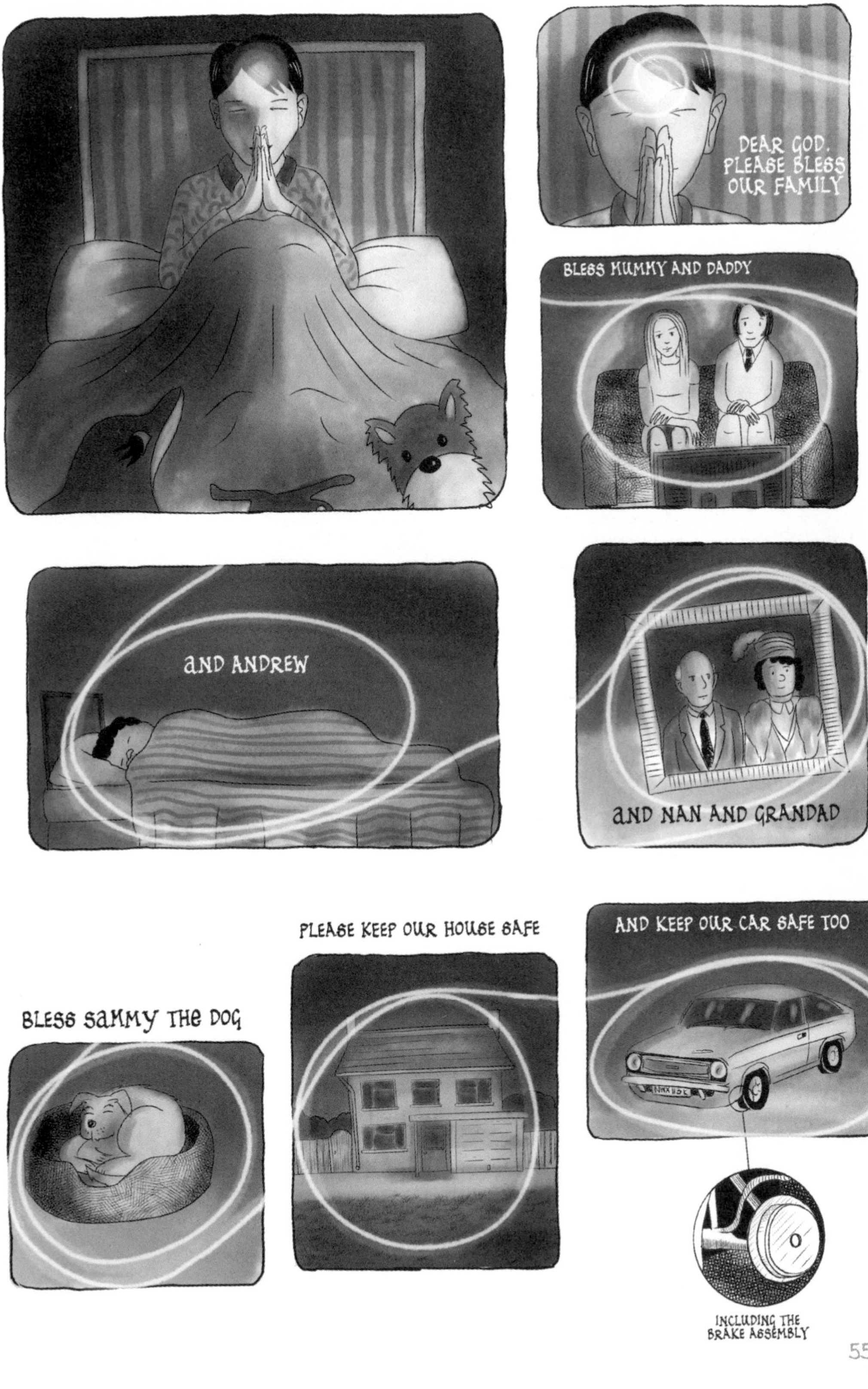
DEAR GOD.
PLEASE BLESS
OUR FAMILY
BLESS MUMMY AND DADDY
AND ANDREW
AND NAN AND GRANDAD
BLESS SAMMY THE DOG
PLEASE KEEP OUR HOUSE SAFE
AND KEEP OUR CAR SAFE TOO
INCLUDING THE
BRAKE ASSEMBLY

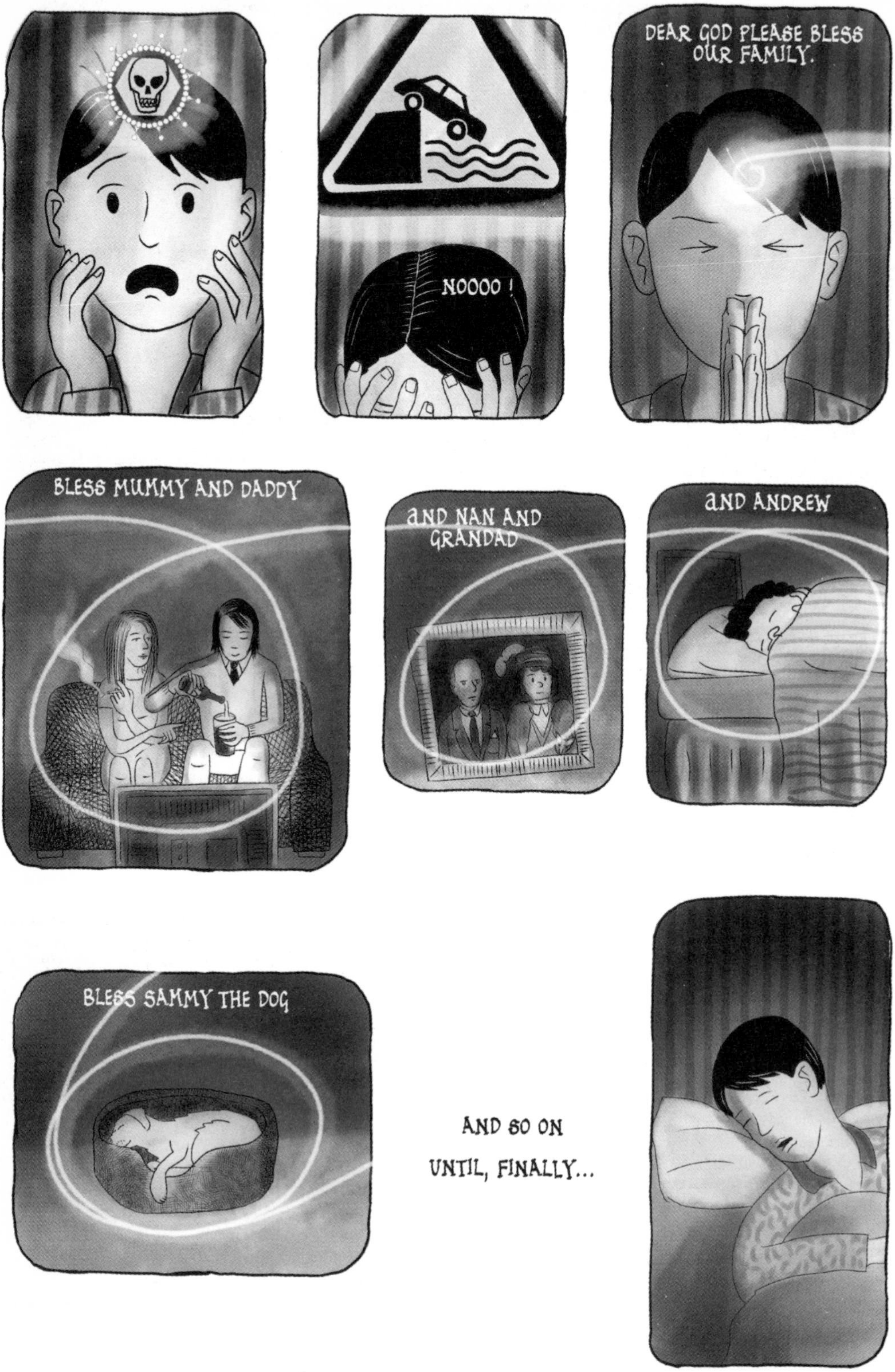
NOOOO !
DEAR GOD PLEASE BLESS OUR FAMILY.
BLESS MUMMY AND DADDY
AND NAN AND GRANDAD
AND ANDREW
BLESS SAMMY THE DOG
AND SO ON
UNTIL, FINALLY...

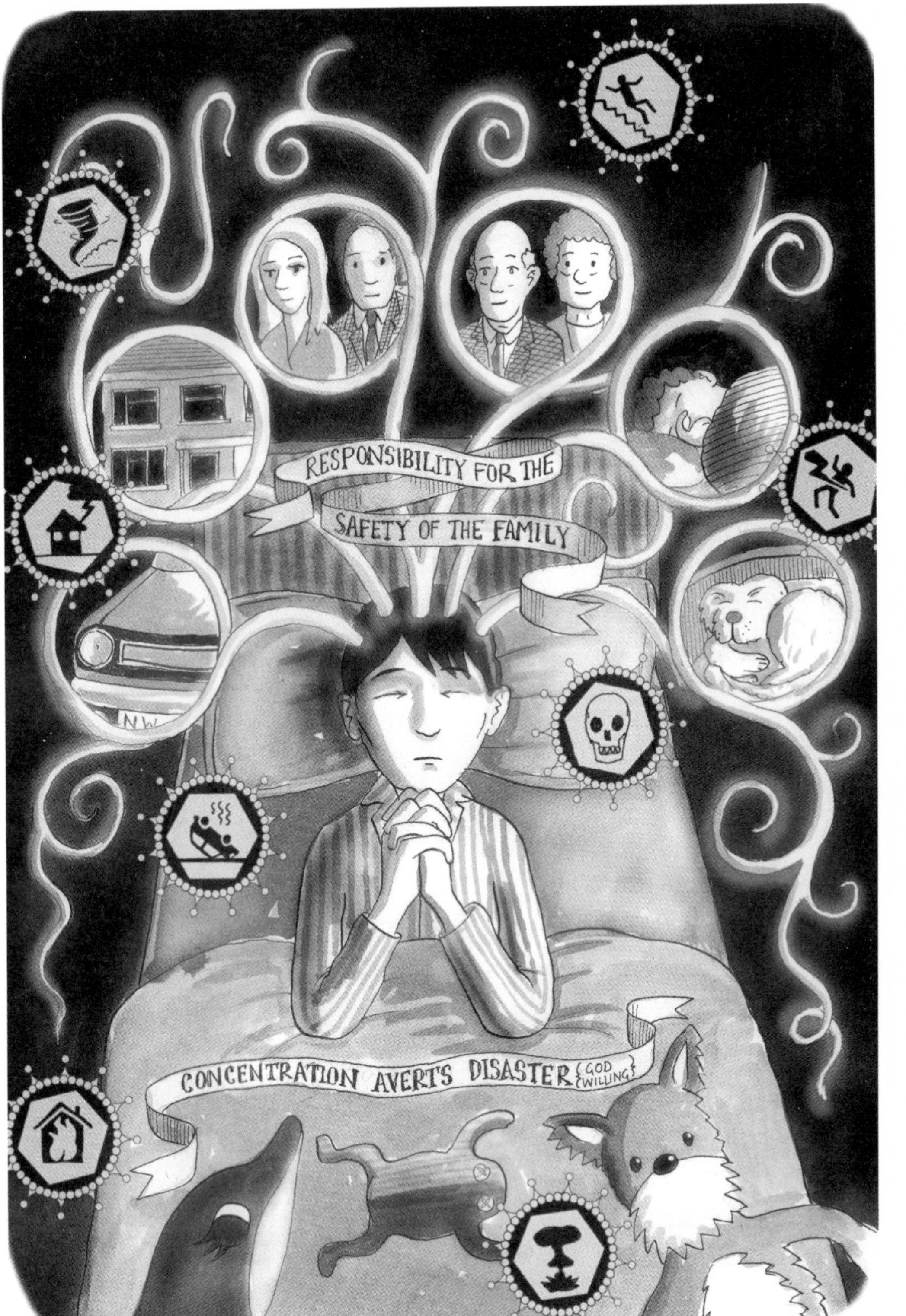
RESPONSIBILITY FOR THE
SAFETY OF THE FAMILY
CONCENTRATION AVERTS DISASTER {GOD WILLING}

66
66
shut
ugh...
66
66
shut
66
66
LOCK
66
ngh...
NNOOOOo!
66
66
66

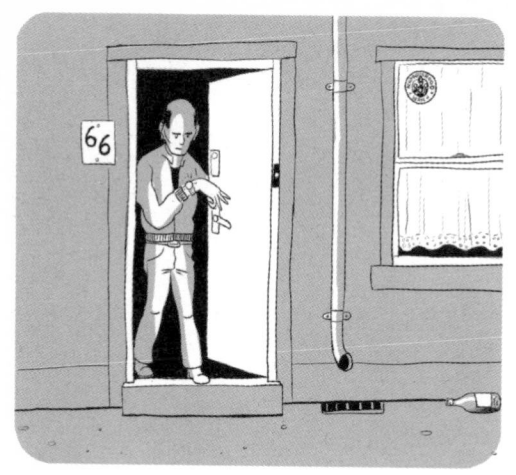

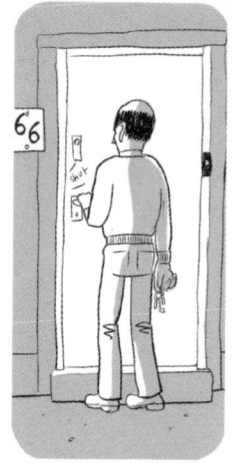

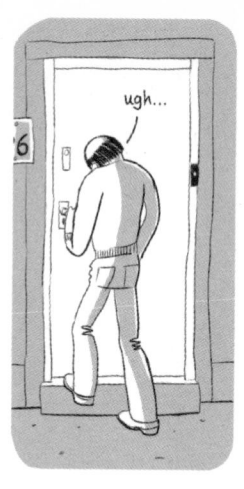

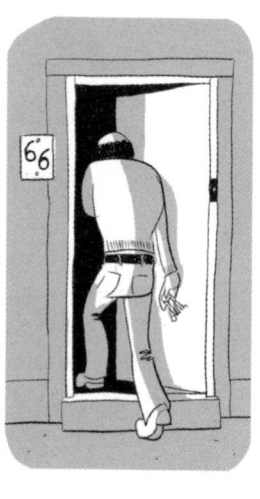

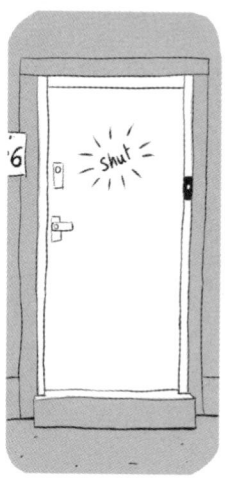

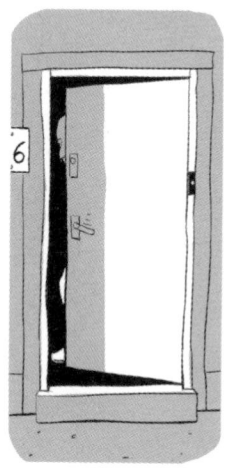

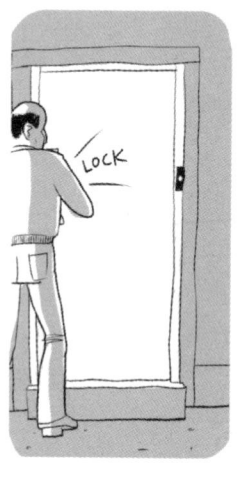

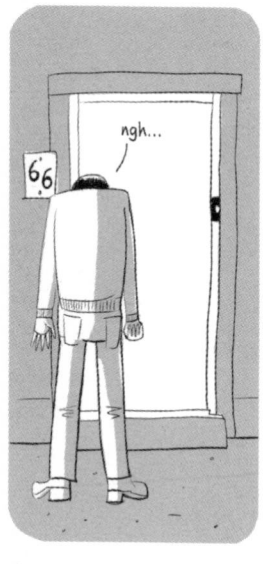

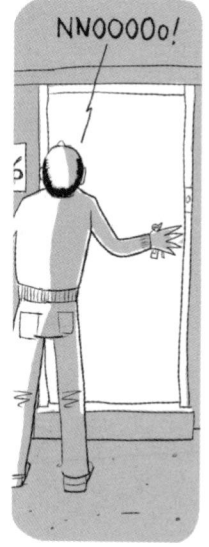

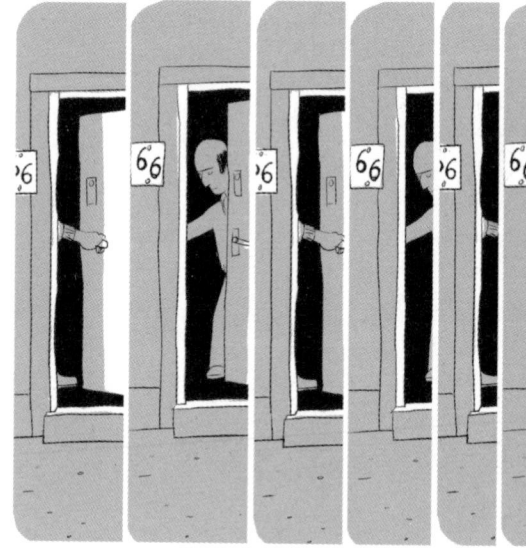

So, how did you get on with the tablets?
Umm... I didn't take them...
I was scared they would make me feel strange.
I've been worrying again...
The usual themes?
Not exactly.
This time it was about my sister's Kids.
Do you think I could be...
slide
a danger to them?

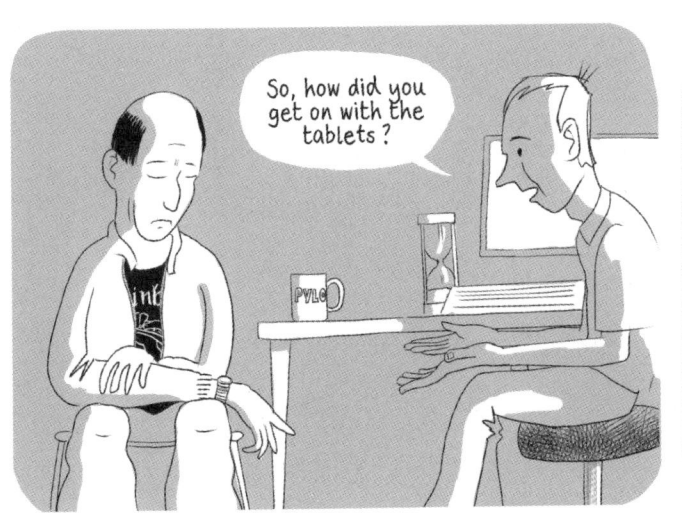

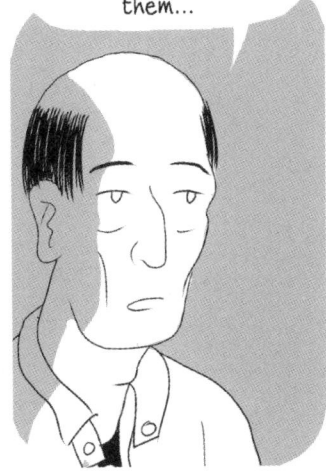

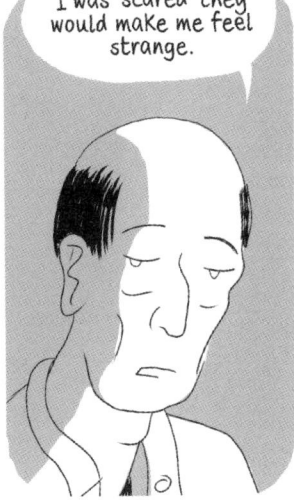

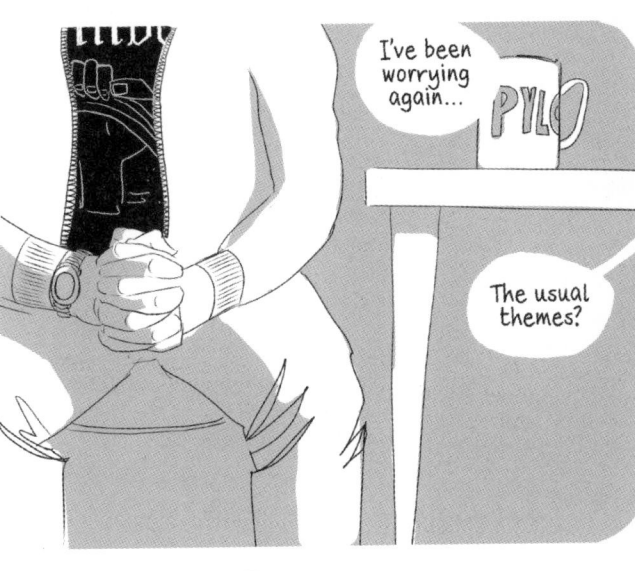

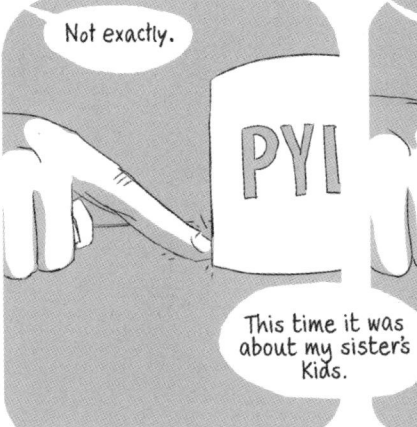

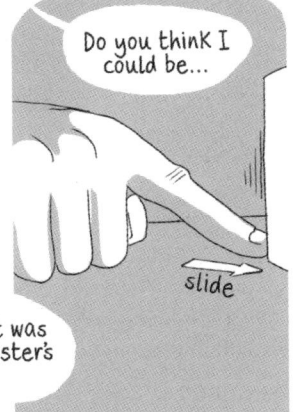

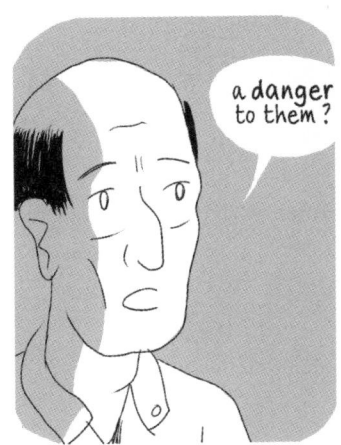

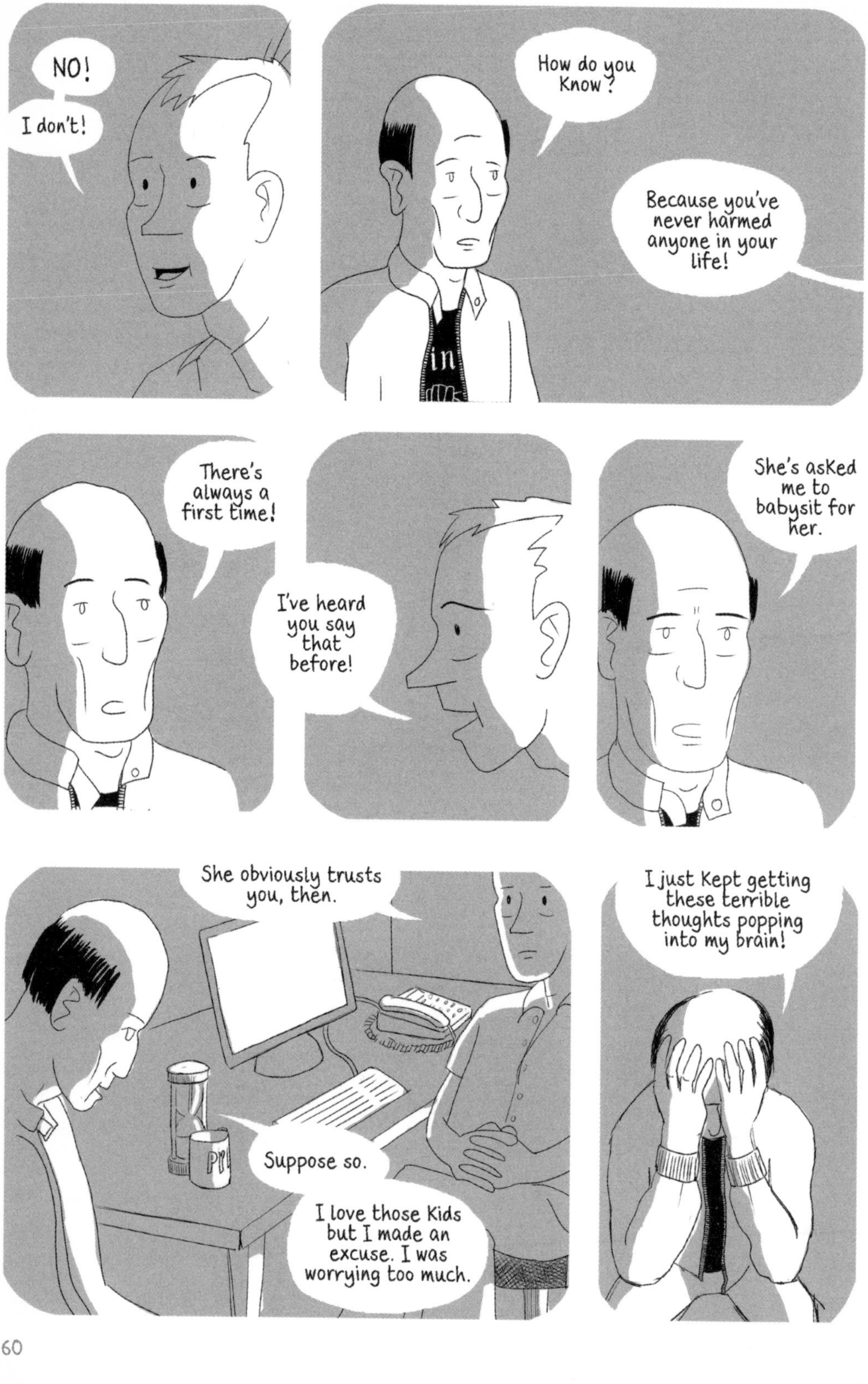
NO!
I don't!
How do you Know?
Because you've never harmed anyone in your life!
There's always a first time!
I've heard you say that before!
She's asKed me to babysit for her.
She obviously trusts you, then.
Suppose so.
I love those Kids but I made an excuse. I was worrying too much.
I just Kept getting these terrible thoughts popping into my brain!

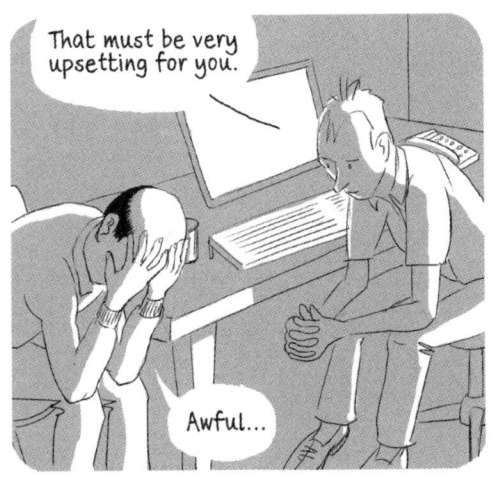

That must be very upsetting for you.

Awful...

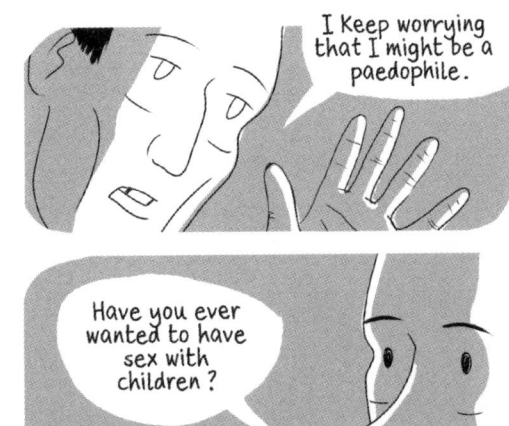

I keep worrying that I might be a paedophile.

Have you ever wanted to have sex with children?

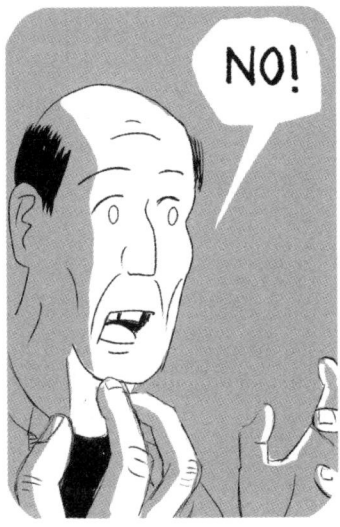

NO!

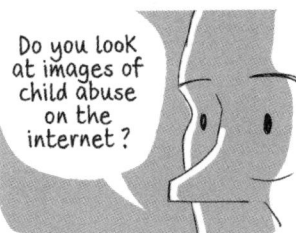

Do you look at images of child abuse on the internet?

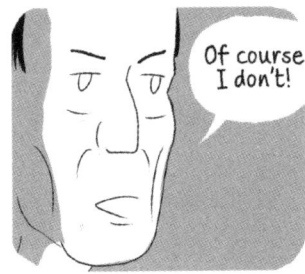

Of course I don't!

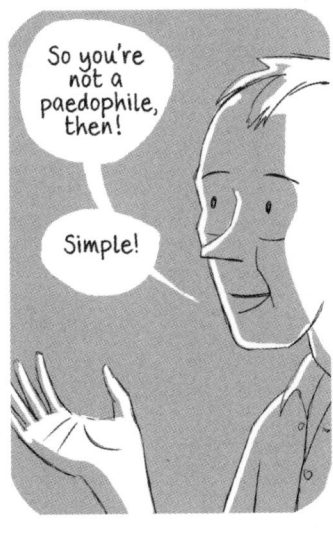

So you're not a paedophile, then!

Simple!

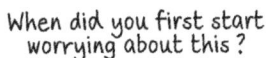

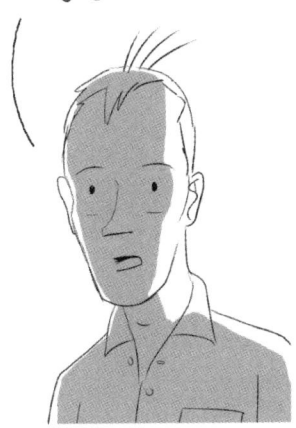

When did you first start worrying about this?

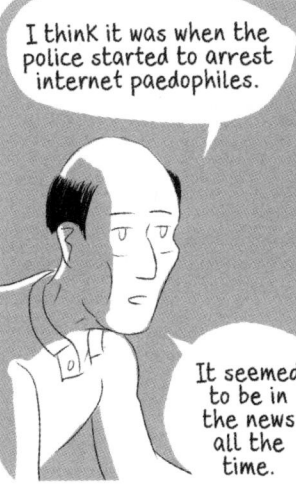

I think it was when the police started to arrest internet paedophiles.

It seemed to be in the news all the time.

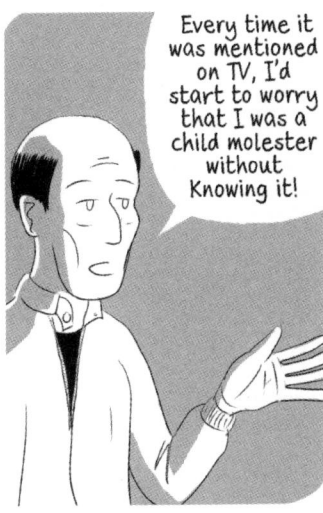

Every time it was mentioned on TV, I'd start to worry that I was a child molester without knowing it!

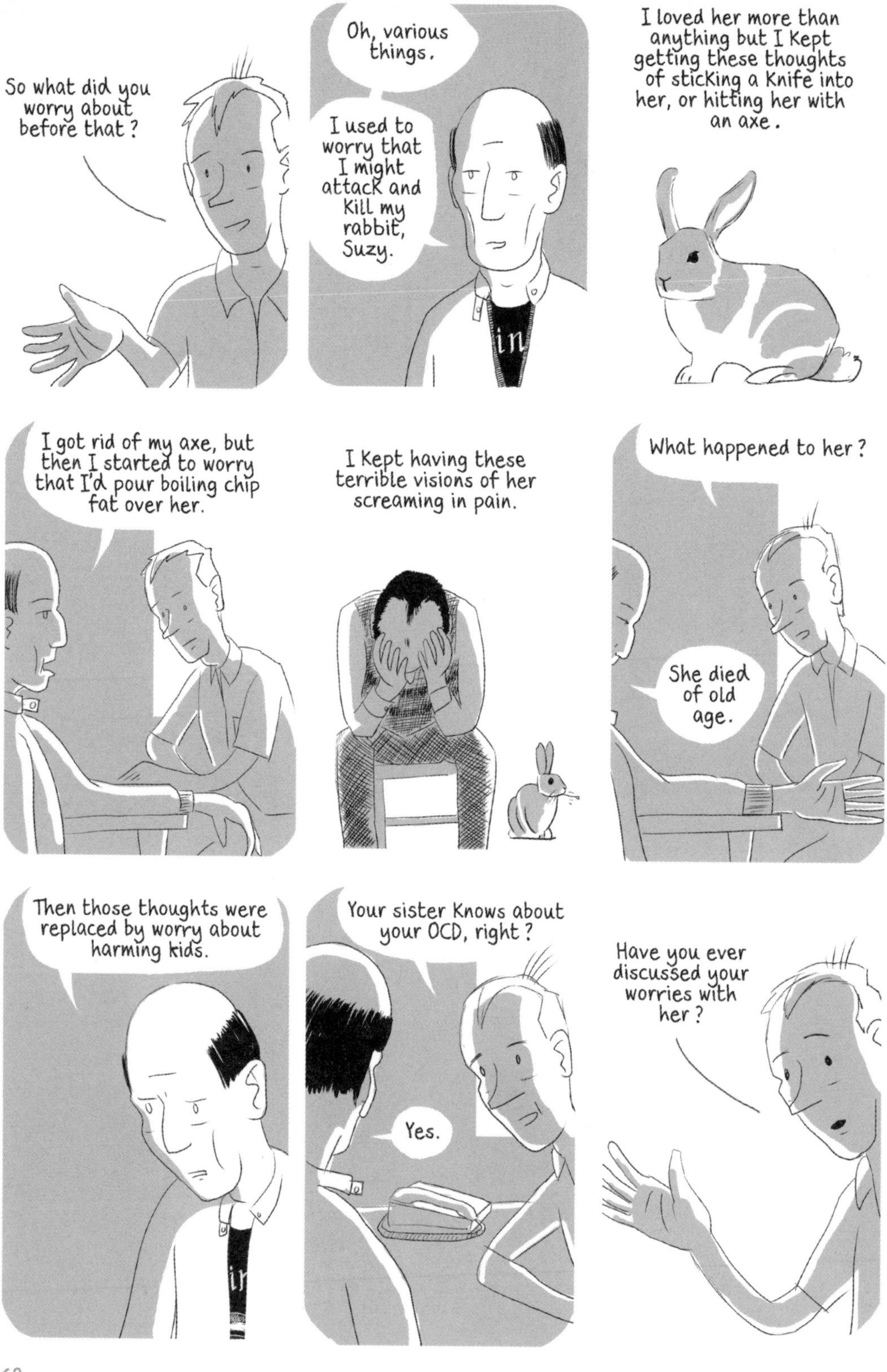
So what did you worry about before that?
Oh, various things.
I used to worry that I might attack and kill my rabbit, Suzy.
I loved her more than anything but I kept getting these thoughts of sticking a knife into her, or hitting her with an axe.
I got rid of my axe, but then I started to worry that I'd pour boiling chip fat over her.
I kept having these terrible visions of her screaming in pain.
What happened to her?
She died of old age.
Then those thoughts were replaced by worry about harming kids.
Your sister knows about your OCD, right?
Yes.
Have you ever discussed your worries with her?

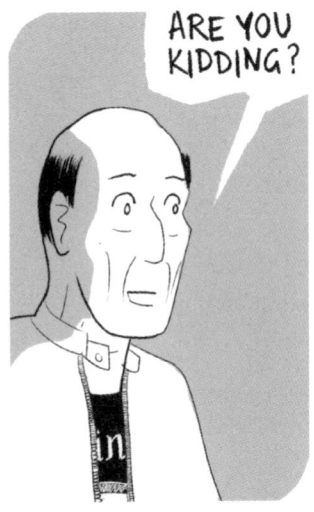

ARE YOU KIDDING?

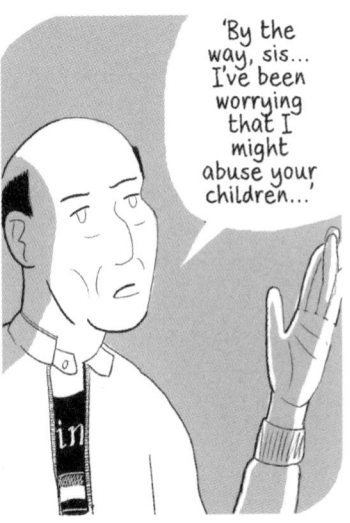

'By the way, sis... I've been worrying that I might abuse your children...'

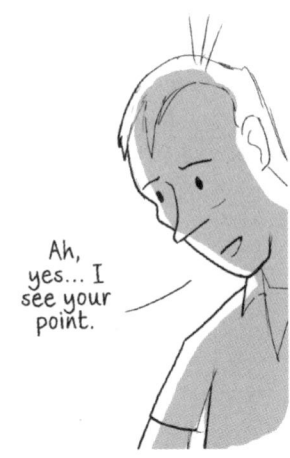

Ah, yes... I see your point.

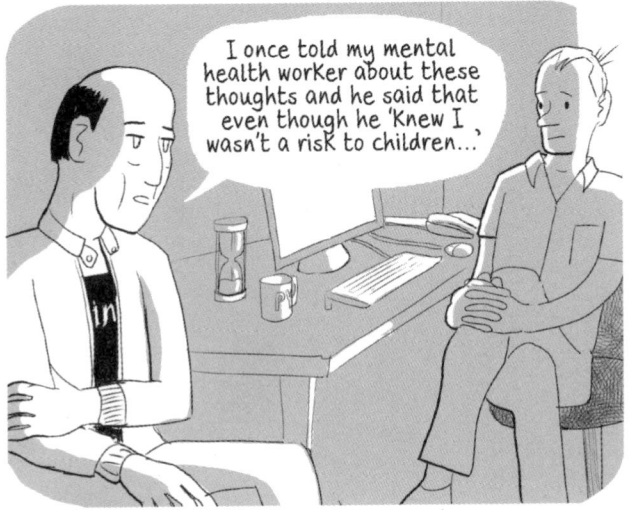

I once told my mental health worker about these thoughts and he said that even though he 'knew I wasn't a risk to children...'

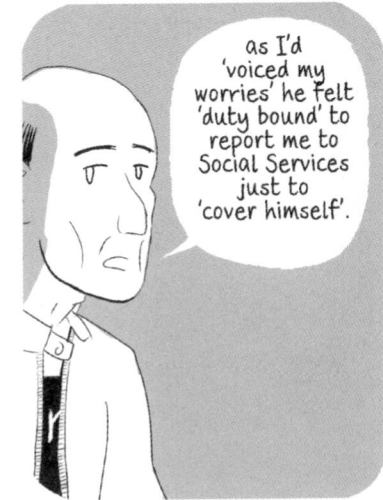

as I'd 'voiced my worries' he felt 'duty bound' to report me to Social Services just to 'cover himself'.

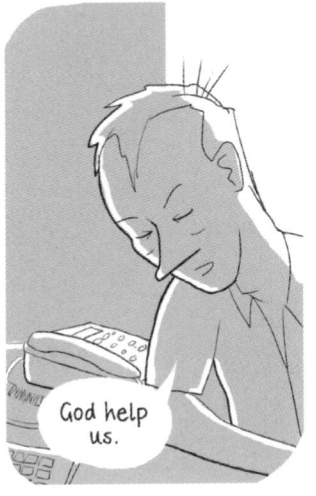

God help us.

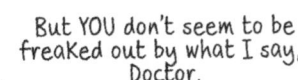

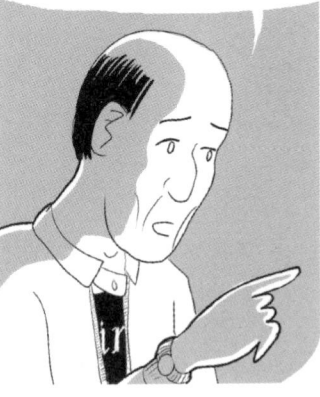

But YOU don't seem to be freaked out by what I say, Doctor.

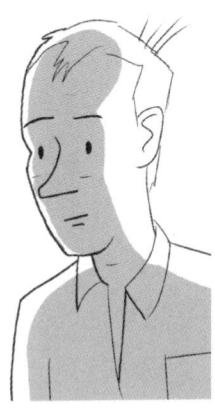

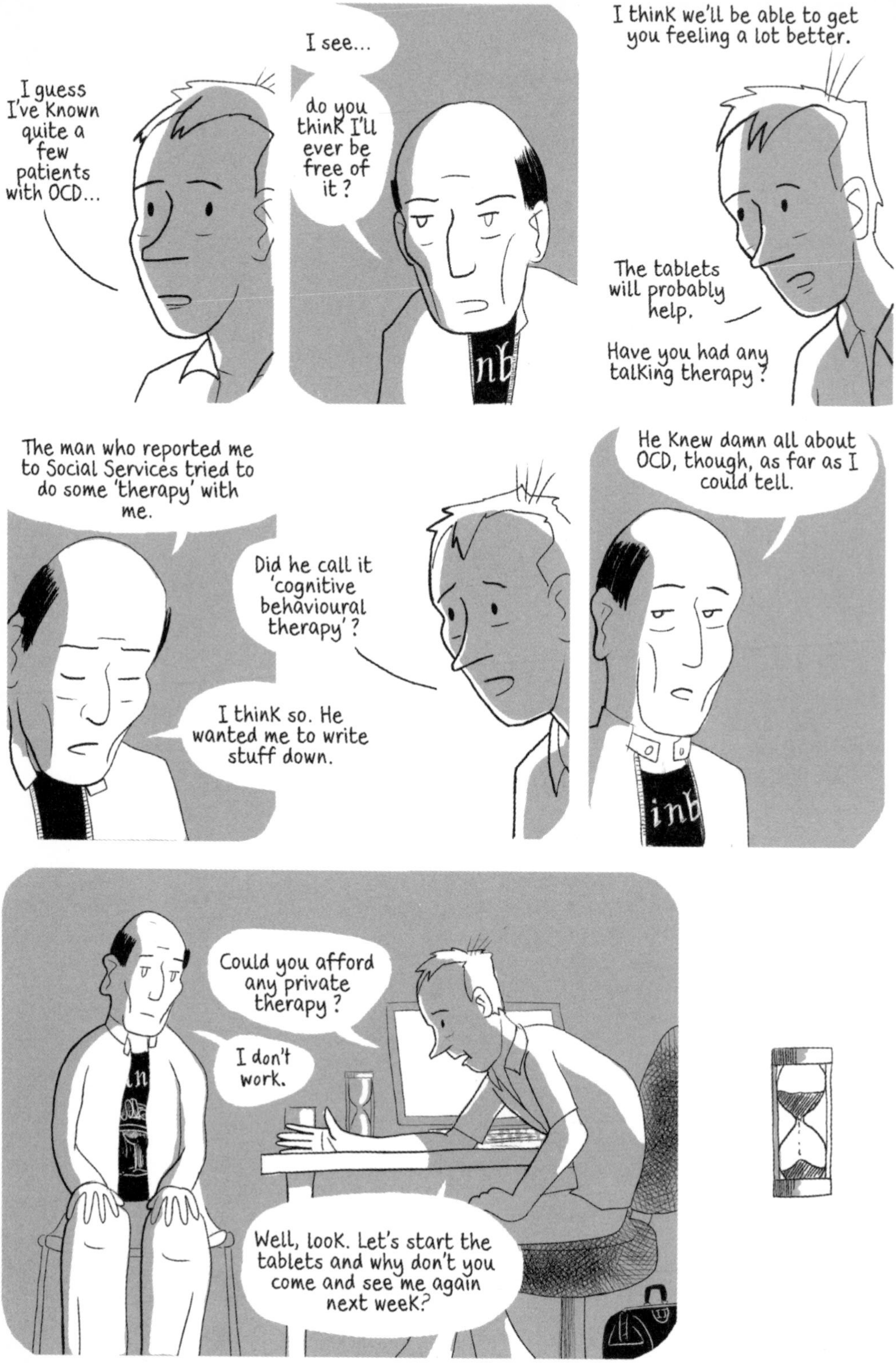
I guess I've Known quite a few patients with OCD...
I see...
do you think I'll ever be free of it?
I think we'll be able to get you feeling a lot better.
The tablets will probably help.
Have you had any talking therapy?
The man who reported me to Social Services tried to do some 'therapy' with me.
Did he call it 'cognitive behavioural therapy'?
I think so. He wanted me to write stuff down.
He Knew damn all about OCD, though, as far as I could tell.
Could you afford any private therapy?
I don't work.
Well, look. Let's start the tablets and why don't you come and see me again next week?

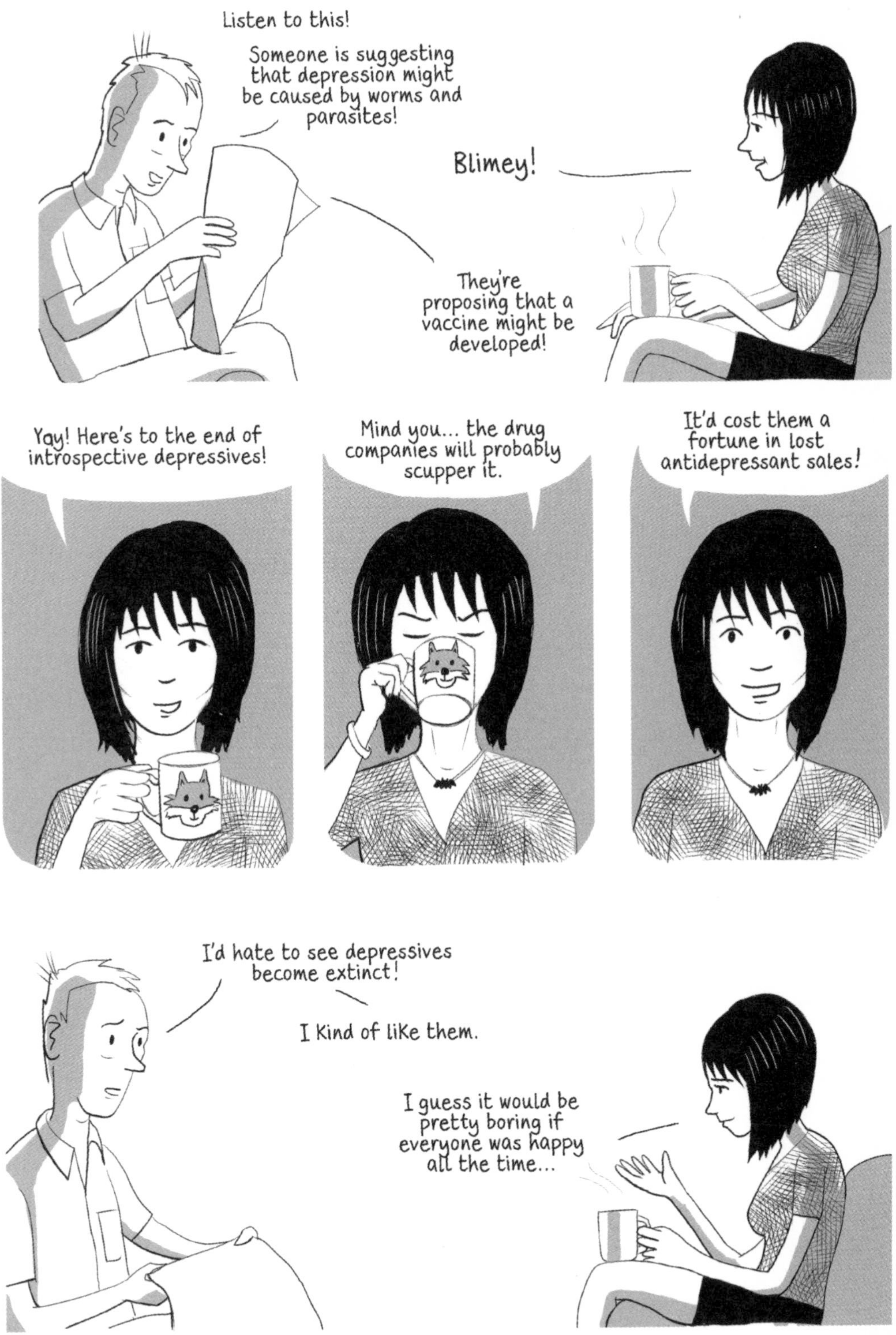
Listen to this!
Someone is suggesting that depression might be caused by worms and parasites!
Blimey!
They're proposing that a vaccine might be developed!
Yay! Here's to the end of introspective depressives!
Mind you... the drug companies will probably scupper it.
It'd cost them a fortune in lost antidepressant sales!
I'd hate to see depressives become extinct!
I kind of like them.
I guess it would be pretty boring if everyone was happy all the time...

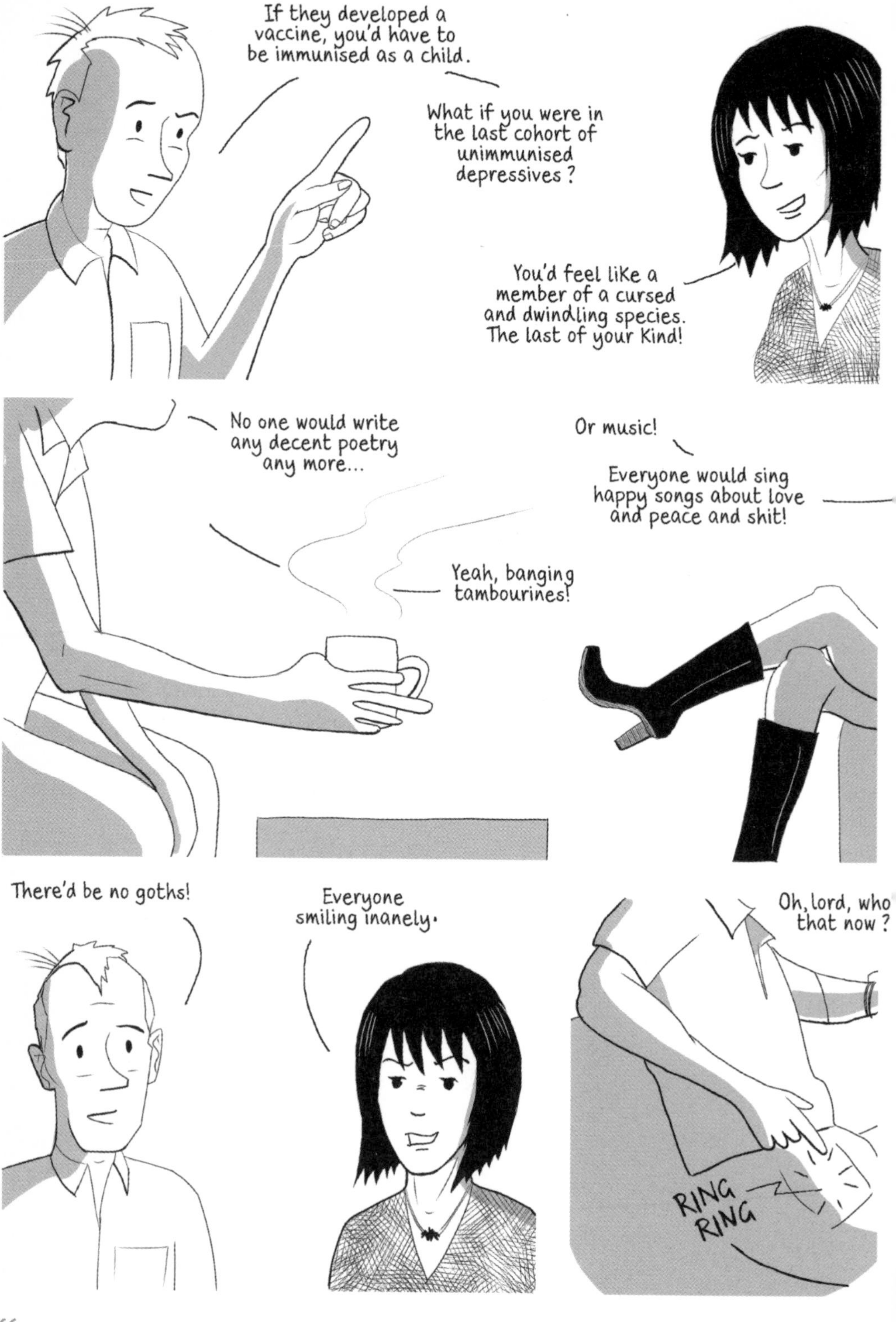
If they developed a vaccine, you'd have to be immunised as a child.
What if you were in the last cohort of unimmunised depressives?
You'd feel like a member of a cursed and dwindling species. The last of your kind!
No one would write any decent poetry any more...
Or music!
Everyone would sing happy songs about love and peace and shit!
Yeah, banging tambourines!
There'd be no goths!
Everyone smiling inanely.
Oh, lord, who that now?
RING RING

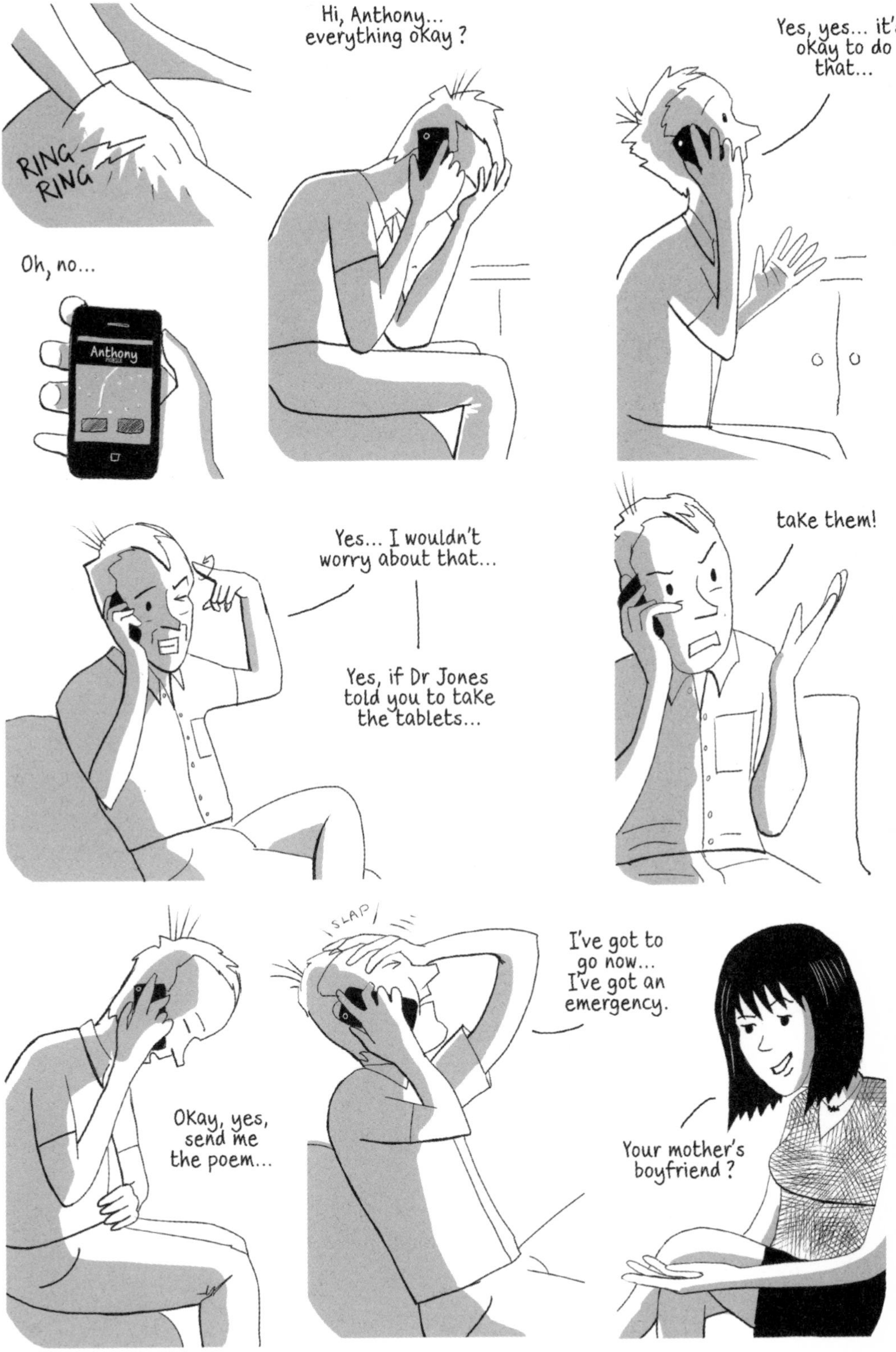
RING RING
Hi, Anthony... everything okay ?
Yes, yes... it's okay to do that...
Oh, no...
Anthony
Yes... I wouldn't worry about that...
Yes, if Dr Jones told you to take the tablets...
take them!
Okay, yes, send me the poem...
SLAP
I've got to go now... I've got an emergency.
Your mother's boyfriend ?

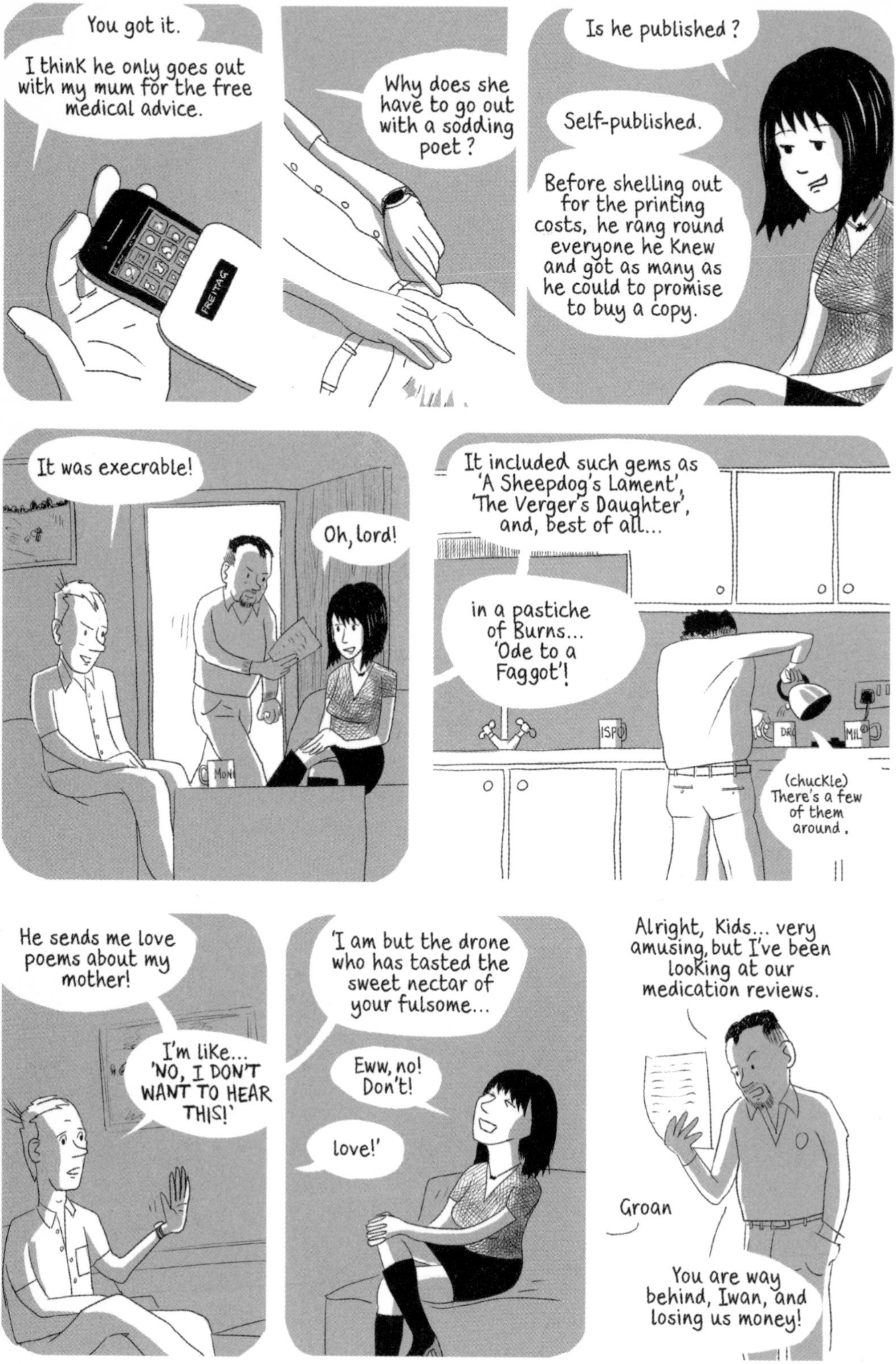
You got it.
I think he only goes out with my mum for the free medical advice.
FREITAG
Why does she have to go out with a sodding poet?
Is he published?
Self-published.
Before shelling out for the printing costs, he rang round everyone he knew and got as many as he could to promise to buy a copy.
It was execrable!
Oh, lord!
It included such gems as 'A Sheepdog's Lament', 'The Verger's Daughter', and, best of all...
in a pastiche of Burns... 'Ode to a Faggot'!
(chuckle) There's a few of them around.
He sends me love poems about my mother!
I'm like... 'NO, I DON'T WANT TO HEAR THIS!'
'I am but the drone who has tasted the sweet nectar of your fulsome...
Eww, no! Don't!
love!'
Alright, kids... very amusing, but I've been looking at our medication reviews.
Groan
You are way behind, Iwan, and losing us money!

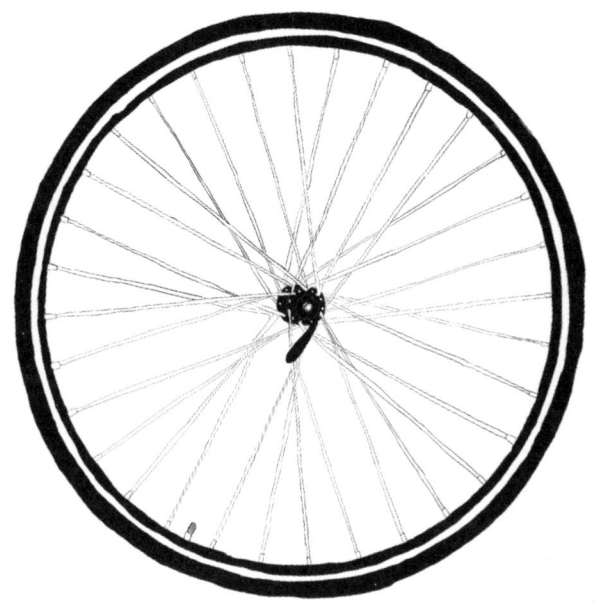

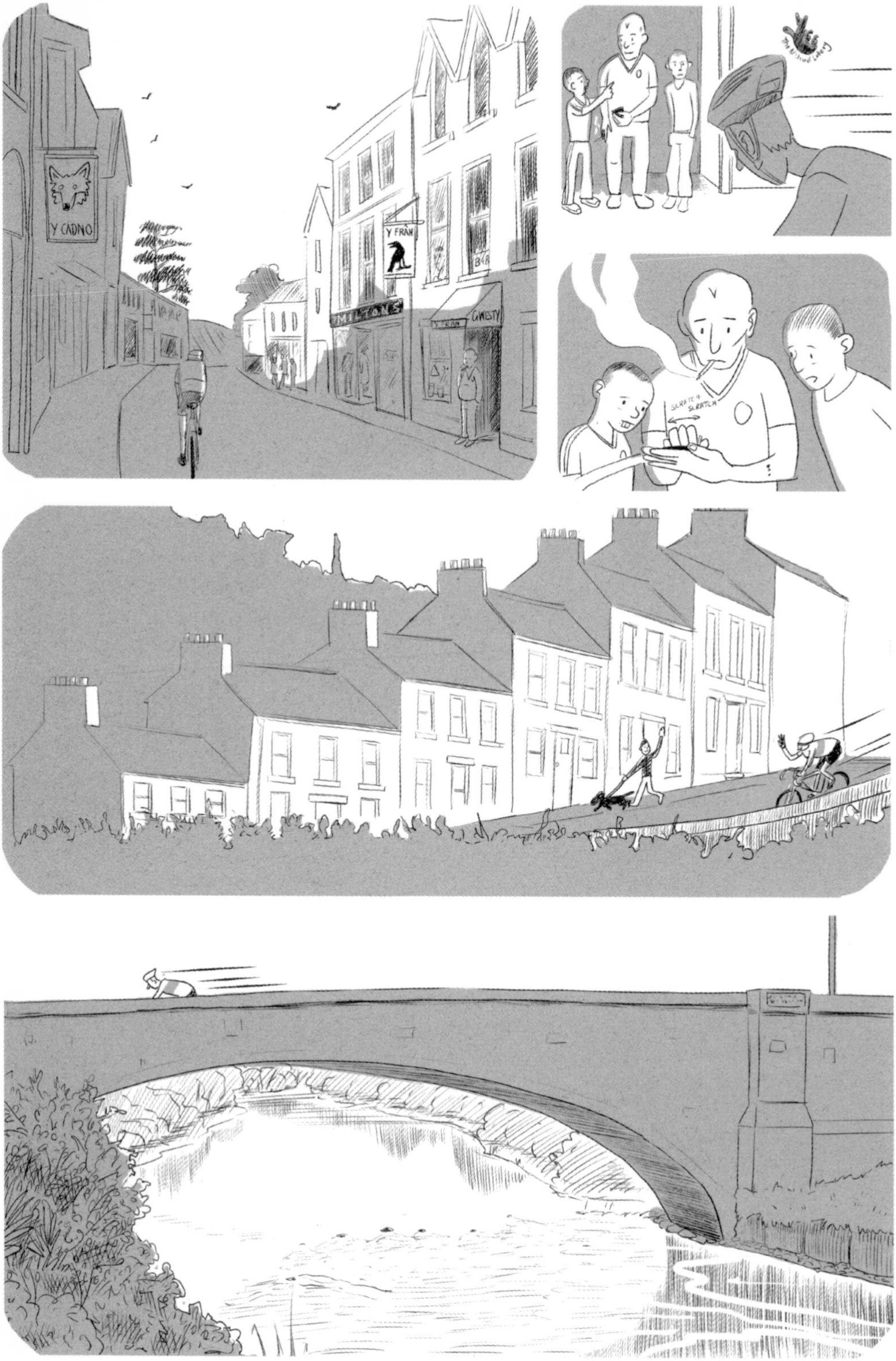
Y CADNO
Y FRÂN
B&B
GWESTY
SCRATCH
SCRATCH

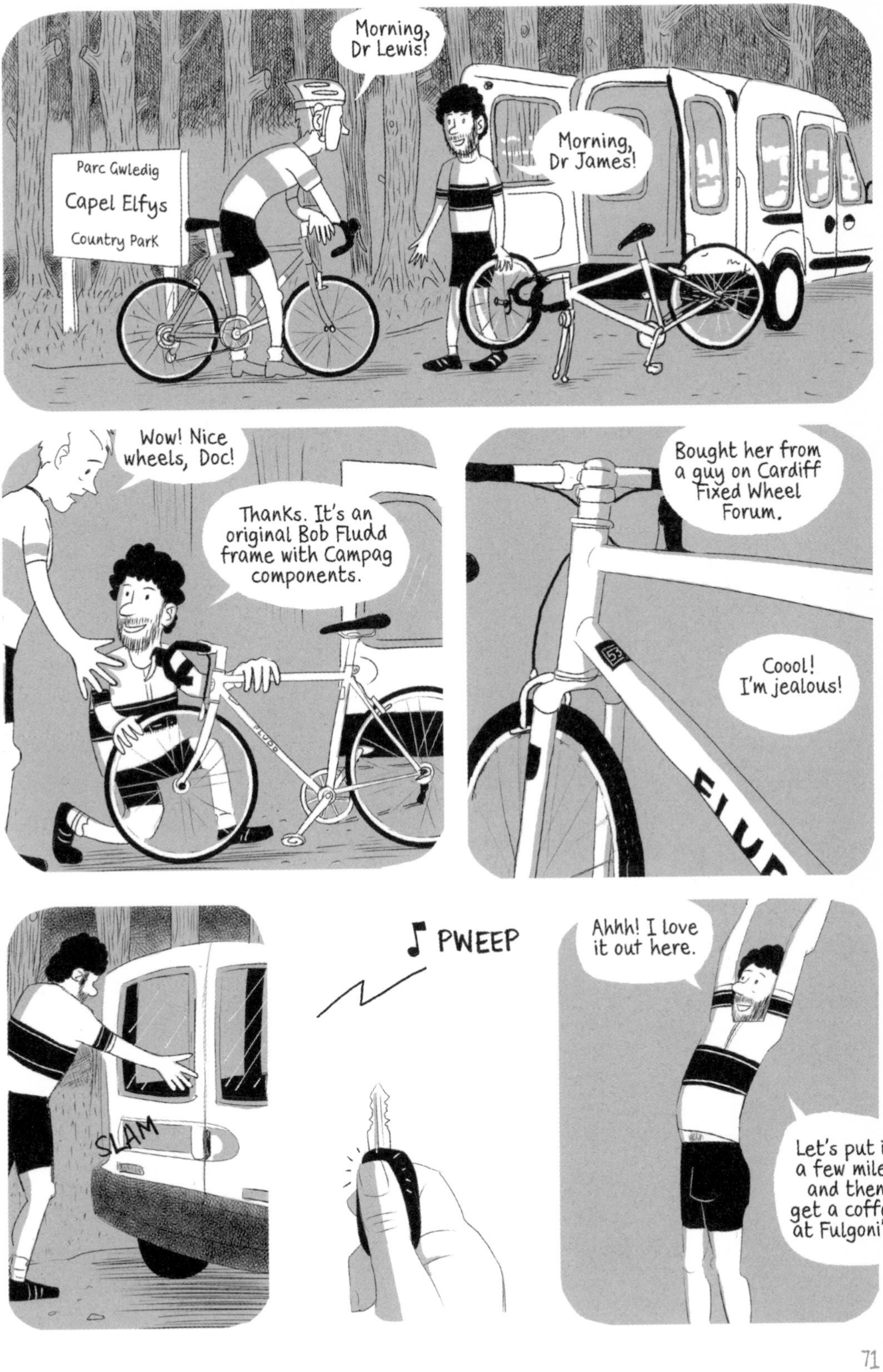
Morning, Dr Lewis!
Parc Gwledig
Capel Elfys
Country Park
Morning, Dr James!
Wow! Nice wheels, Doc!
Thanks. It's an original Bob Fludd frame with Campag components.
Bought her from a guy on Cardiff Fixed Wheel Forum.
Coool! I'm jealous!
SLAM
PWEEP
Ahhh! I love it out here.
Let's put in a few miles and then get a coffee at Fulgoni's.

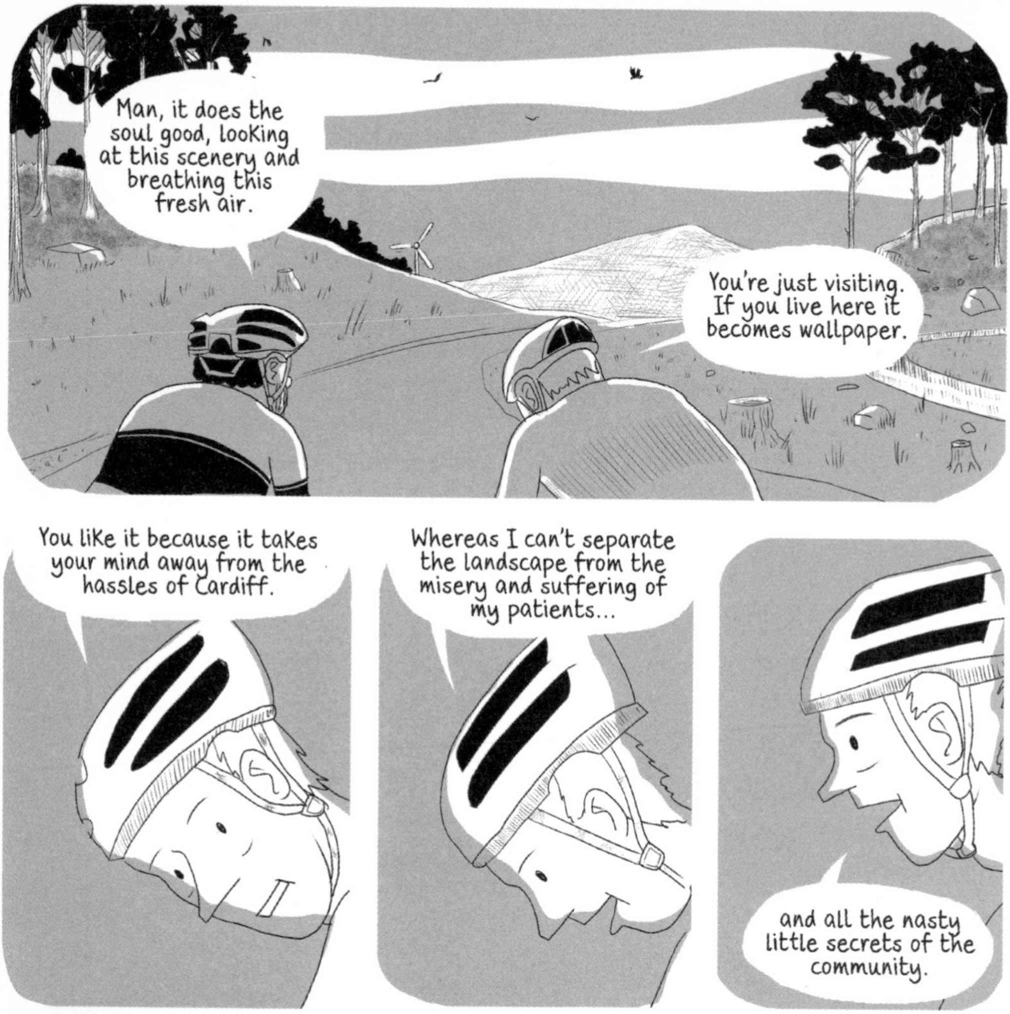

Man, it does the soul good, looking at this scenery and breathing this fresh air.
You're just visiting. If you live here it becomes wallpaper.
You like it because it takes your mind away from the hassles of Cardiff.
Whereas I can't separate the landscape from the misery and suffering of my patients...
and all the nasty little secrets of the community.
Wow! who lives there ?
Local businessman.
Owns a couple of mini-markets.
Thinks he's a Lord !
Nightmare.

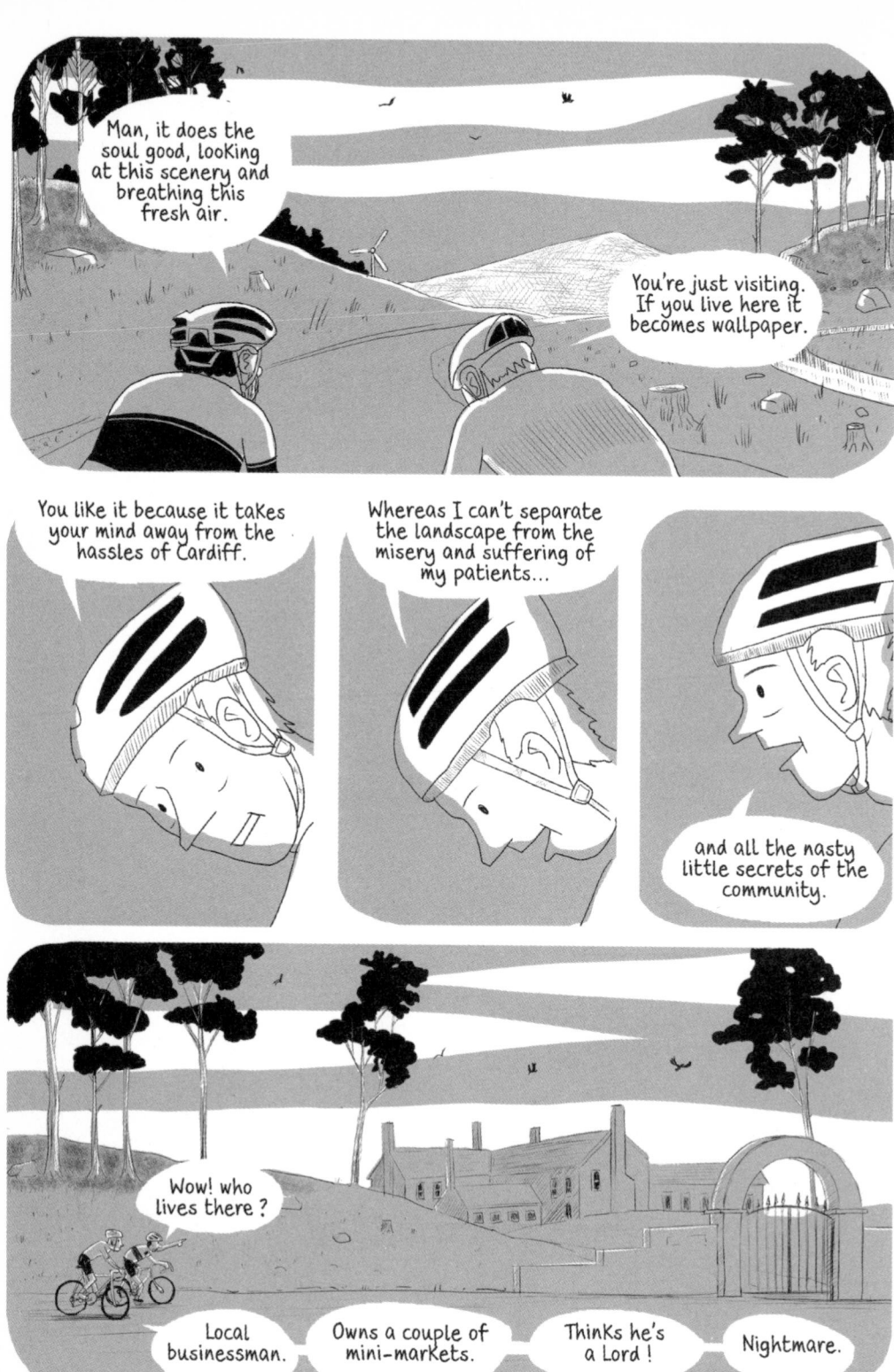

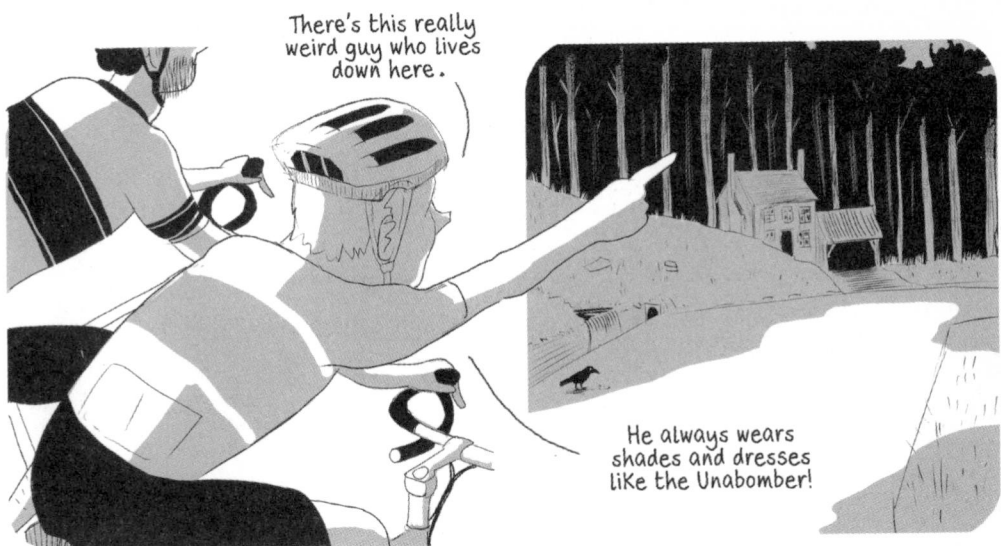

There's this really weird guy who lives down here.

He always wears shades and dresses like the Unabomber!

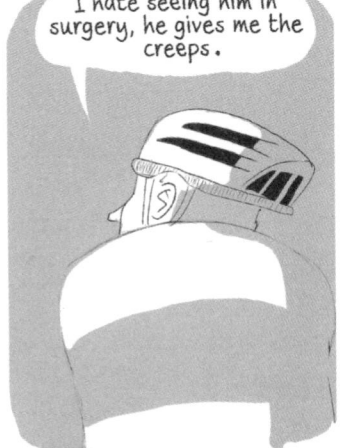

I hate seeing him in surgery, he gives me the creeps.

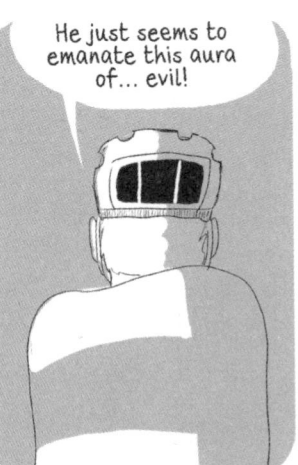

He just seems to emanate this aura of... evil!

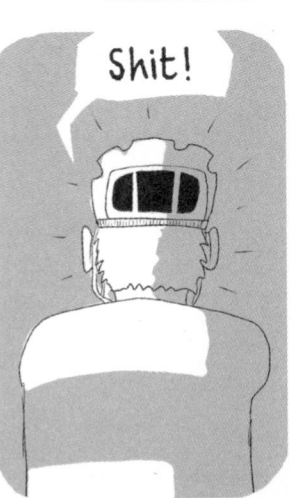

Shit!

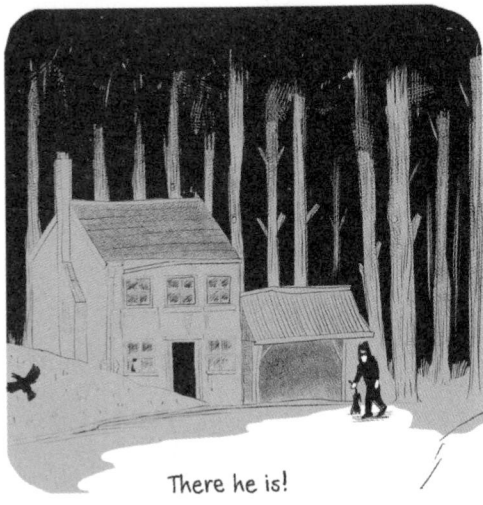

There he is!

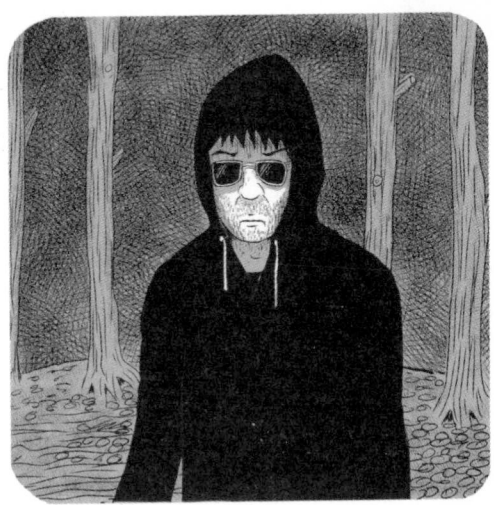

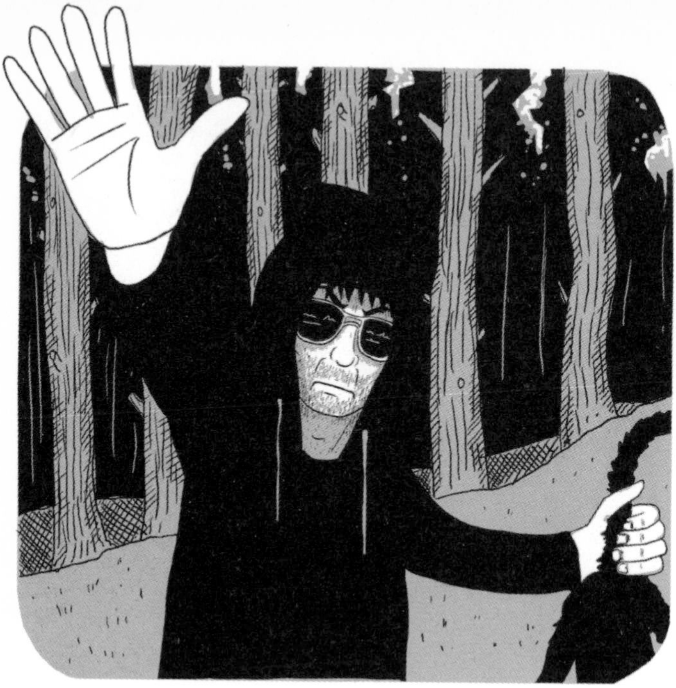

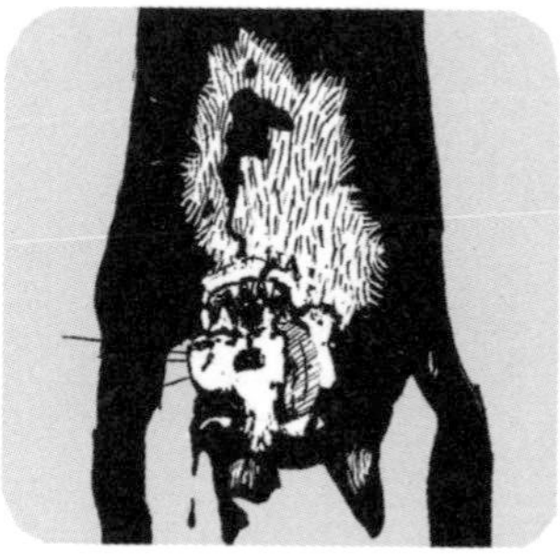

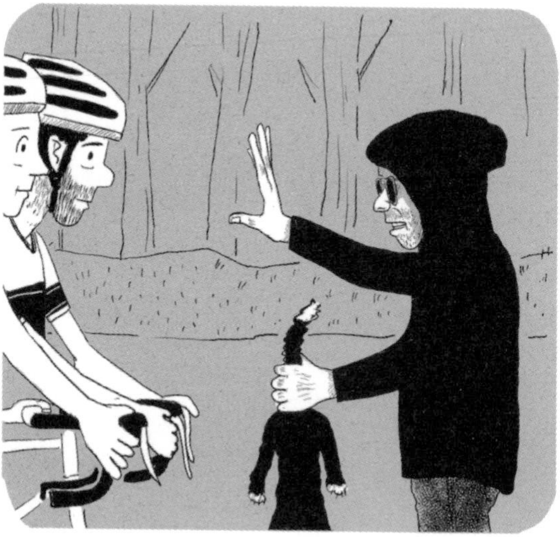

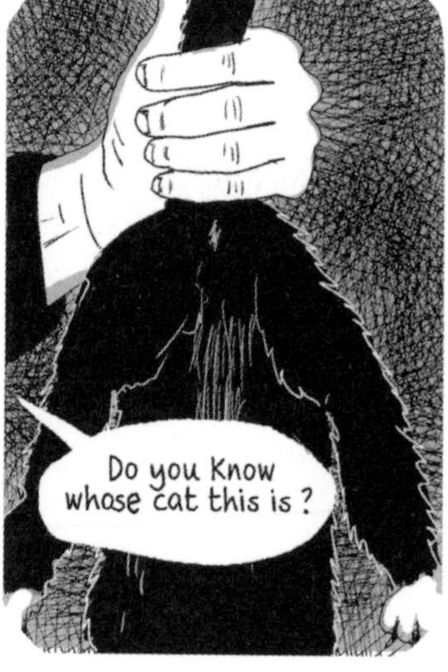
Do you Know whose cat this is ?

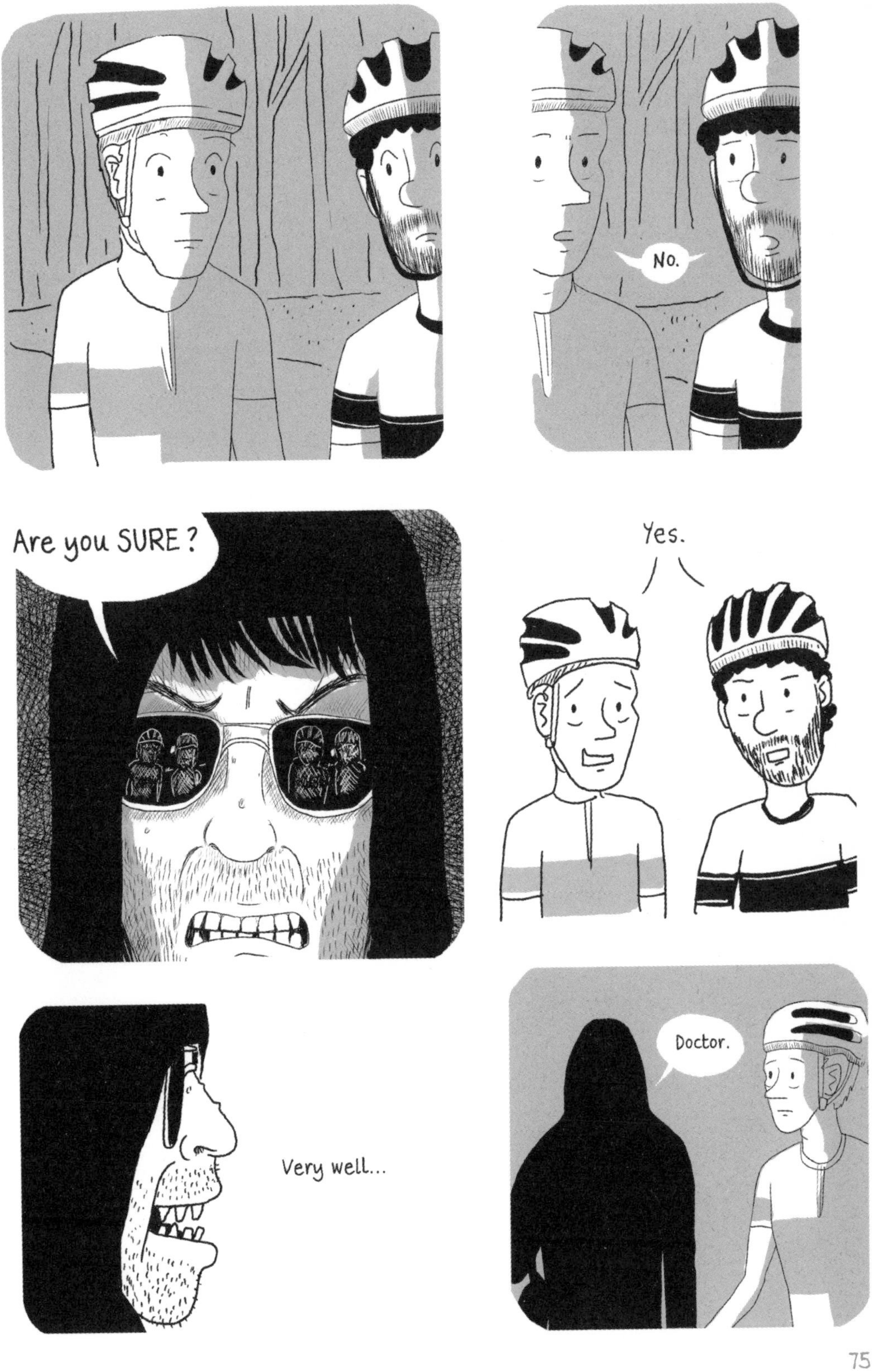
No.
Are you SURE?
Yes.
Very well...
Doctor.

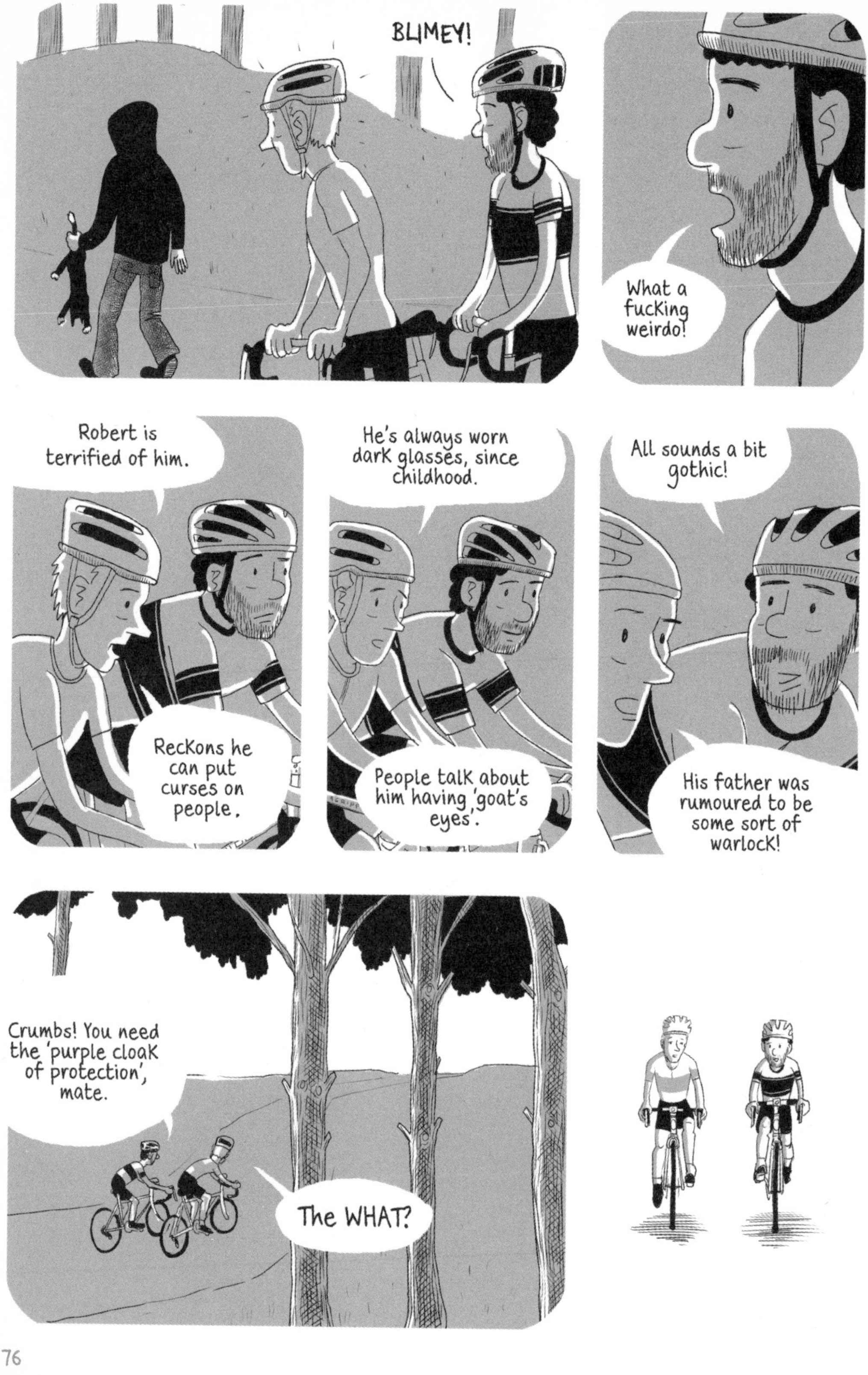
BLIMEY!
What a fucking weirdo!
Robert is terrified of him.
Reckons he can put curses on people.
He's always worn dark glasses, since childhood.
People talk about him having 'goat's eyes'.
All sounds a bit gothic!
His father was rumoured to be some sort of warlock!
Crumbs! You need the 'purple cloak of protection', mate.
The WHAT?

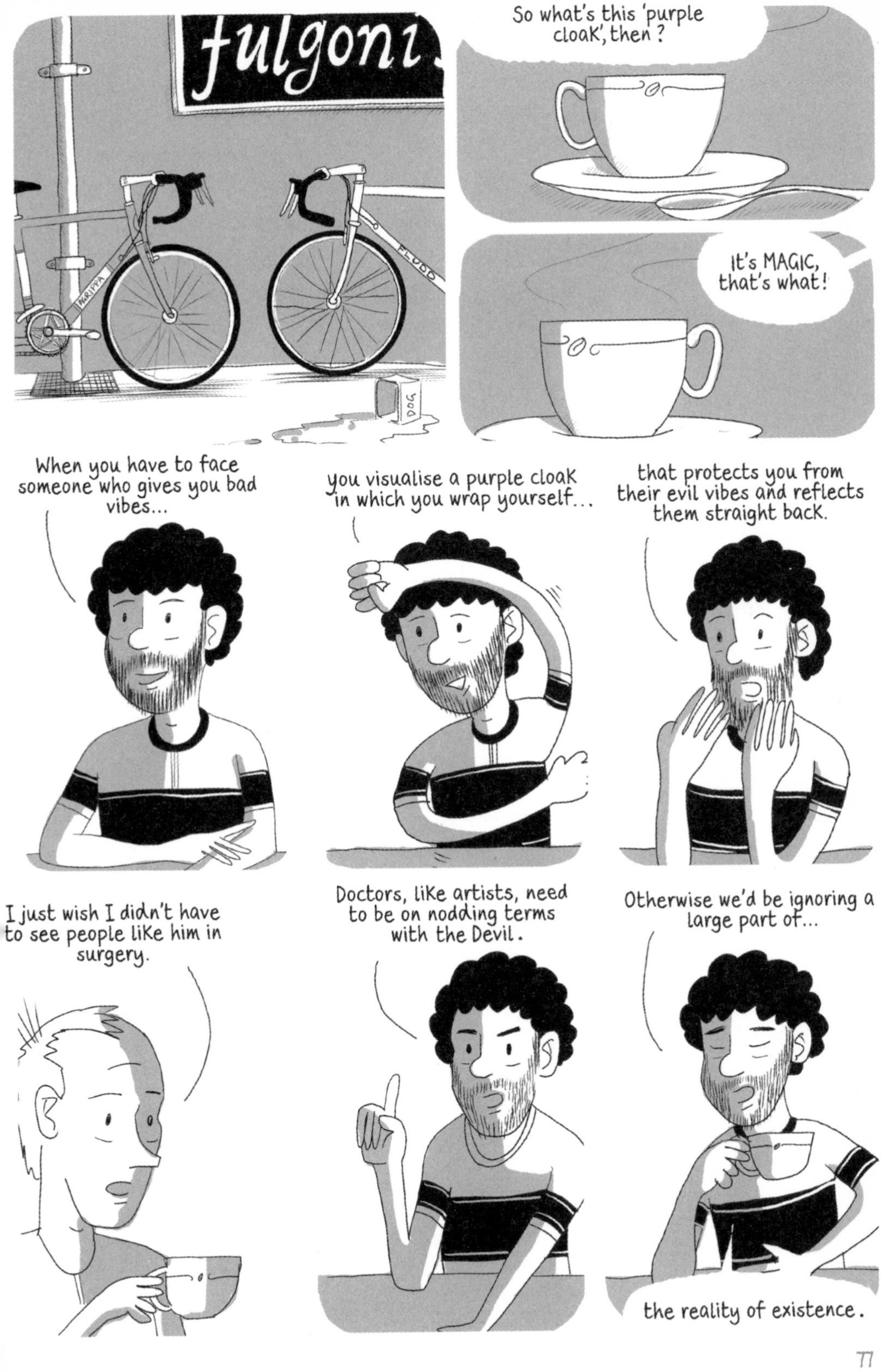
fulgoni
AGRIPPA
FLUDD
DOG
So what's this 'purple cloak', then?
It's MAGIC, that's what!
When you have to face someone who gives you bad vibes...
you visualise a purple cloak in which you wrap yourself...
that protects you from their evil vibes and reflects them straight back.
I just wish I didn't have to see people like him in surgery.
Doctors, like artists, need to be on nodding terms with the Devil.
Otherwise we'd be ignoring a large part of...
the reality of existence.

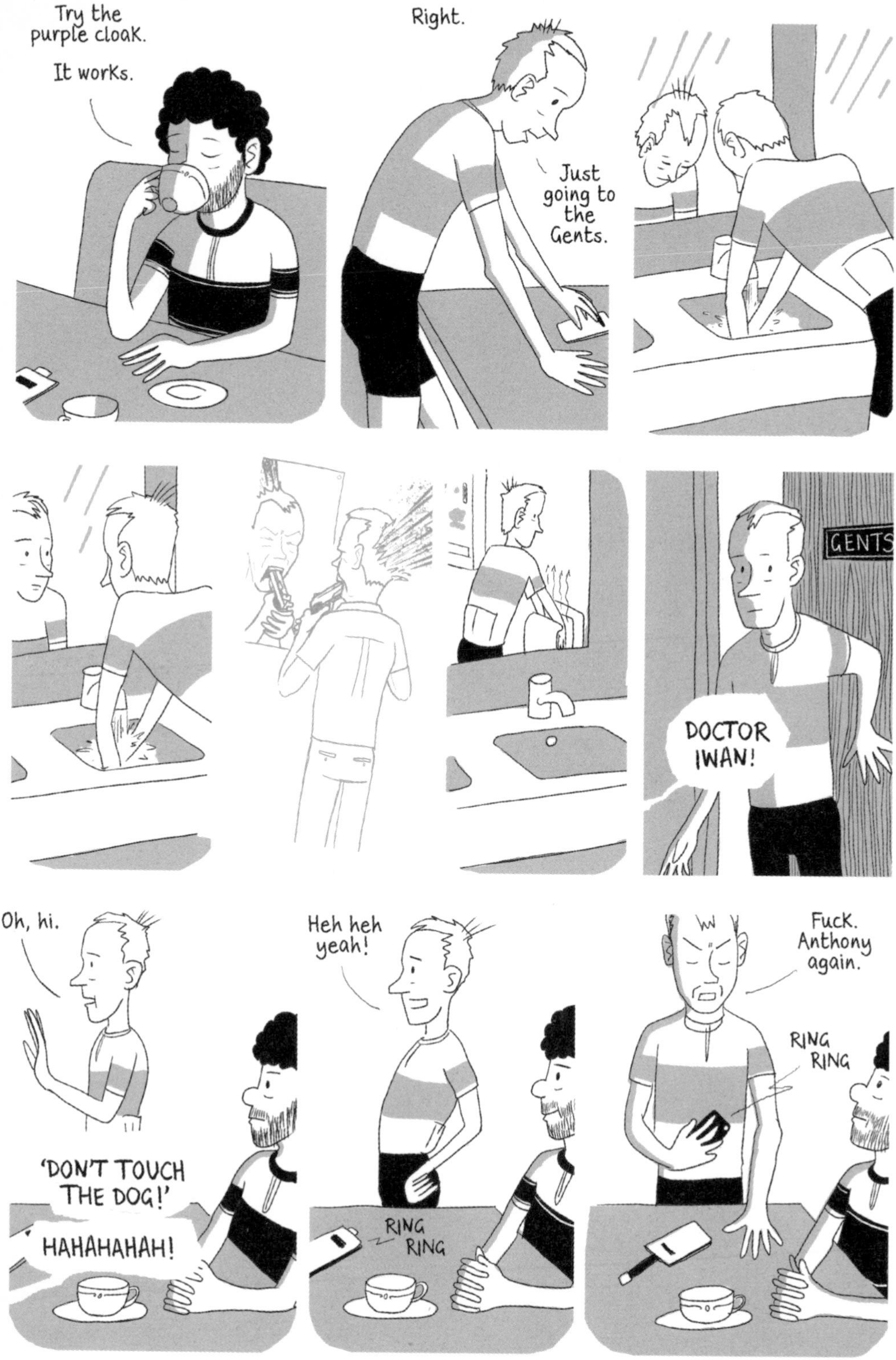
Try the purple cloak.
It works.
Right.
Just going to the Gents.
GENTS
DOCTOR IWAN!
Oh, hi.
'DON'T TOUCH THE DOG!'
HAHAHAHAH!
Heh heh yeah!
RING RING
Fuck. Anthony again.
RING RING

Ignis
Calor
Sicci.
Aer
Terra
Humor
Frigi.
Aqua
Sym
bola
A sym
bo la

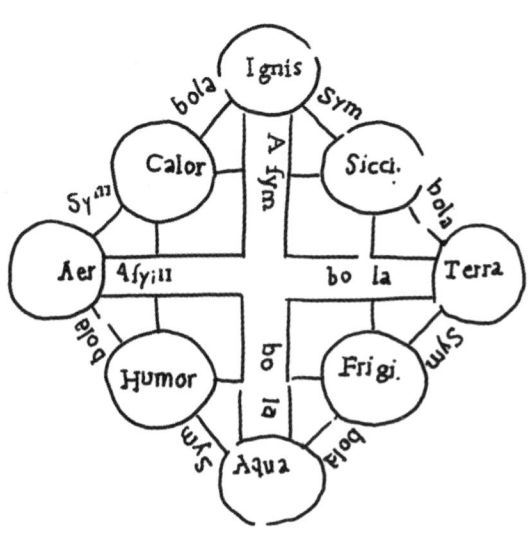

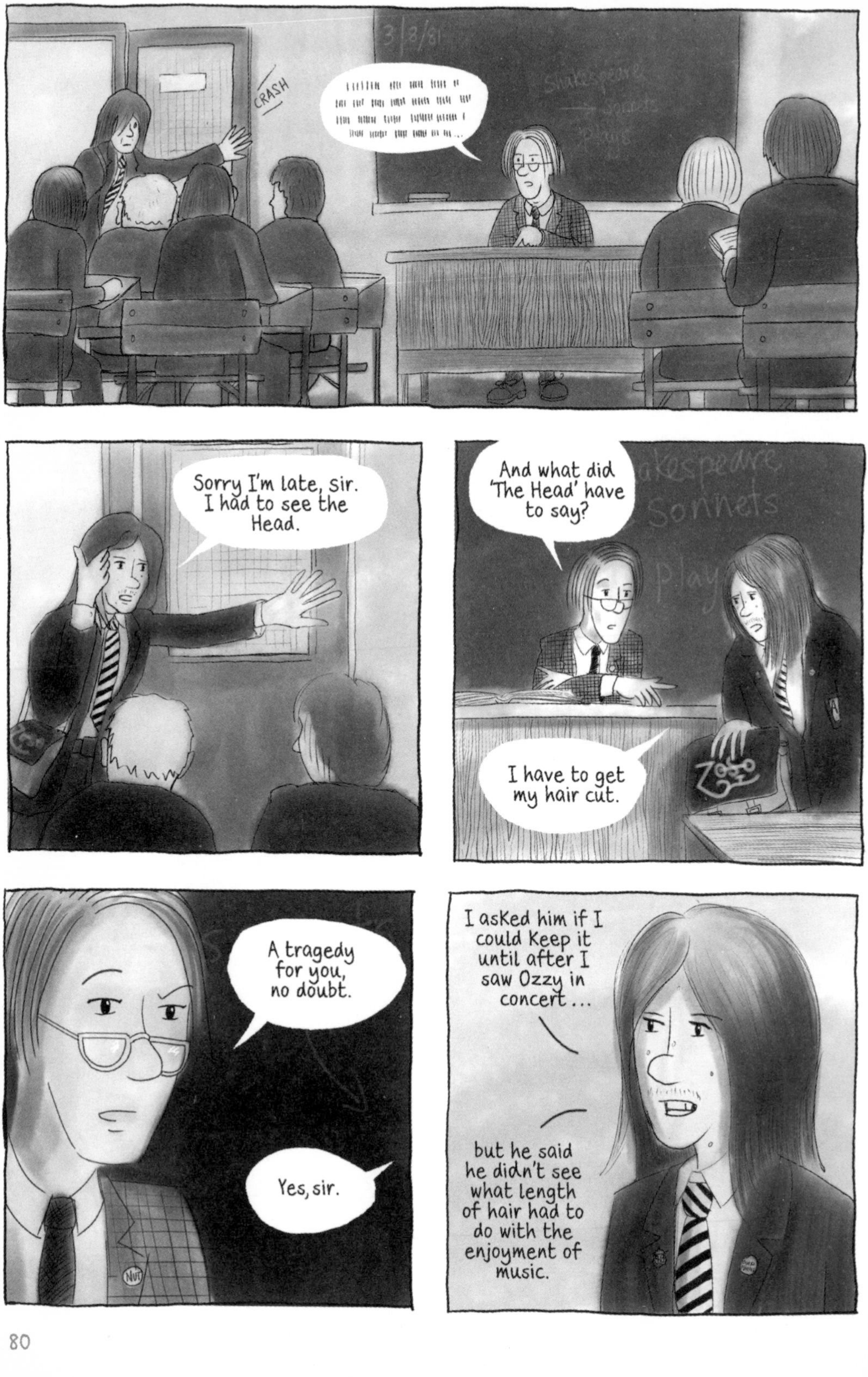

CRASH
3/8/81
Shakespeare
Sonnets
Plays
Sorry I'm late, sir. I had to see the Head.
And what did 'The Head' have to say?
I have to get my hair cut.
A tragedy for you, no doubt.
Yes, sir.
I asked him if I could keep it until after I saw Ozzy in concert...
but he said he didn't see what length of hair had to do with the enjoyment of music.

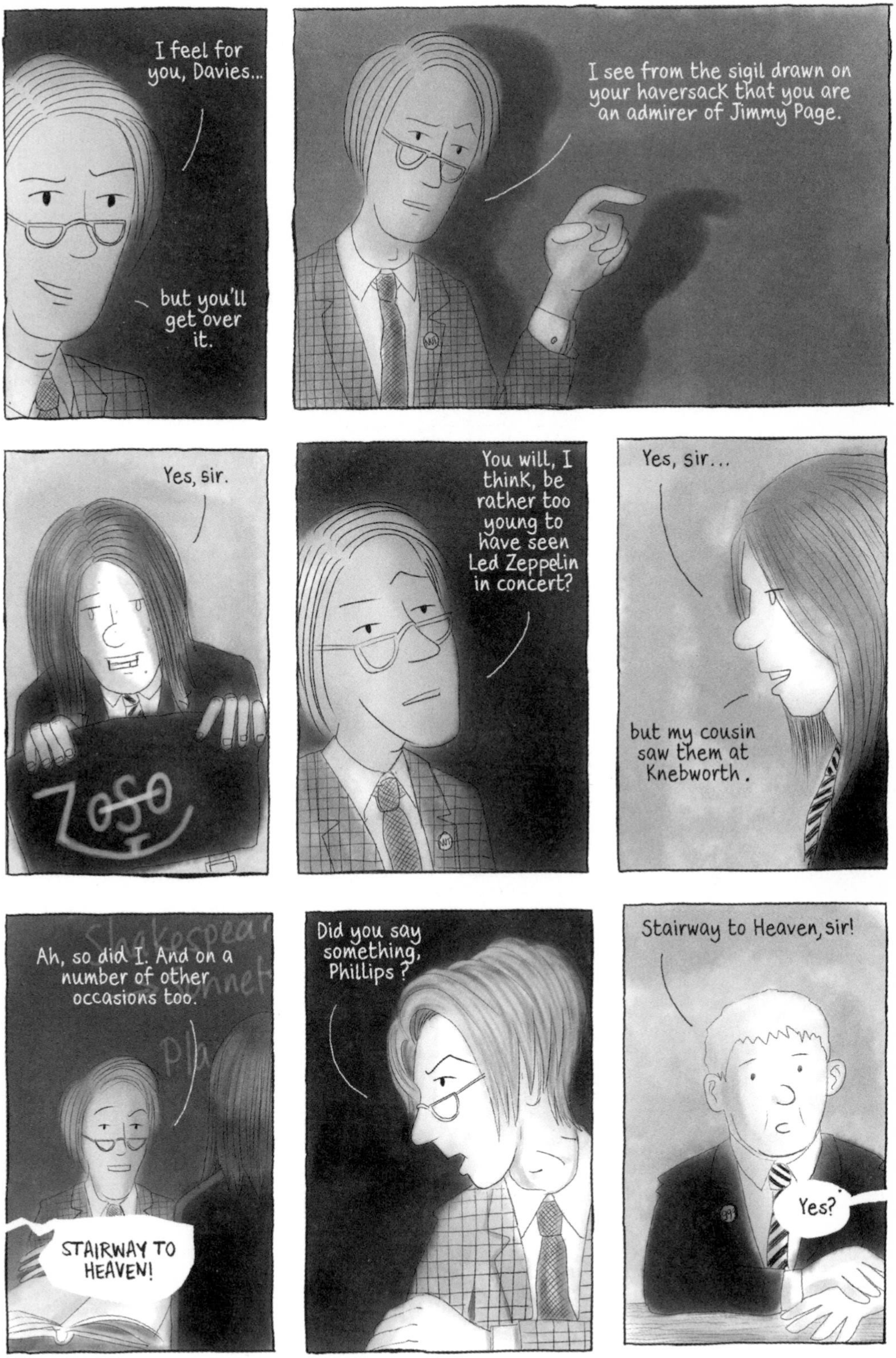
I feel for you, Davies...
but you'll get over it.
I see from the sigil drawn on your haversack that you are an admirer of Jimmy Page.
Yes, sir.
ZOSO
You will, I think, be rather too young to have seen Led Zeppelin in concert?
Yes, sir...
but my cousin saw them at Knebworth.
Ah, so did I. And on a number of other occasions too.
STAIRWAY TO HEAVEN!
Did you say something, Phillips?
Stairway to Heaven, sir!
Yes?

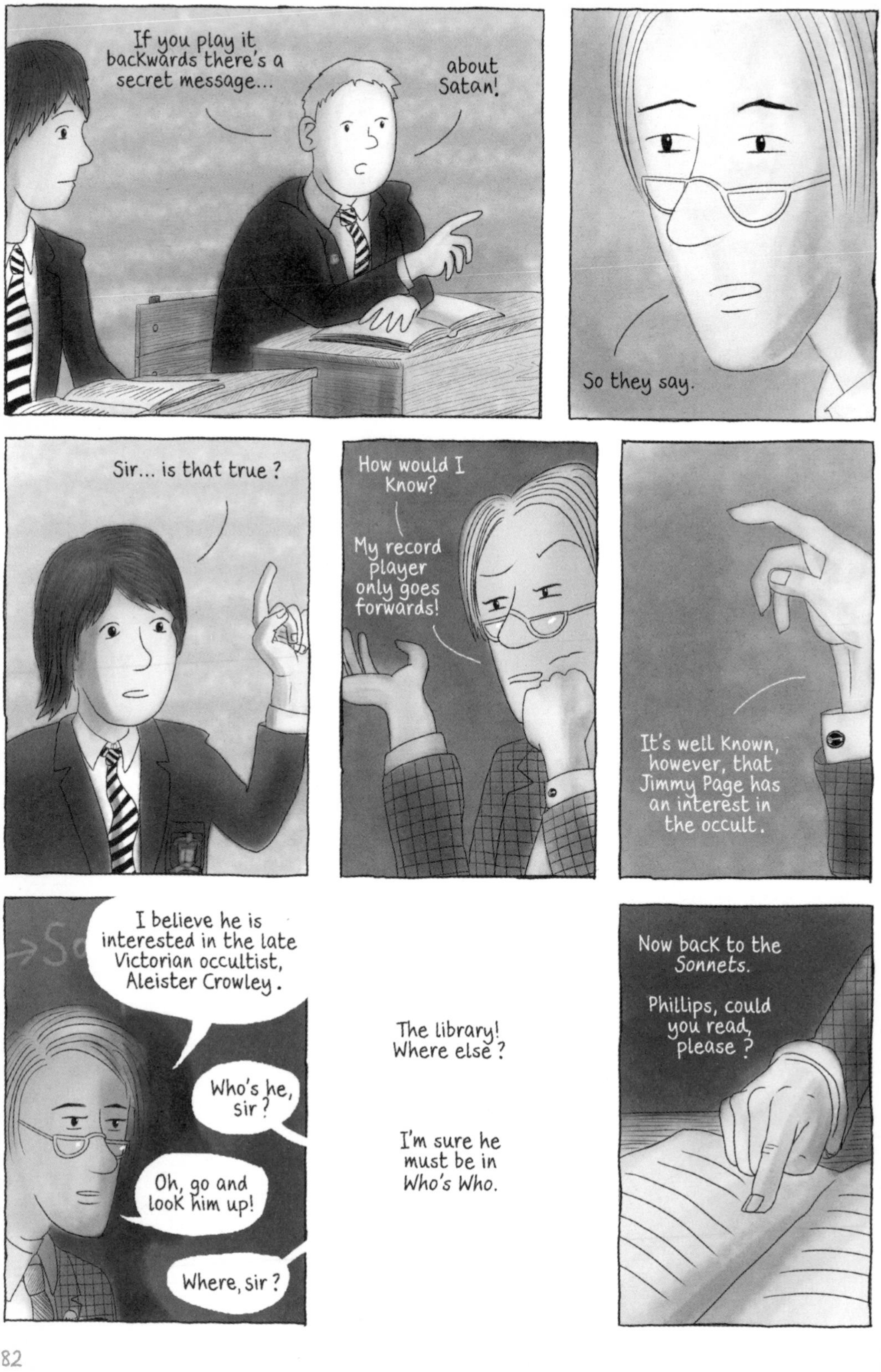
If you play it backwards there's a secret message...
about Satan!
So they say.
Sir... is that true?
How would I know?
My record player only goes forwards!
It's well known, however, that Jimmy Page has an interest in the occult.
I believe he is interested in the late Victorian occultist, Aleister Crowley.
Who's he, sir?
Oh, go and look him up!
Where, sir?
The library! Where else?
I'm sure he must be in *Who's Who*.
Now back to the *Sonnets*.
Phillips, could you read, please?

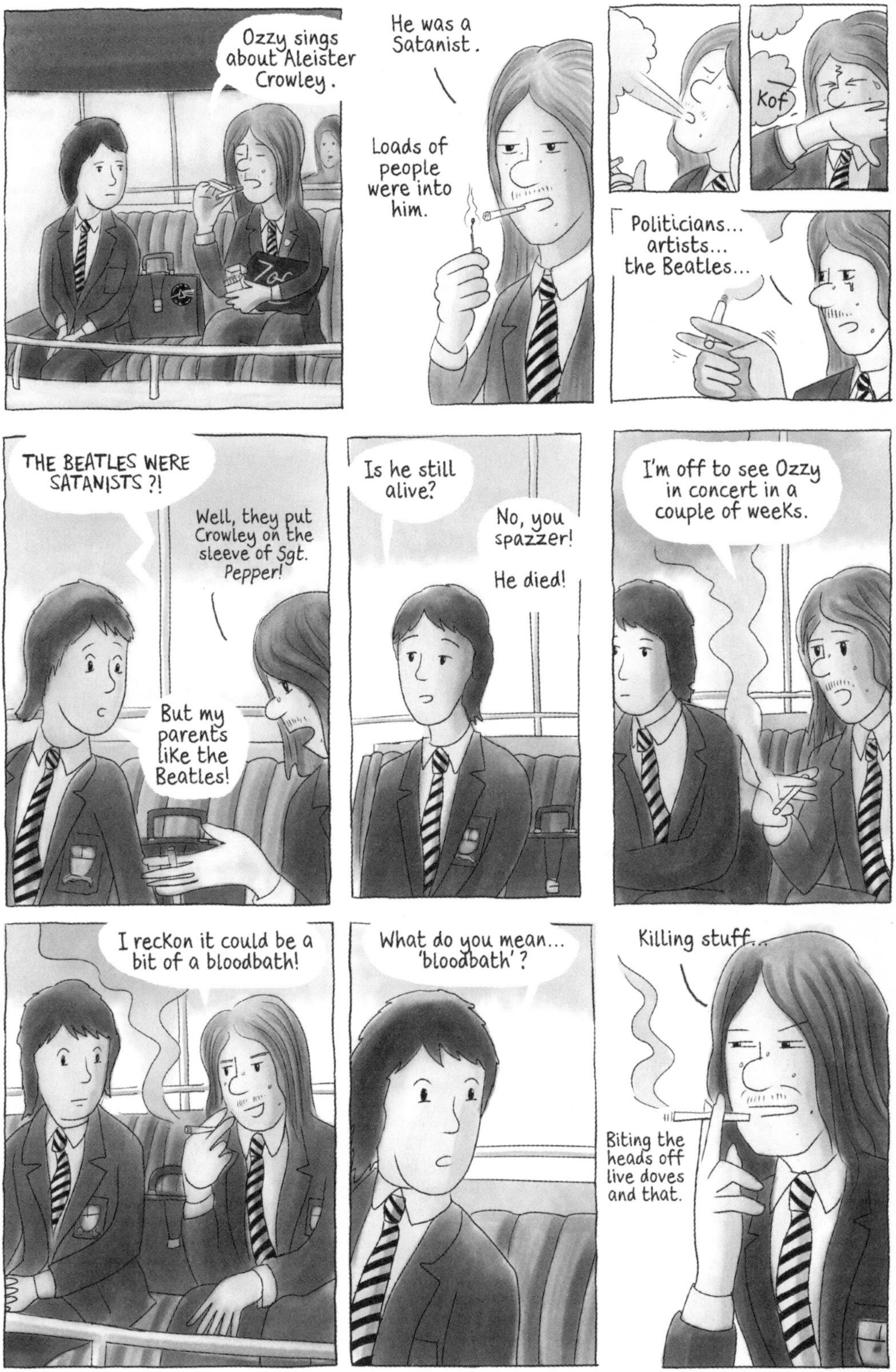
Ozzy sings about Aleister Crowley.
He was a Satanist.
Loads of people were into him.
Kof
Politicians... artists... the Beatles...
THE BEATLES WERE SATANISTS ?!
Well, they put Crowley on the sleeve of Sgt. Pepper!
But my parents like the Beatles!
Is he still alive?
No, you spazzer!
He died!
I'm off to see Ozzy in concert in a couple of weeks.
I reckon it could be a bit of a bloodbath!
What do you mean... 'bloodbath'?
Killing stuff...
Biting the heads off live doves and that.

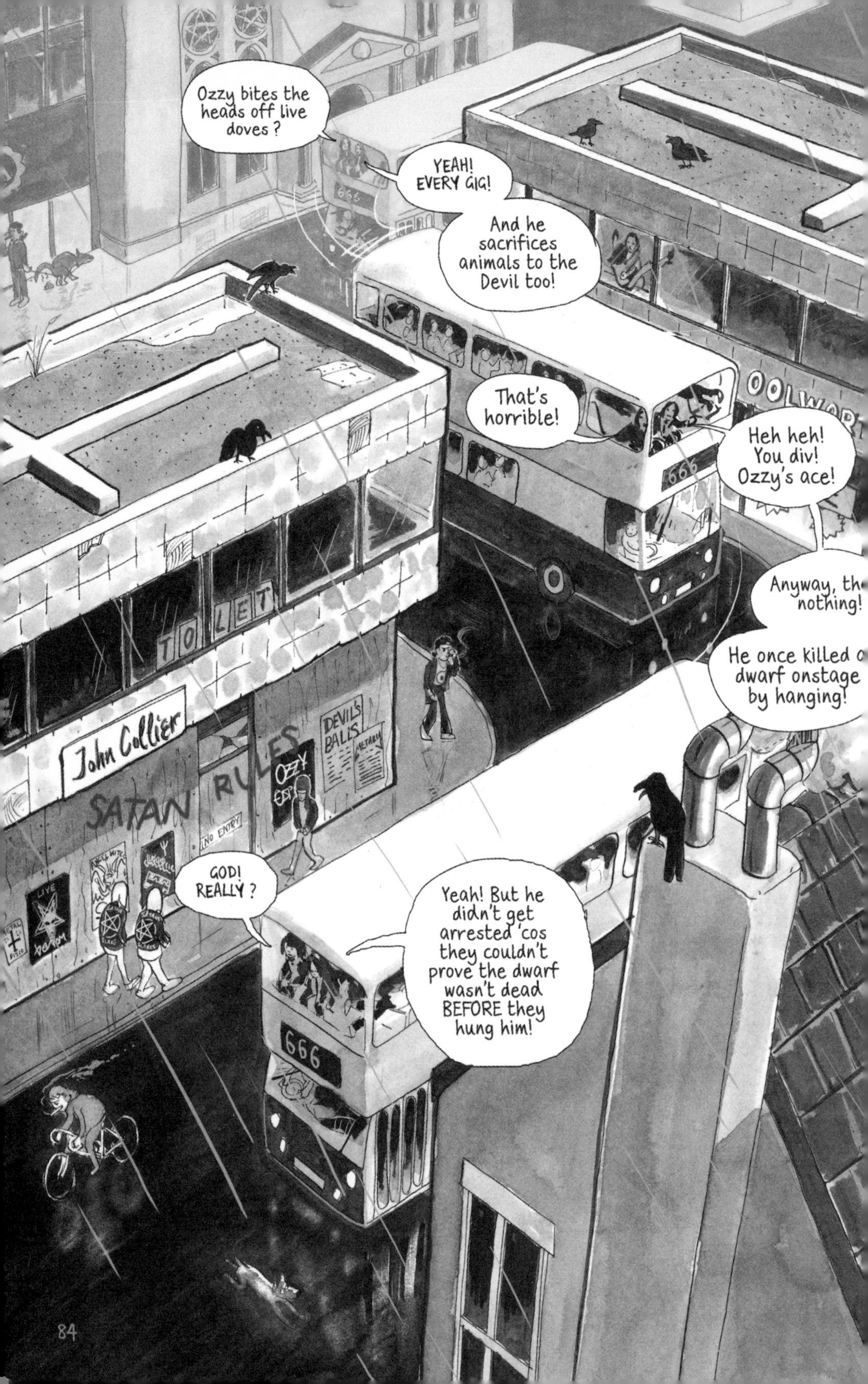
Ozzy bites the heads off live doves?
YEAH! EVERY GIG!
And he sacrifices animals to the Devil too!
That's horrible!
Heh heh! You div! Ozzy's ace!
Anyway, th nothing!
He once killed a dwarf onstage by hanging!
GOD! REALLY?
Yeah! But he didn't get arrested 'cos they couldn't prove the dwarf wasn't dead BEFORE they hung him!
666
TO LET
John Collier
SATAN RULES
DEVIL'S BALLS
OZZY
NO ENTRY

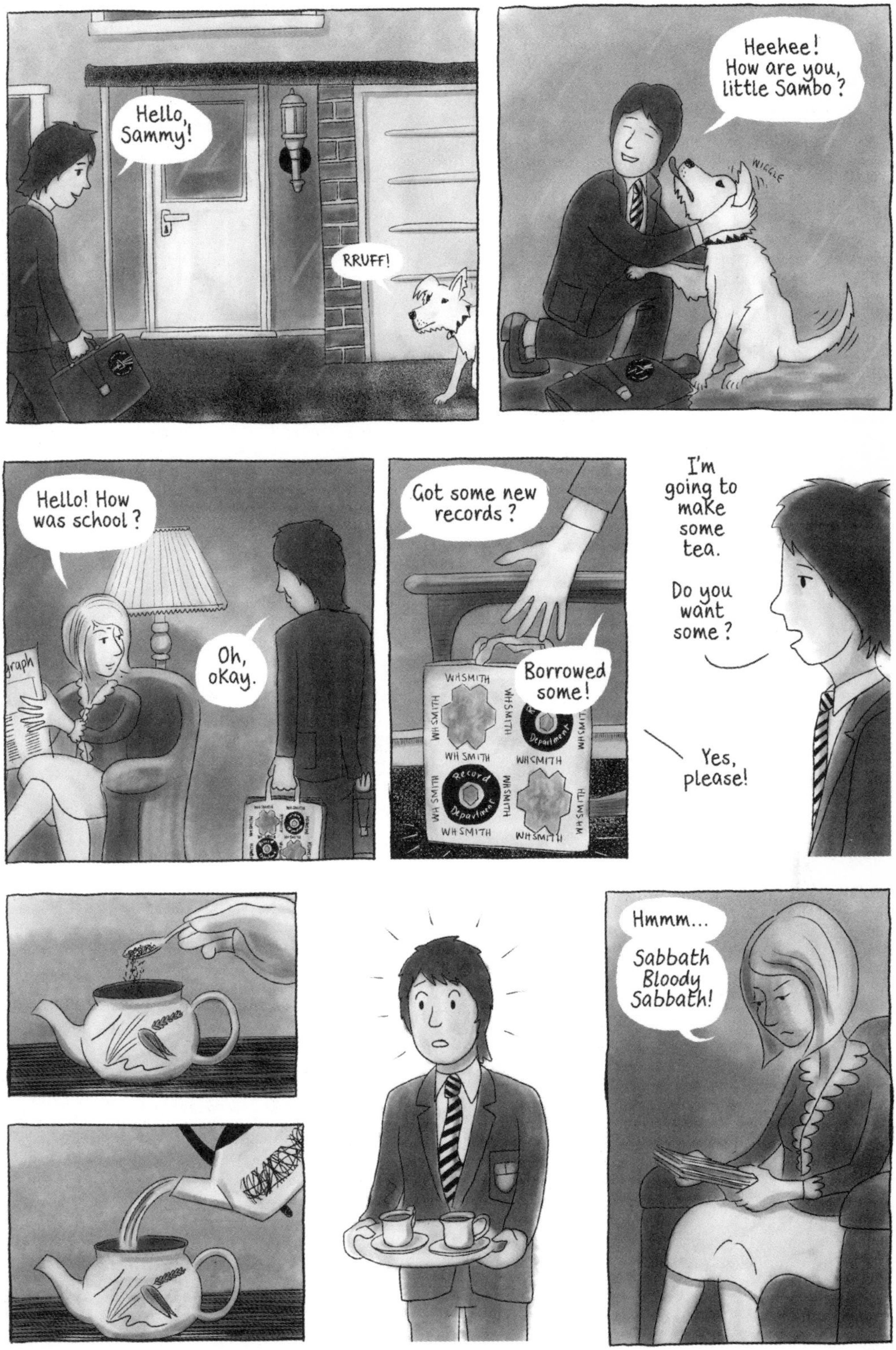
Hello, Sammy!
RRUFF!
Heehee! How are you, little Sambo?
WIGGLE
Hello! How was school?
Oh, okay.
Got some new records?
Borrowed some!
WHSMITH
Record Department
I'm going to make some tea.
Do you want some?
Yes, please!
Hmmm...
Sabbath Bloody Sabbath!

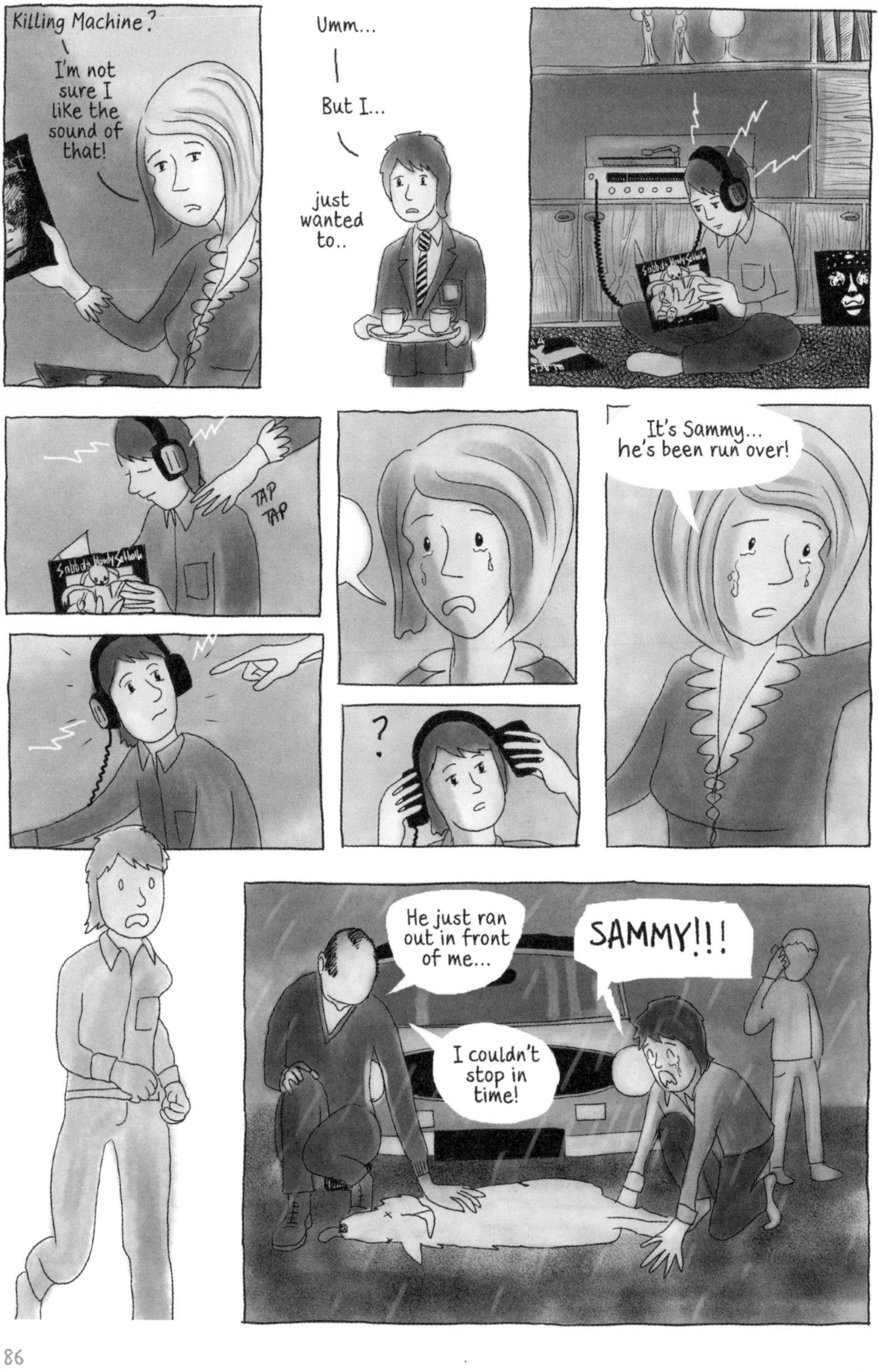
Killing Machine?
I'm not sure I like the sound of that!
Umm...
But I...
just wanted to..
TAP TAP
?
It's Sammy... he's been run over!
He just ran out in front of me...
SAMMY!!!
I couldn't stop in time!

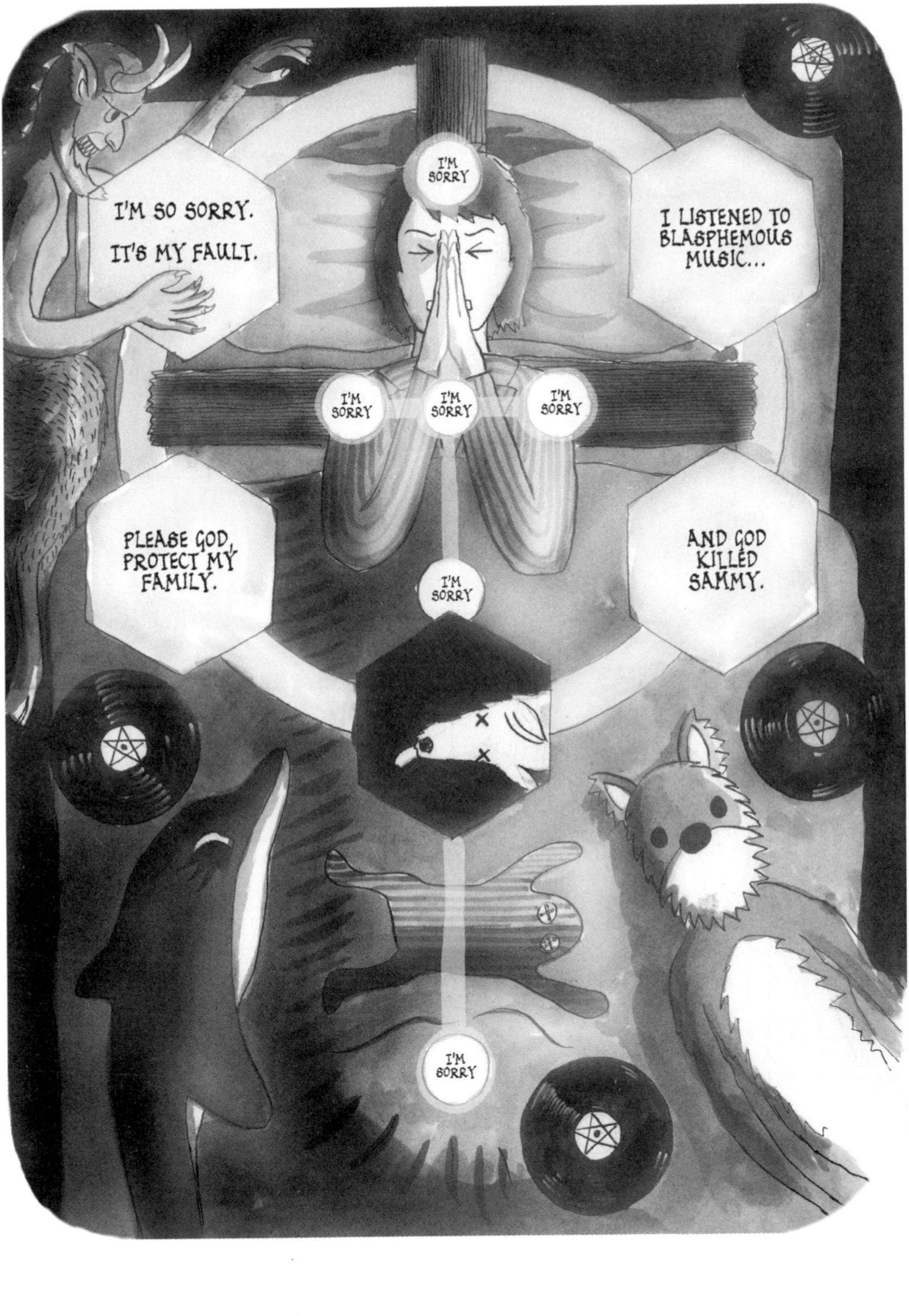
I'M SORRY
I'M SO SORRY. IT'S MY FAULT.
I LISTENED TO BLASPHEMOUS MUSIC...
I'M SORRY
I'M SORRY
I'M SORRY
PLEASE GOD, PROTECT MY FAMILY.
AND GOD KILLED SAMMY.
I'M SORRY
I'M SORRY

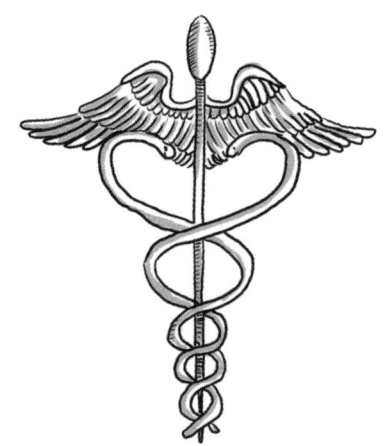

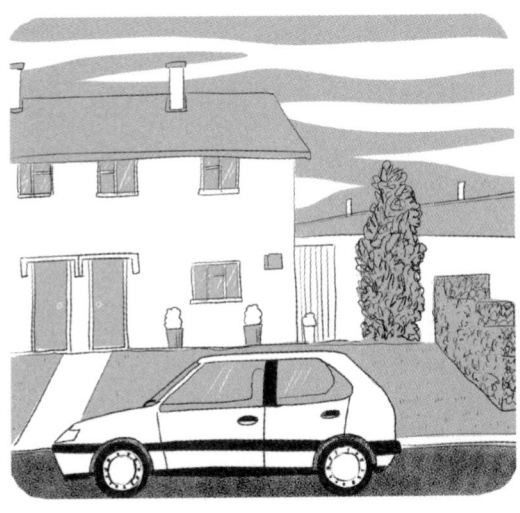

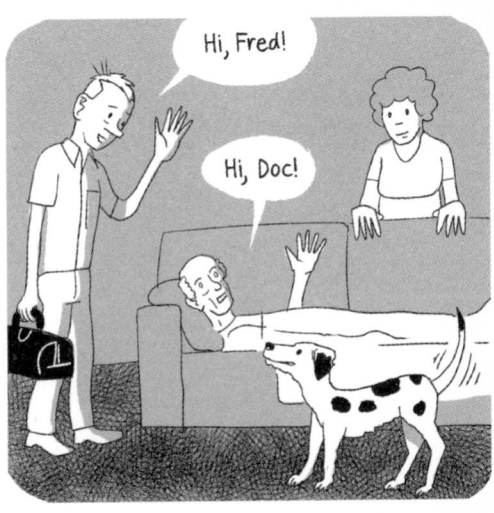

Hi, Fred!

Hi, Doc!

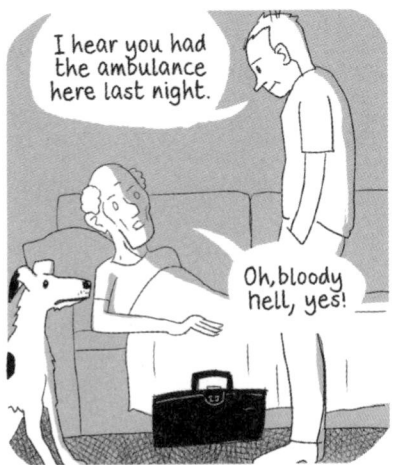

I hear you had the ambulance here last night.

Oh, bloody hell, yes!

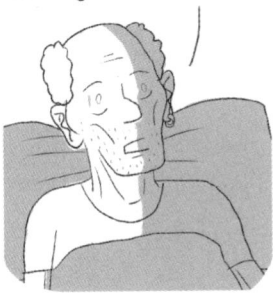

I had more pain. I phoned the out-of-hours service. I wanted a doctor but as soon as I mentioned pain in my chest they insisted on sending an ambulance.

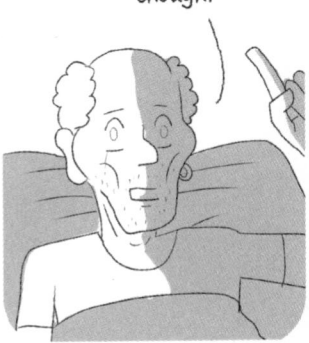

I told 'em... I'm dying of bloody lung cancer, THATS why I've got chest pain! They wouldn't have it, though.

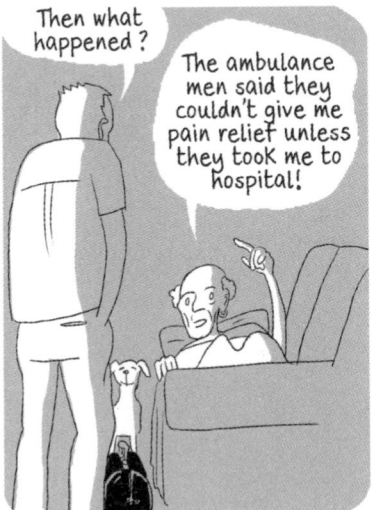

Then what happened?

The ambulance men said they couldn't give me pain relief unless they took me to hospital!

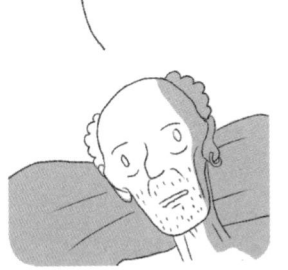

I told 'em I wasn't going to go into hospital and they said, 'Oh... so you're refusing treatment, are you?'

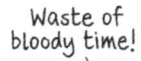

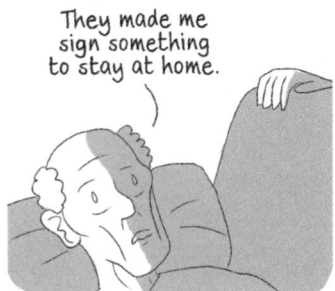

They didn't say it quite like that, Doctor!

Waste of bloody time!

They made me sign something to stay at home.

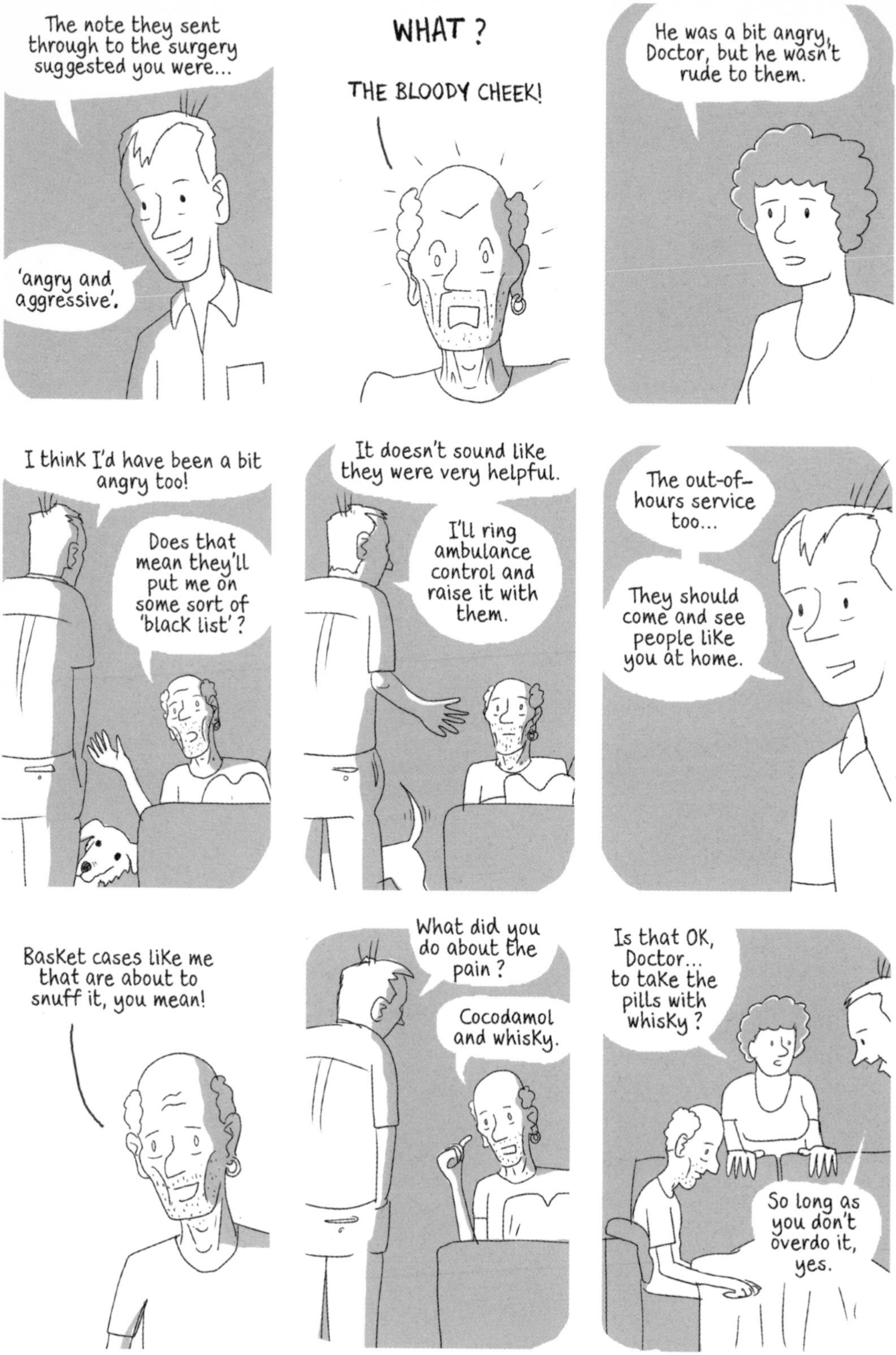

The note they sent through to the surgery suggested you were...
'angry and aggressive'.
WHAT ?
THE BLOODY CHEEK!
He was a bit angry, Doctor, but he wasn't rude to them.
I think I'd have been a bit angry too!
Does that mean they'll put me on some sort of 'black list'?
It doesn't sound like they were very helpful.
I'll ring ambulance control and raise it with them.
The out-of-hours service too...
They should come and see people like you at home.
Basket cases like me that are about to snuff it, you mean!
What did you do about the pain ?
Cocodamol and whisky.
Is that OK, Doctor... to take the pills with whisky ?
So long as you don't overdo it, yes.

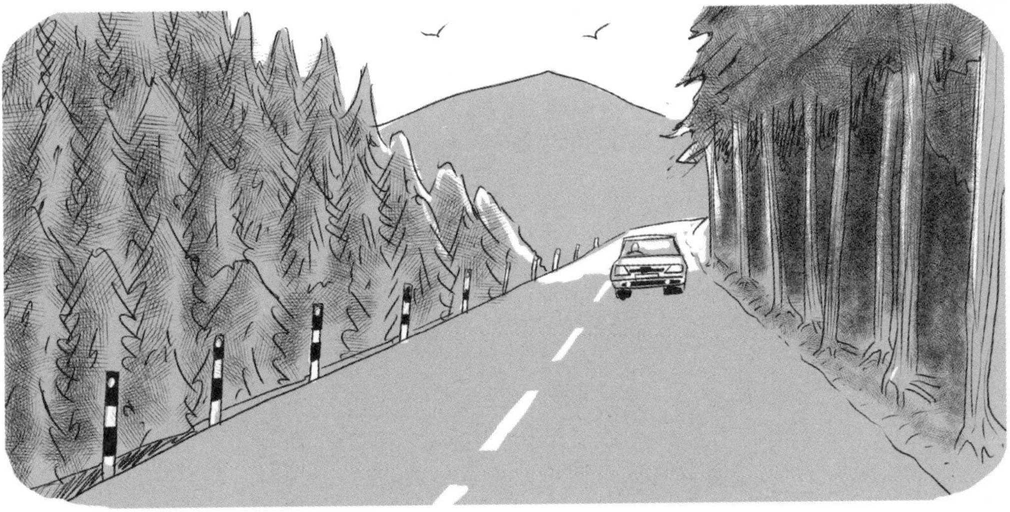
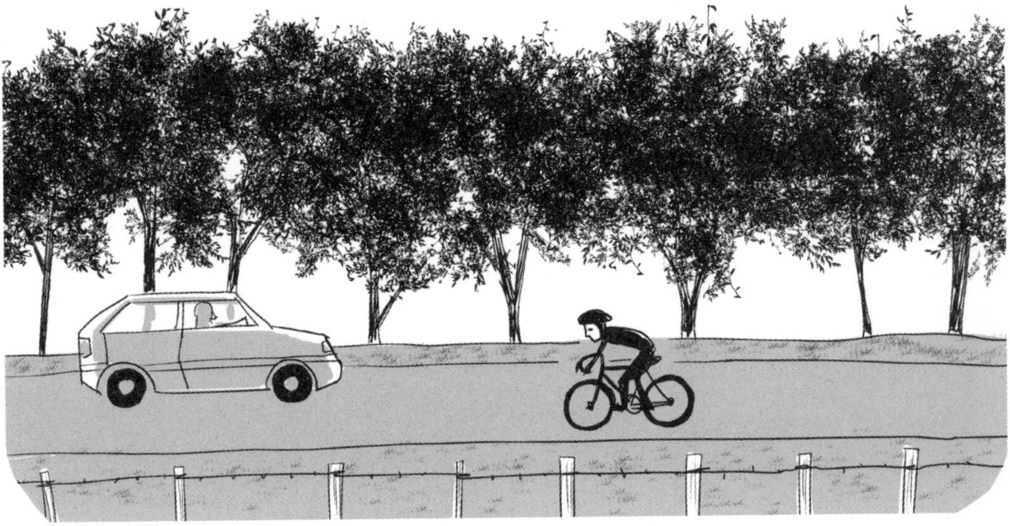
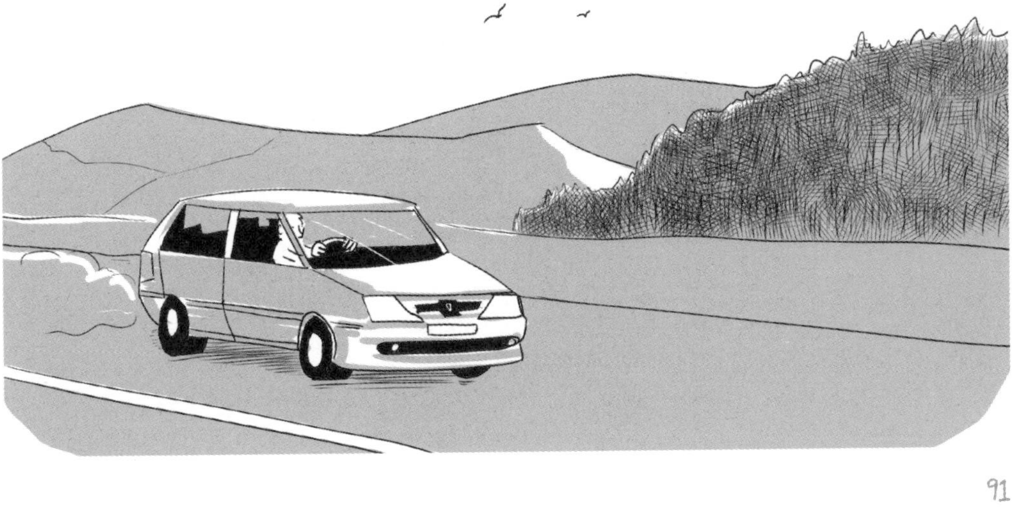

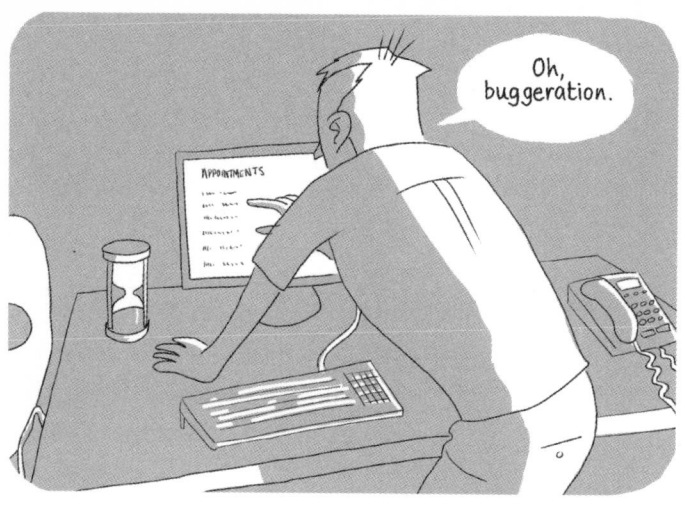

Oh, buggeration.

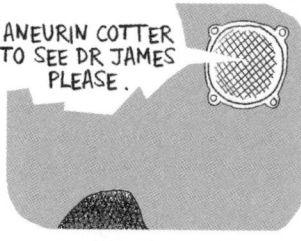

ANEURIN COTTER TO SEE DR JAMES PLEASE.

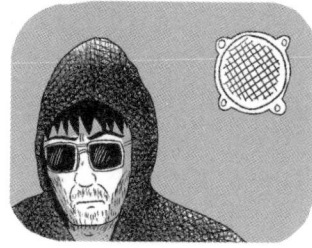

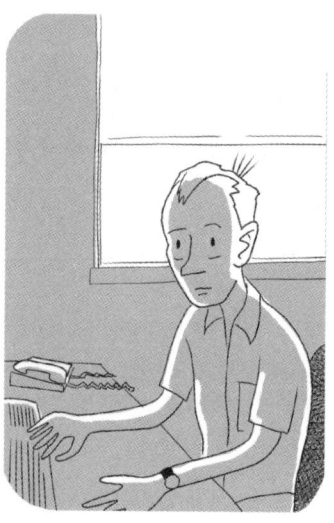

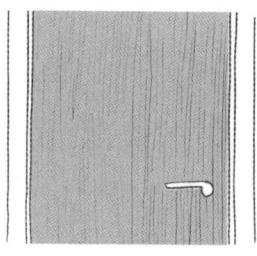

KNOCK

KNOCK

KNOCK

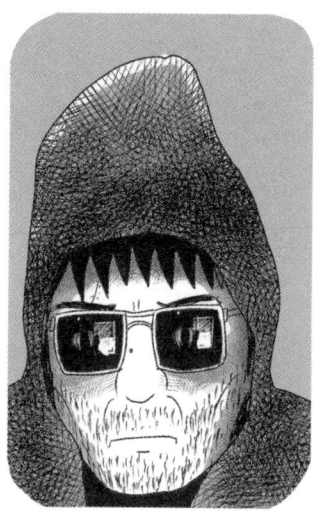

What can I do for you?

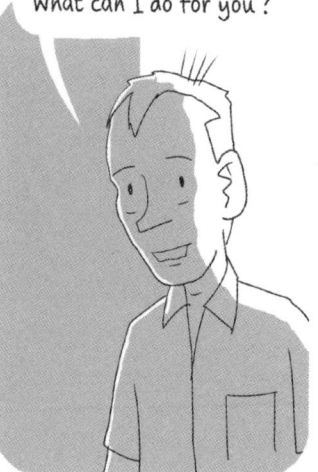

I want you to sign my shotgun licence.

I need to renew it.

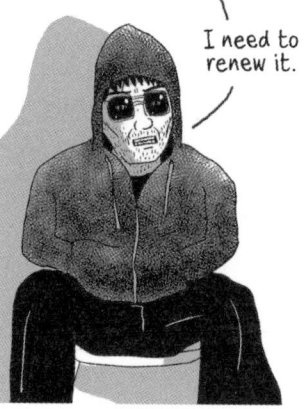

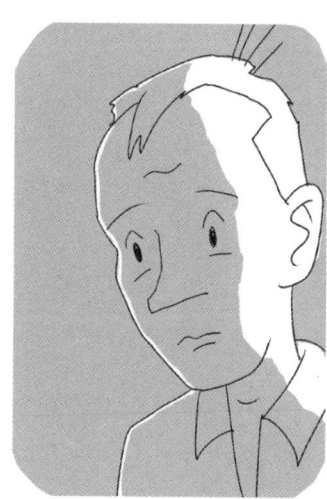

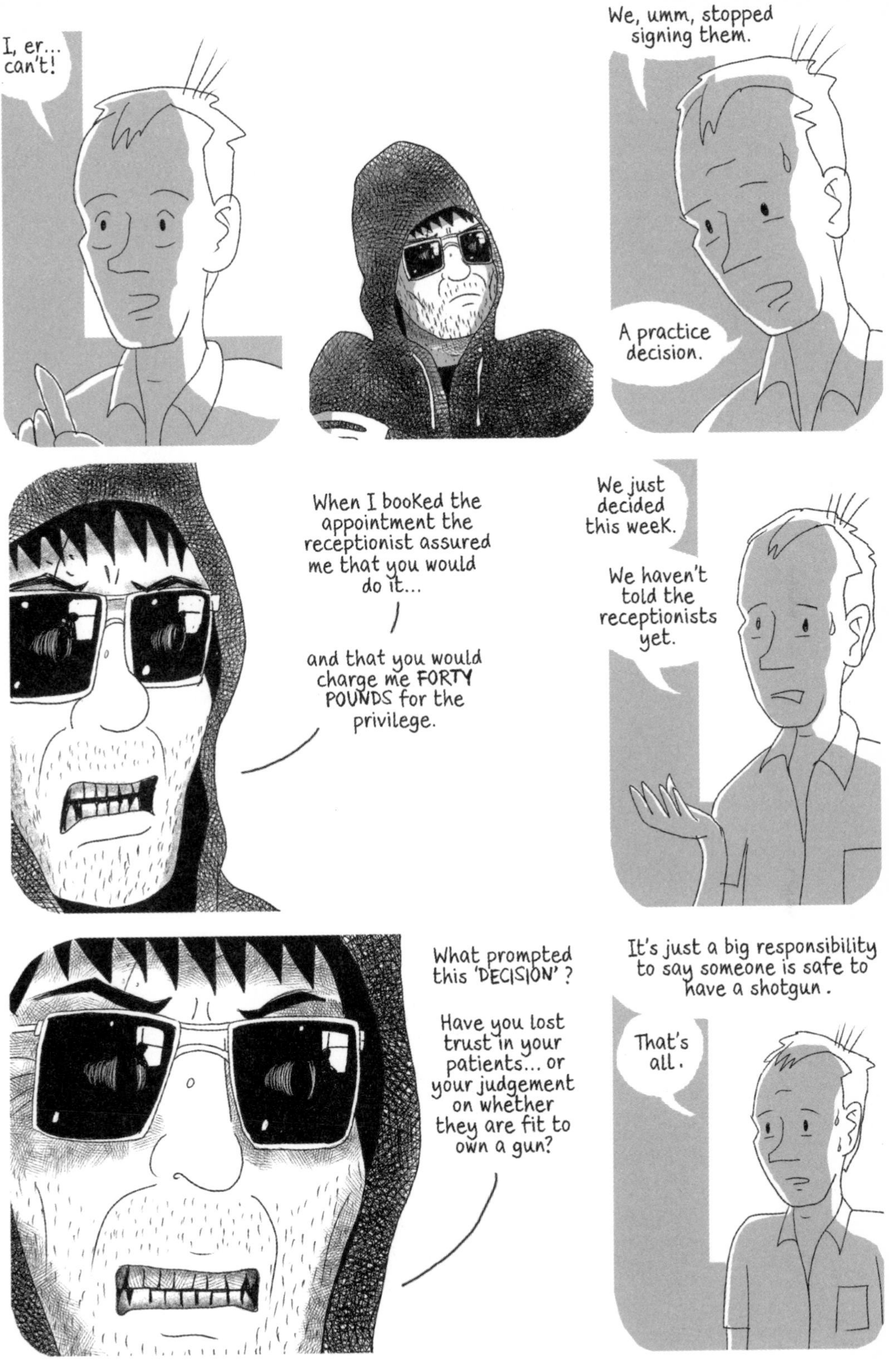
I, er... can't!
We, umm, stopped signing them.
A practice decision.
When I booked the appointment the receptionist assured me that you would do it...
and that you would charge me FORTY POUNDS for the privilege.
We just decided this week.
We haven't told the receptionists yet.
What prompted this 'DECISION'?
Have you lost trust in your patients... or your judgement on whether they are fit to own a gun?
It's just a big responsibility to say someone is safe to have a shotgun.
That's all.

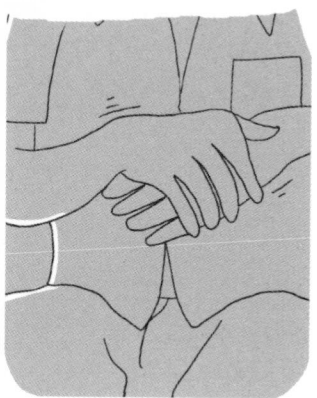

We just don't know some patients very well and it can be difficult to say no...

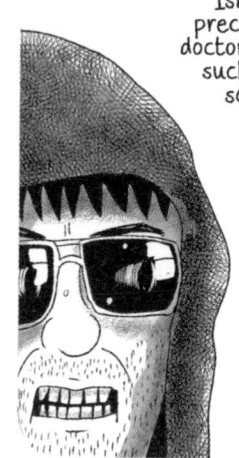

Isn't that precisely why doctors are paid such a huge salary?

To take responsibility?

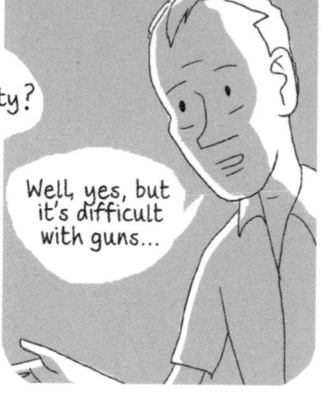

Well, yes, but it's difficult with guns...

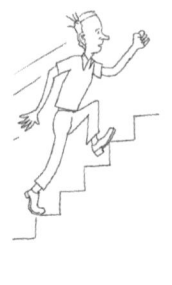

Robert! Lois!

I've just made an executive decision!

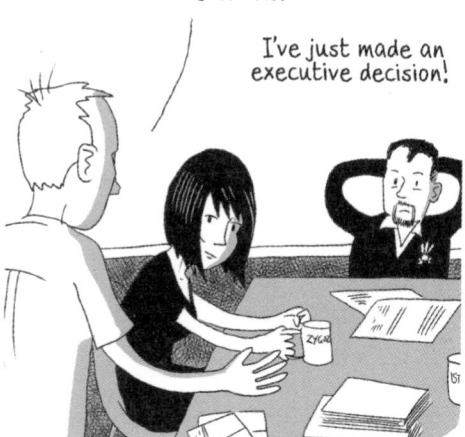

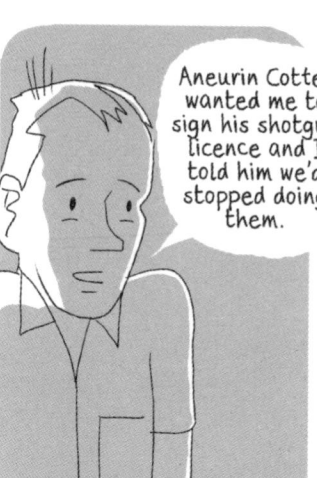

Aneurin Cotter wanted me to sign his shotgun licence and I told him we'd stopped doing them.

Great! Why did you do that?

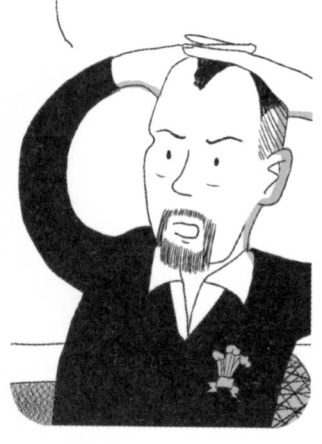

Well, I'd be happy to stop signing them.

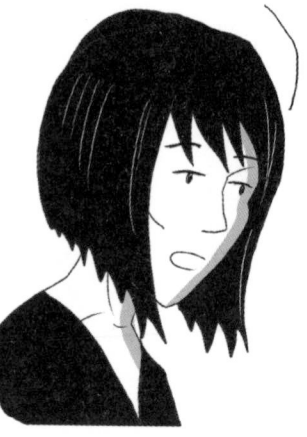

They can get the licence form signed by a police officer or a J.P.

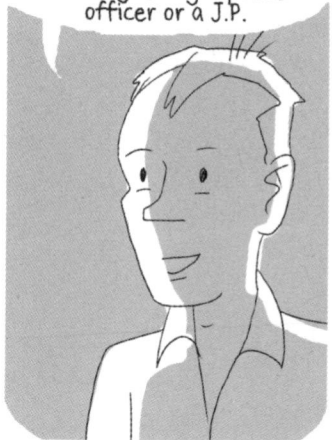

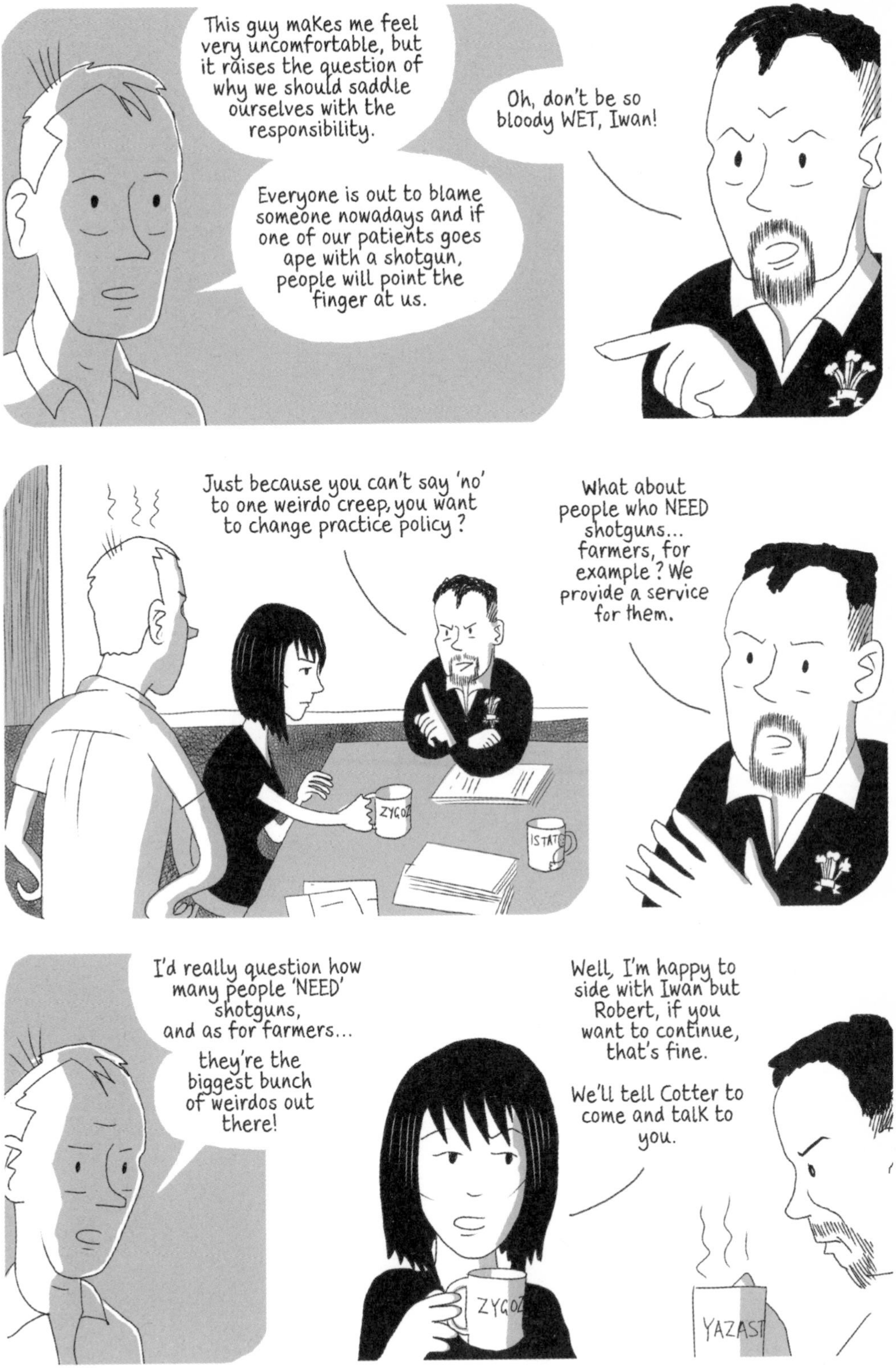
This guy makes me feel very uncomfortable, but it raises the question of why we should saddle ourselves with the responsibility.
Everyone is out to blame someone nowadays and if one of our patients goes ape with a shotgun, people will point the finger at us.
Oh, don't be so bloody WET, Iwan!
Just because you can't say 'no' to one weirdo creep, you want to change practice policy ?
ZYGOZ
ISTAT
What about people who NEED shotguns... farmers, for example ? We provide a service for them.
I'd really question how many people 'NEED' shotguns, and as for farmers...
they're the biggest bunch of weirdos out there!
Well, I'm happy to side with Iwan but Robert, if you want to continue, that's fine.
We'll tell Cotter to come and talk to you.
ZYGOZ
YAZAST

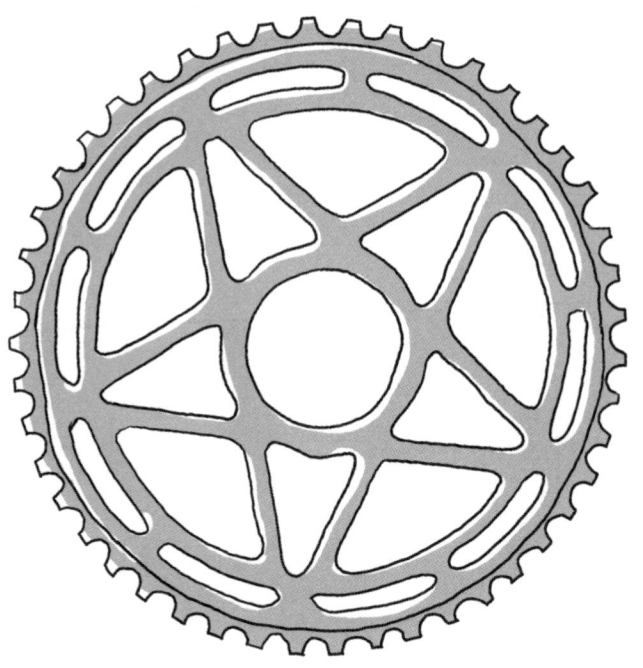

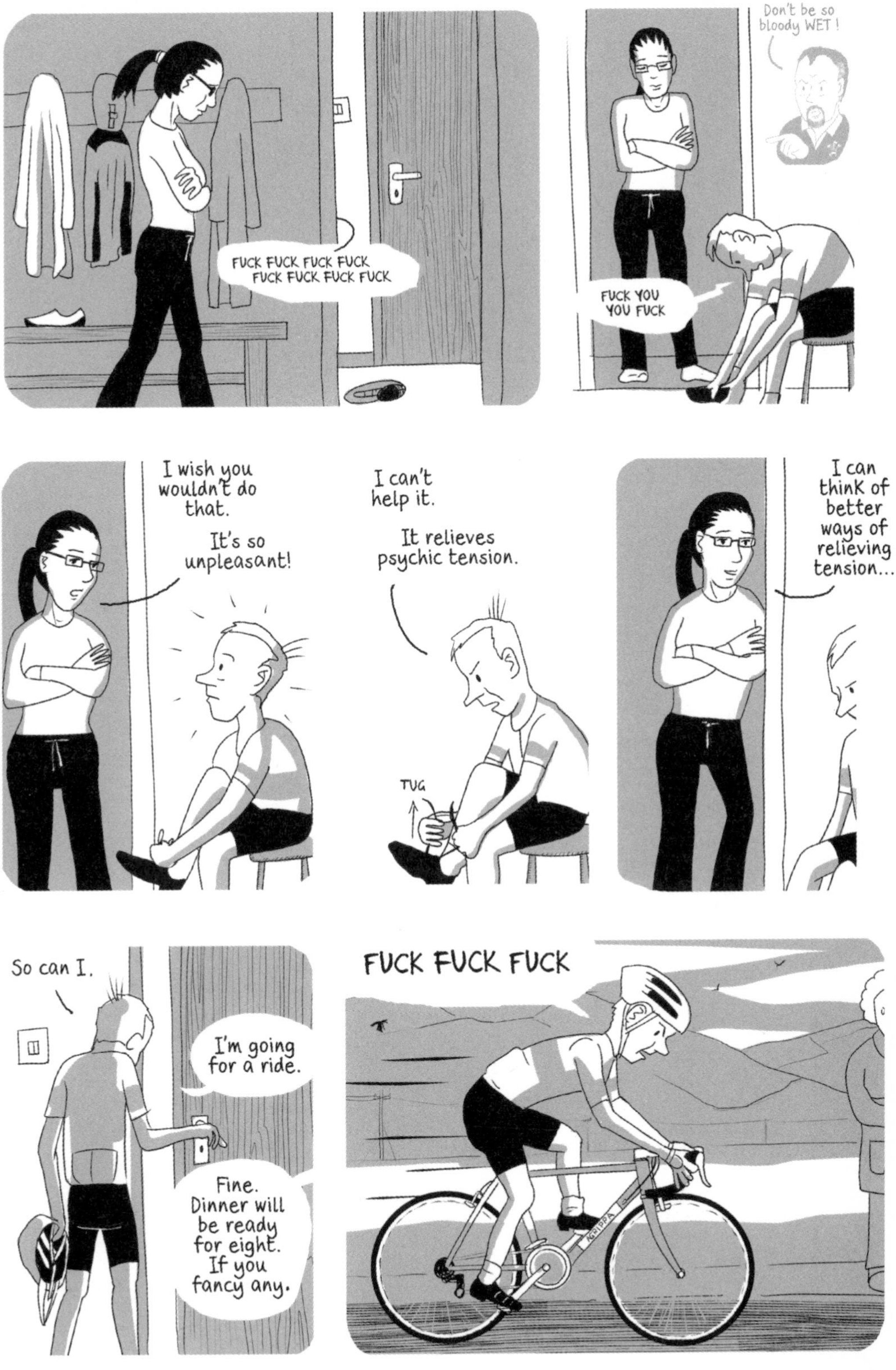

FUCK FUCK FUCK FUCK FUCK FUCK FUCK FUCK
Don't be so bloody WET!
FUCK YOU YOU FUCK
I wish you wouldn't do that.
It's so unpleasant!
I can't help it.
It relieves psychic tension.
TUG
I can think of better ways of relieving tension...
So can I.
I'm going for a ride.
Fine. Dinner will be ready for eight. If you fancy any.
FUCK FUCK FUCK
AGRIPPA

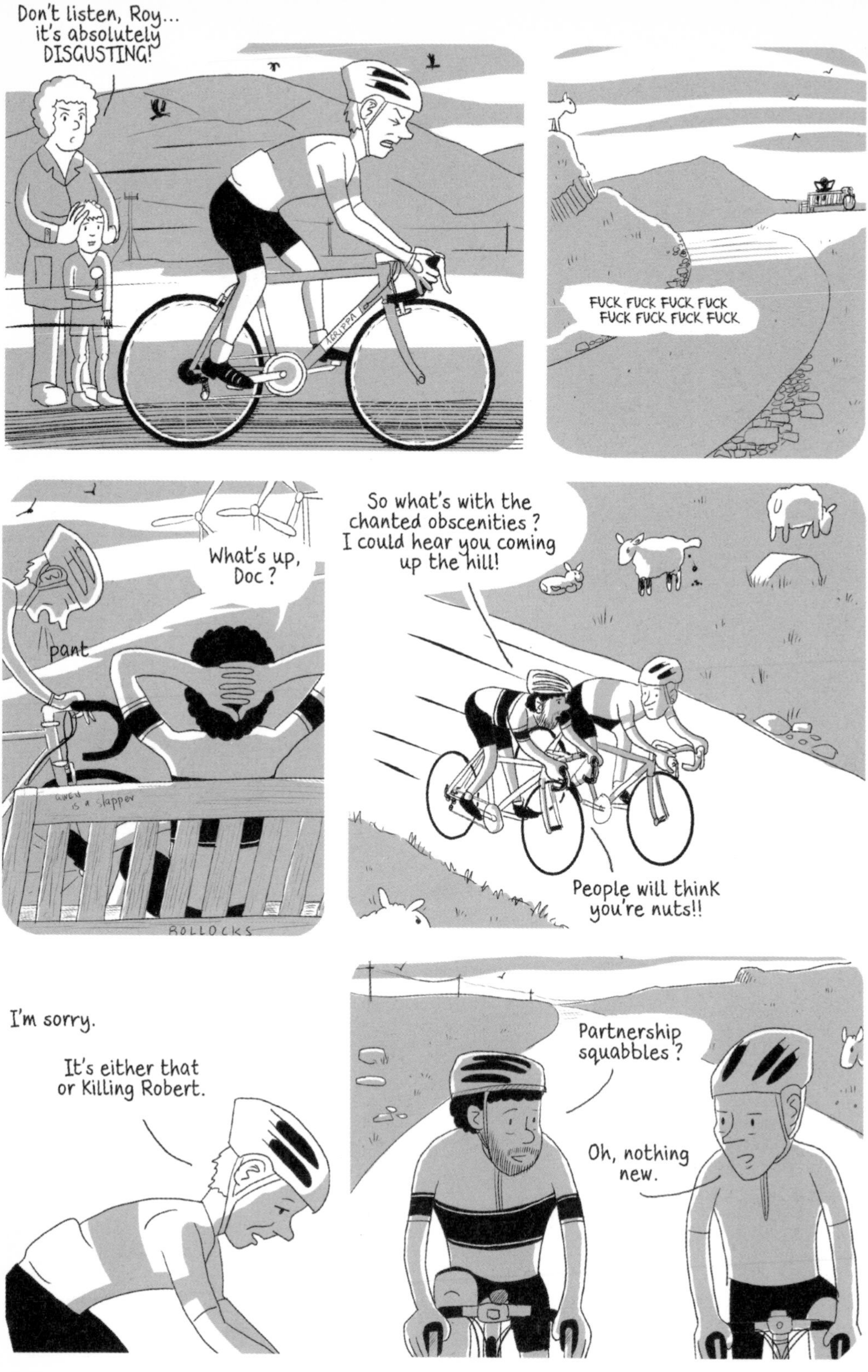
Don't listen, Roy... it's absolutely DISGUSTING!
AGRIPPA
FUCK FUCK FUCK FUCK
FUCK FUCK FUCK FUCK
What's up, Doc?
pant
Gwen is a slapper
BOLLOCKS
So what's with the chanted obscenities? I could hear you coming up the hill!
People will think you're nuts!!
I'm sorry.
It's either that or Killing Robert.
Partnership squabbles?
Oh, nothing new.

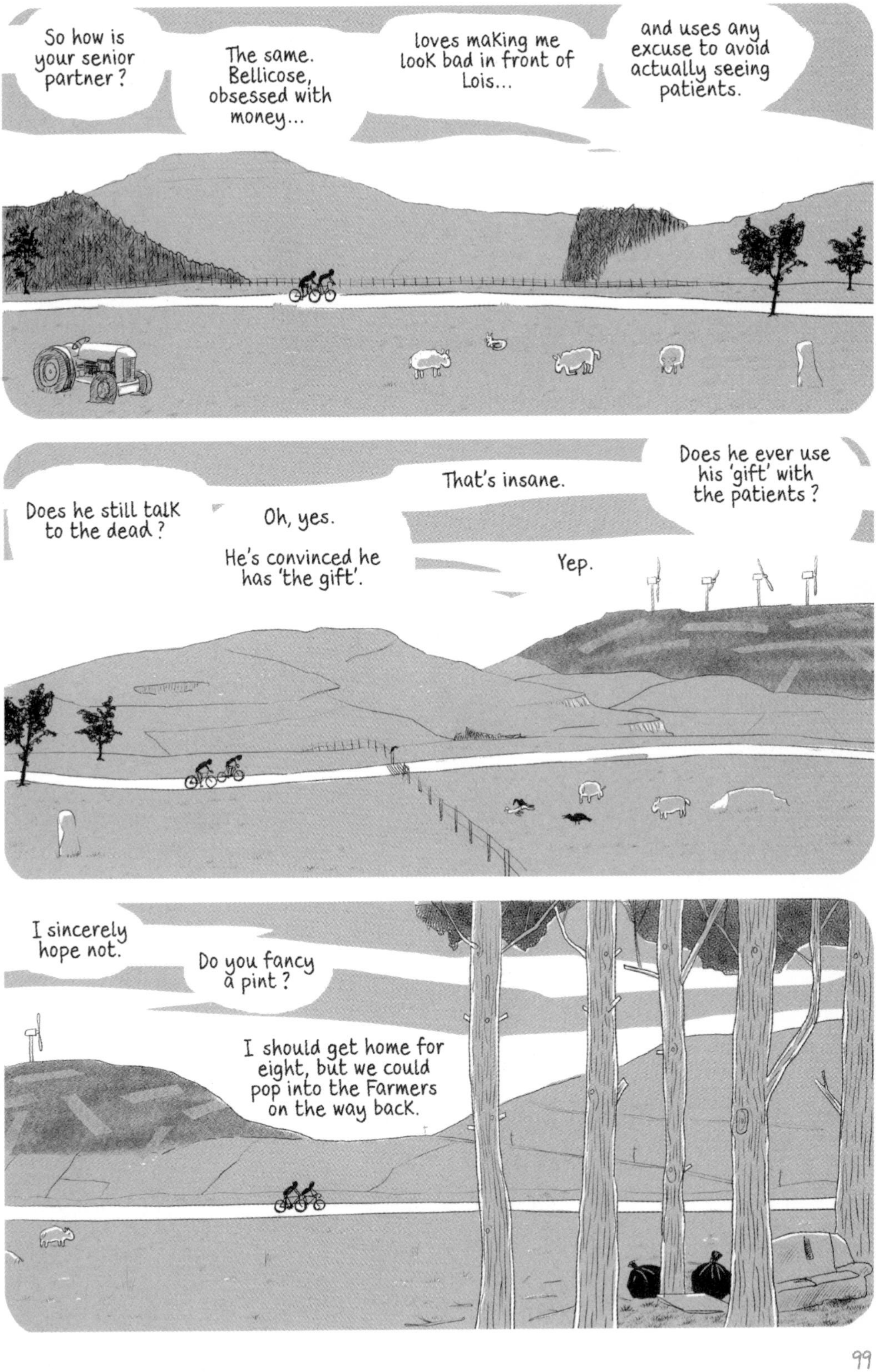
So how is your senior partner?
The same. Bellicose, obsessed with money...
loves making me look bad in front of Lois...
and uses any excuse to avoid actually seeing patients.
Does he still talk to the dead?
Oh, yes.
He's convinced he has 'the gift'.
That's insane.
Yep.
Does he ever use his 'gift' with the patients?
I sincerely hope not.
Do you fancy a pint?
I should get home for eight, but we could pop into the Farmers on the way back.

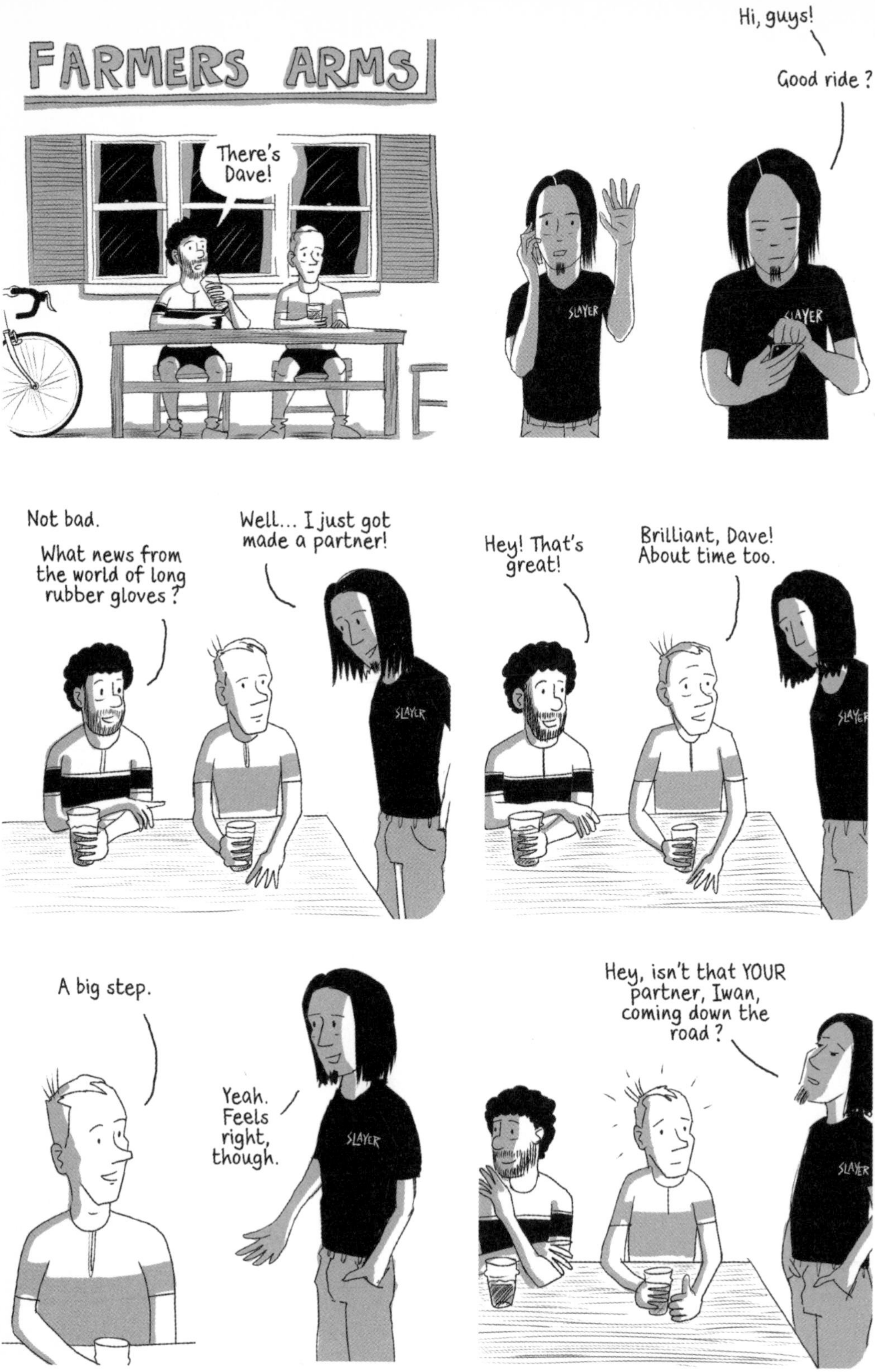
FARMERS ARMS
There's Dave!
Hi, guys!
Good ride?
SLAYER
Not bad.
What news from the world of long rubber gloves?
Well... I just got made a partner!
Hey! That's great!
Brilliant, Dave! About time too.
A big step.
Yeah. Feels right, though.
Hey, isn't that YOUR partner, Iwan, coming down the road?

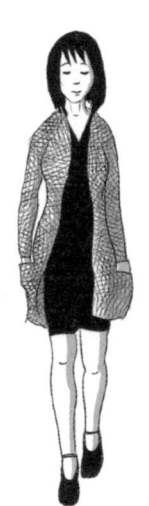

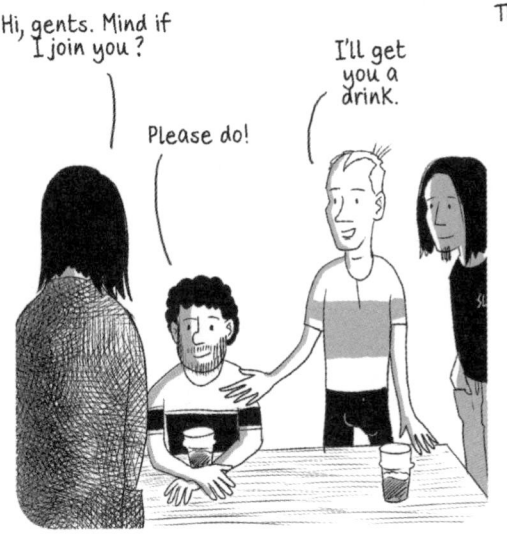

Hi, gents. Mind if I join you?

Please do!

I'll get you a drink.

Thanks, Iwan, I'll have a vodka and tonic.

Nice shorts!

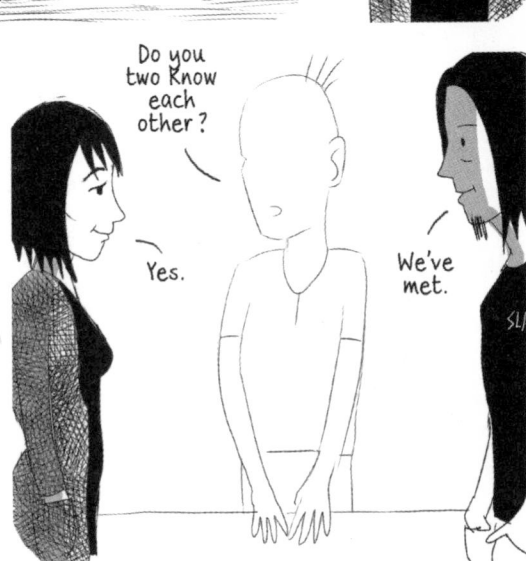

How about you, Dave? Celebratory drink?

Cheers Iwan!

I'll have an IPA.

Do you two know each other?

Yes.

We've met.

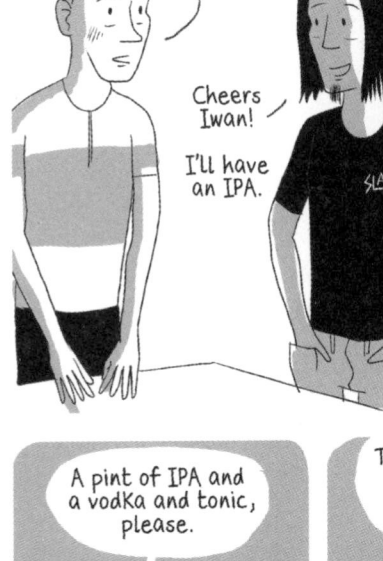

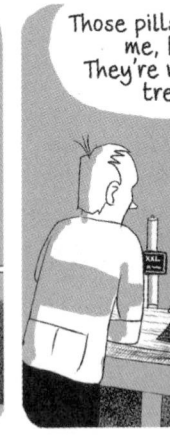

A pint of IPA and a vodka and tonic, please.

Those pills you gave me, Doc... They're working a treat!

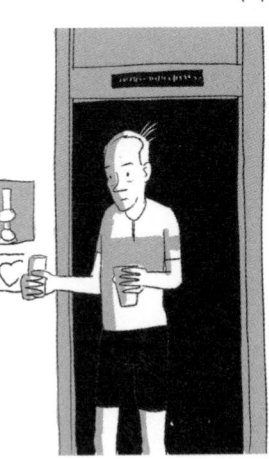

101

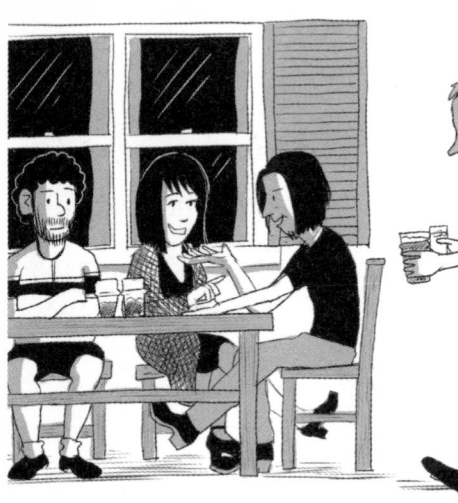
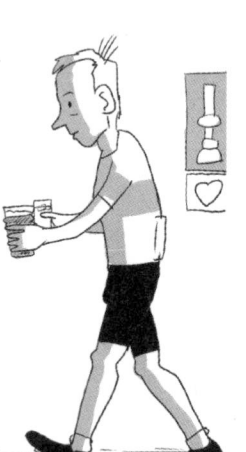
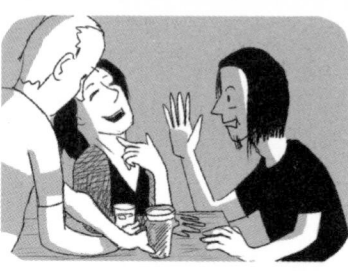

Thanks, Iwan.

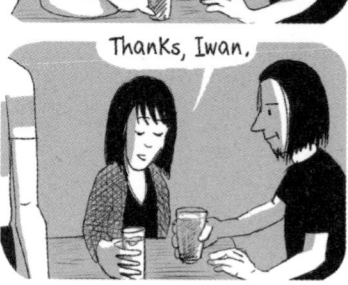

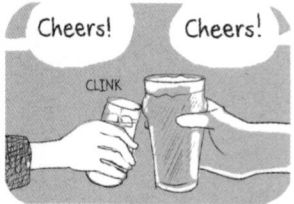

Cheers! Cheers!

CLINK

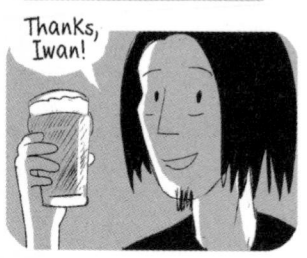

Thanks, Iwan!

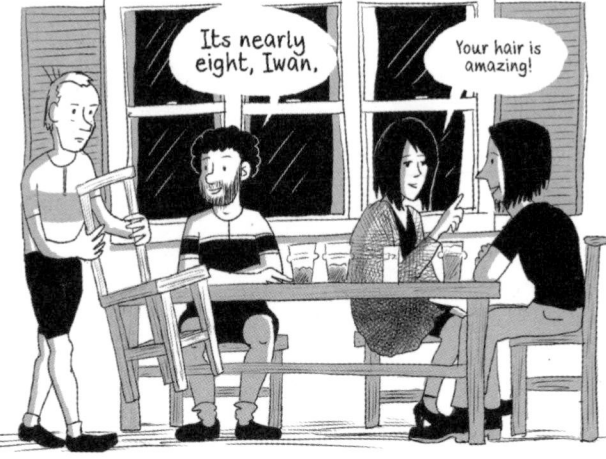

Its nearly eight, Iwan.

Your hair is amazing!

We'd better head off soon.

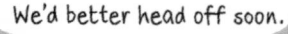

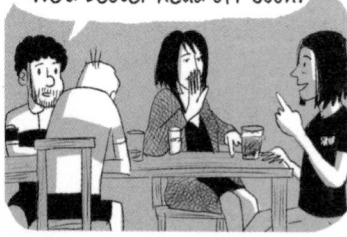

But Lois only just arrived.

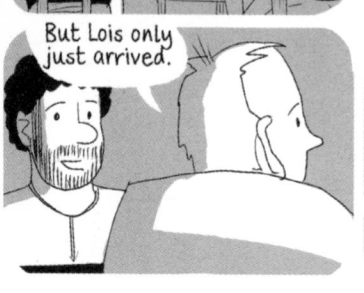

Don't worry, Iwan. You head off.

I'll look after her.

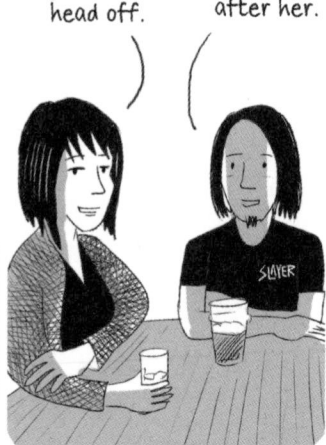

HAHAHAHAHA

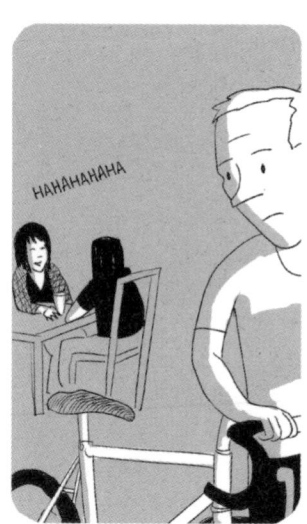

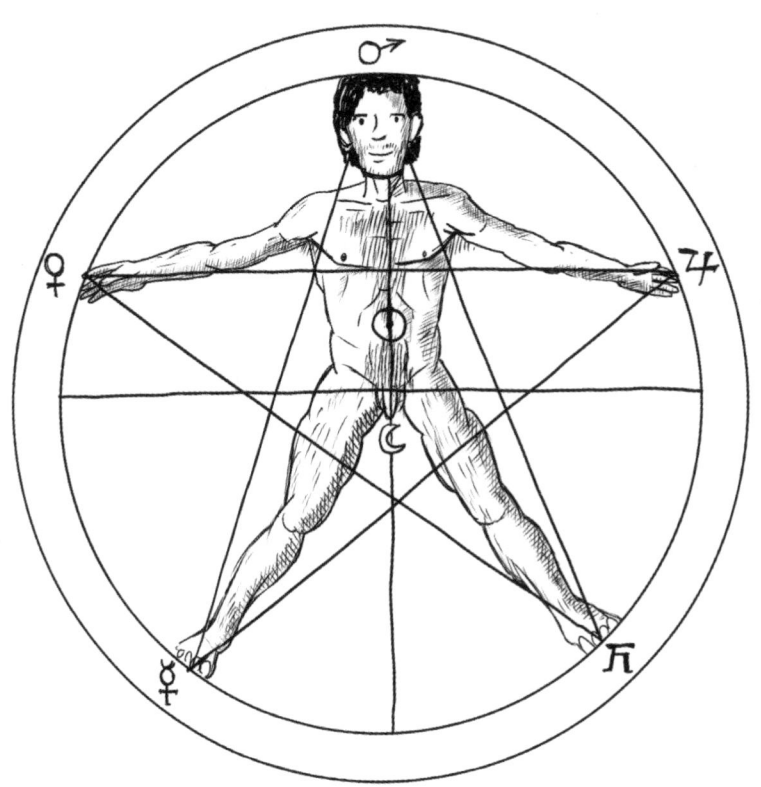

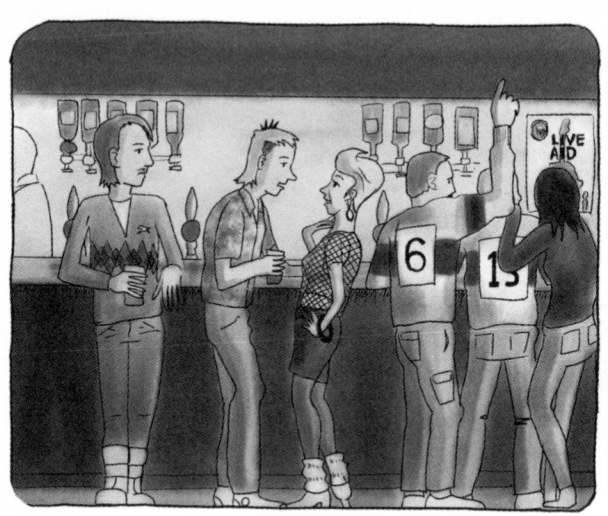

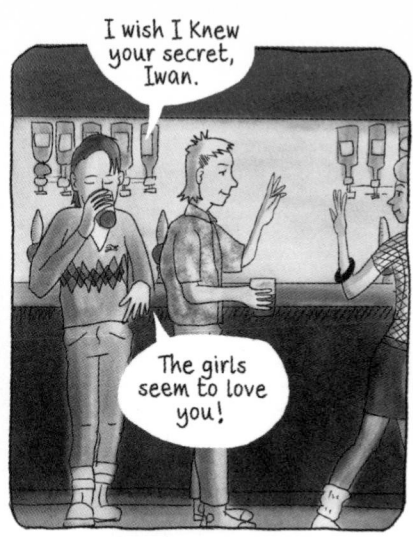

I wish I knew your secret, Iwan.

The girls seem to love you!

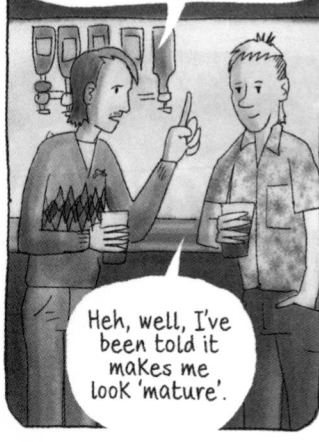

Maybe it's your hair! That 'silver fox' look is cool.

Heh, well, I've been told it makes me look 'mature'.

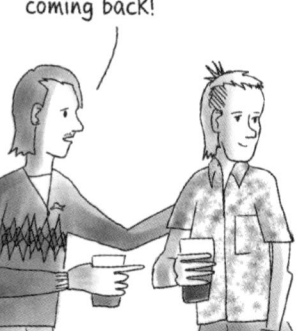

Look, she's coming back!

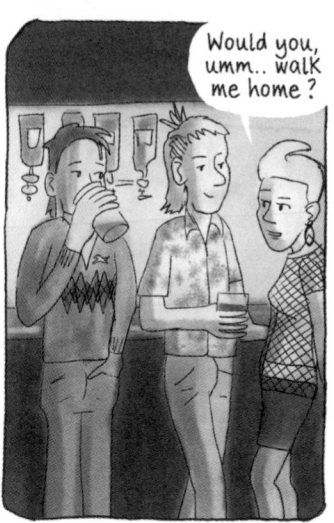

Would you, umm.. walk me home?

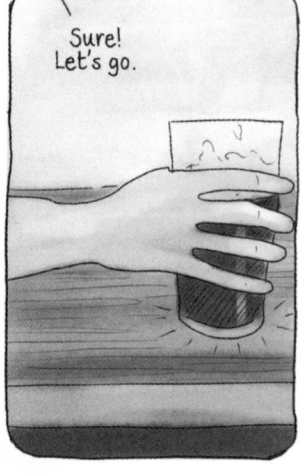

Sure! Let's go.

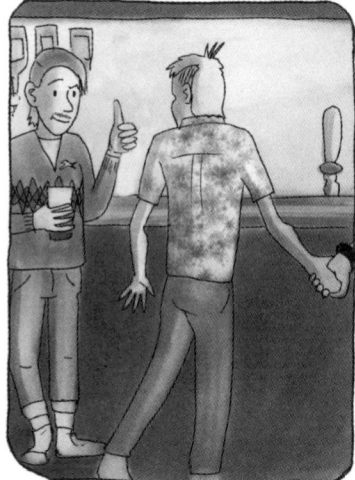

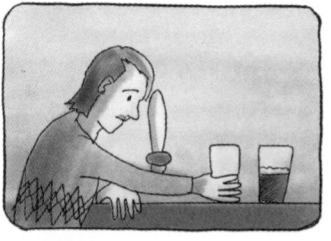

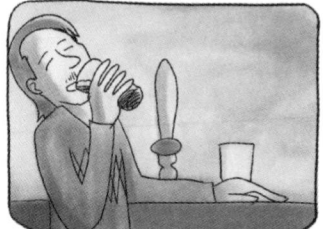

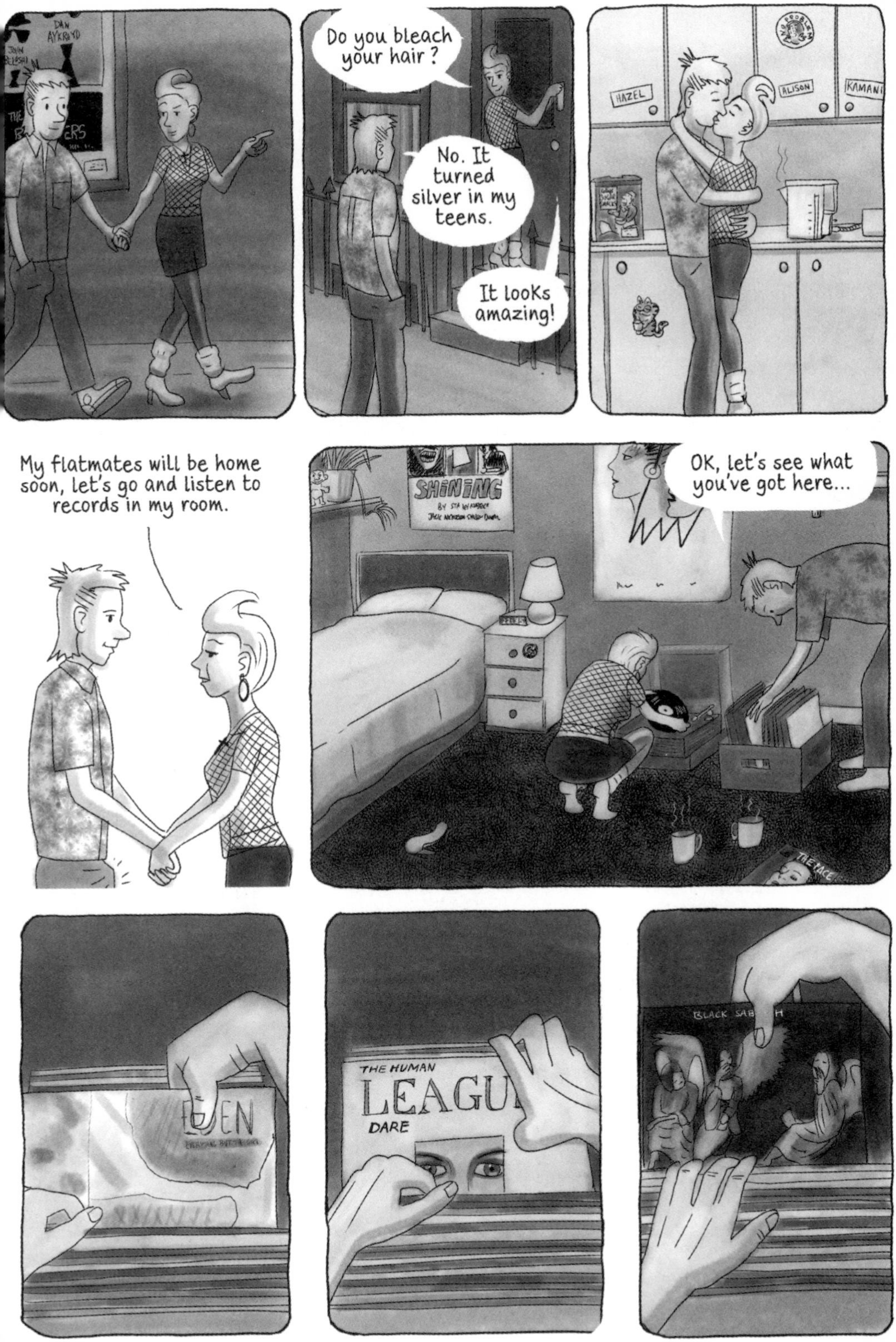
DAN AYKROYD
Do you bleach your hair?
No. It turned silver in my teens.
It looks amazing!
HAZEL
ALISON
KAMANI
My flatmates will be home soon, let's go and listen to records in my room.
SHINING
OK, let's see what you've got here...
THE FACE
THE HUMAN
DARE

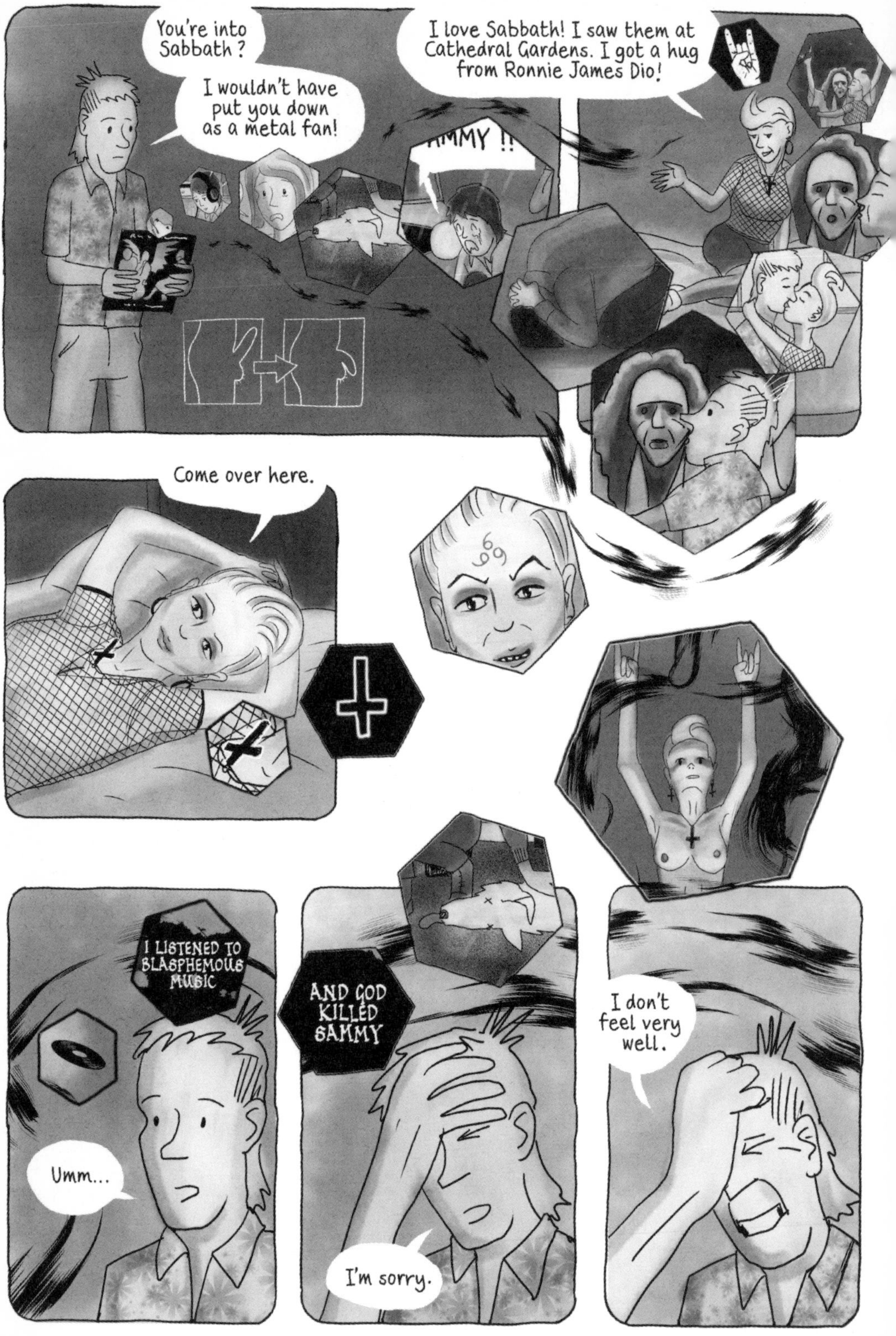
You're into Sabbath ?
I wouldn't have put you down as a metal fan!
AMMY !!
I love Sabbath! I saw them at Cathedral Gardens. I got a hug from Ronnie James Dio!
Come over here.
I LISTENED TO BLASPHEMOUS MUSIC
Umm...
AND GOD KILLED SAMMY
I'm sorry.
I don't feel very well.

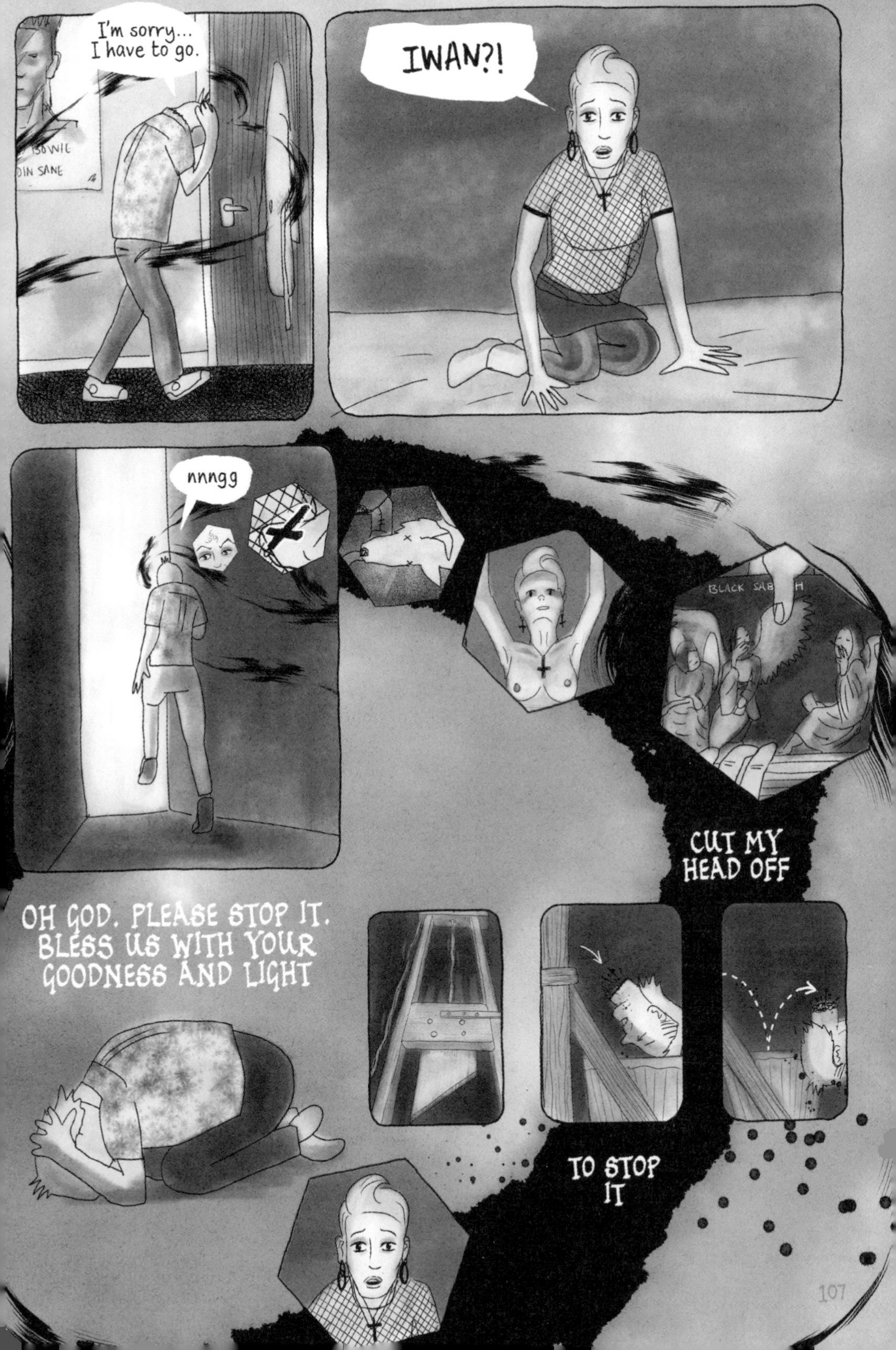

I'm sorry...
I have to go.
BOWIE
DIN SANE
IWAN?!
nnngg
BLACK SAB
CUT MY HEAD OFF
OH GOD. PLEASE STOP IT. BLESS US WITH YOUR GOODNESS AND LIGHT
TO STOP IT

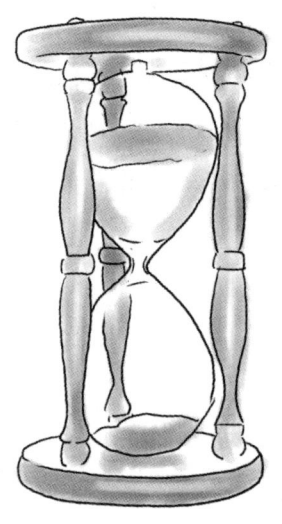

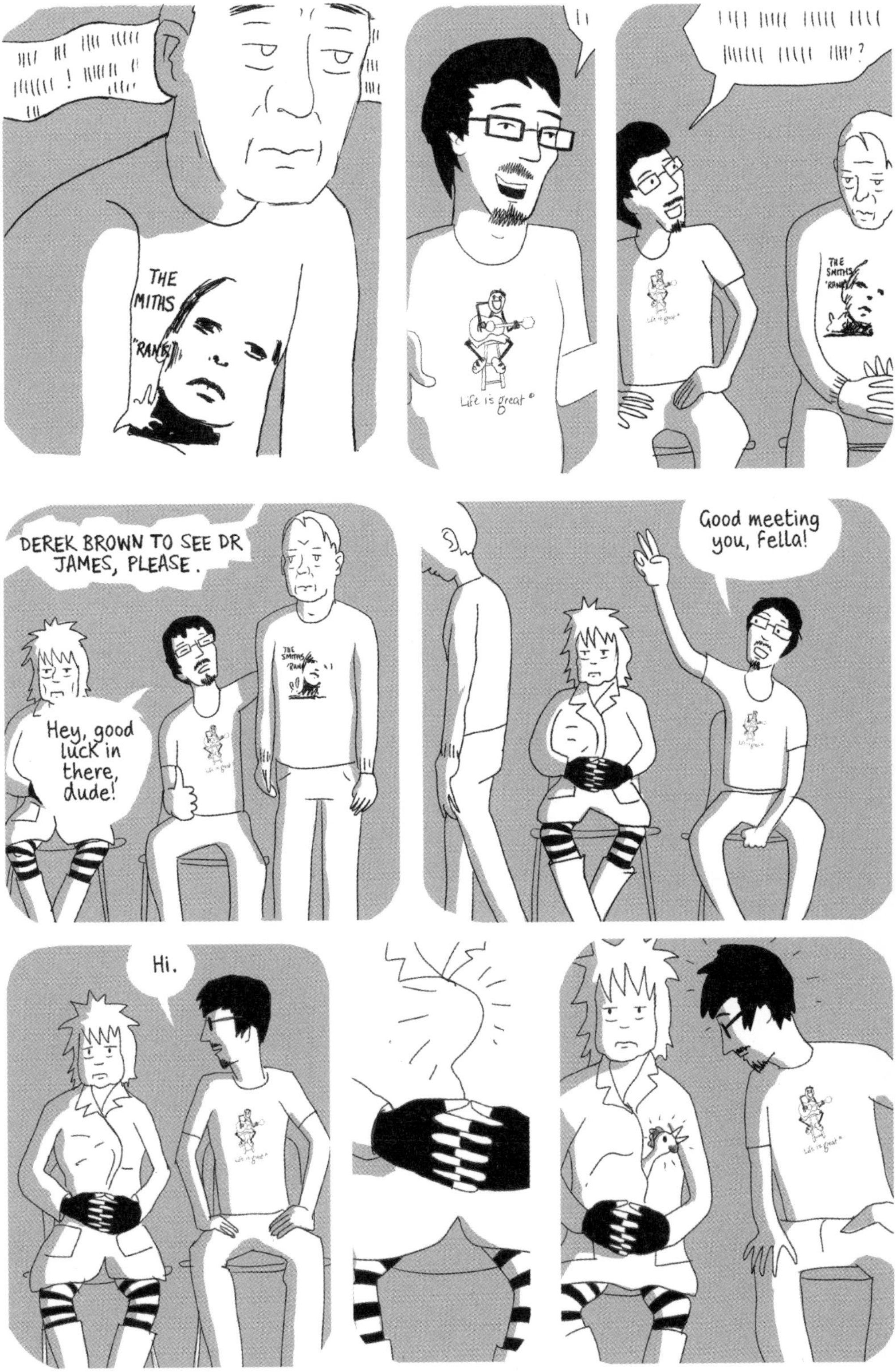
THE MITHS
"RANK"
Life is great
THE SMITHS "RANK"
DEREK BROWN TO SEE DR JAMES, PLEASE.
Hey, good luck in there, dude!
Good meeting you, fella!
Hi.

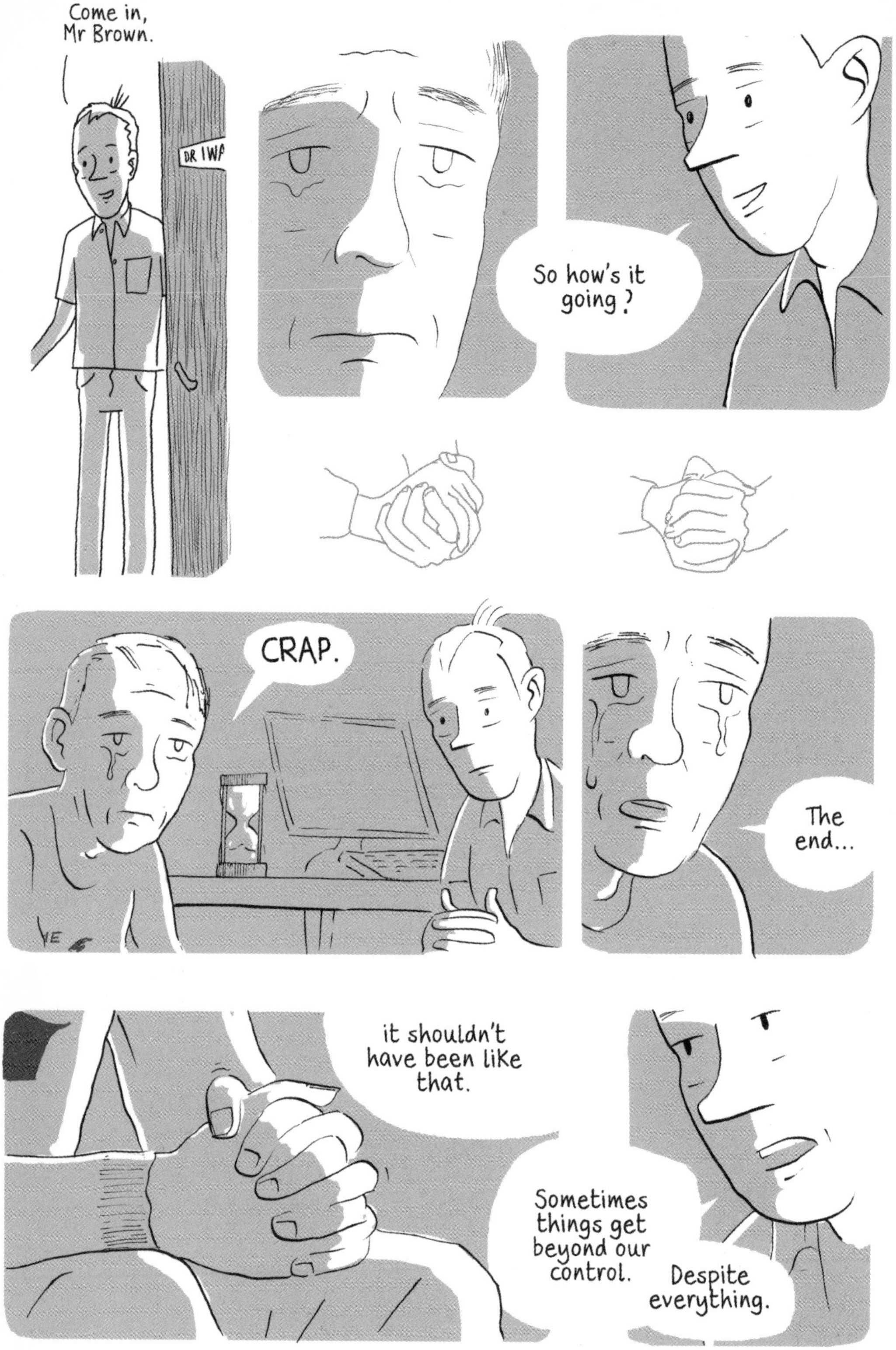
Come in, Mr Brown.
DR IWA
So how's it going ?
CRAP.
The end...
it shouldn't have been like that.
Sometimes things get beyond our control.
Despite everything.

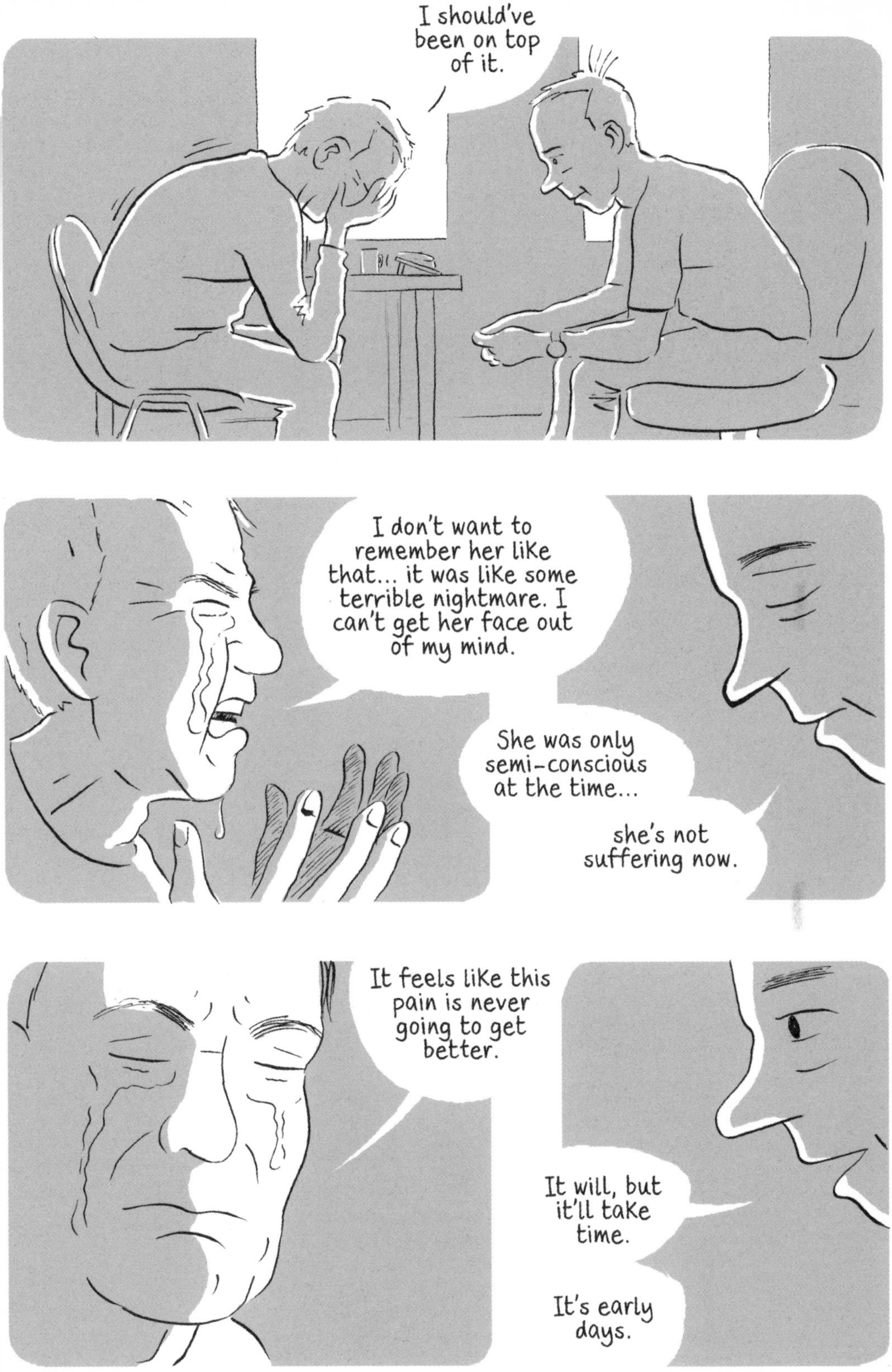
I should've been on top of it.
I don't want to remember her like that... it was like some terrible nightmare. I can't get her face out of my mind.
She was only semi-conscious at the time...
she's not suffering now.
It feels like this pain is never going to get better.
It will, but it'll take time.
It's early days.

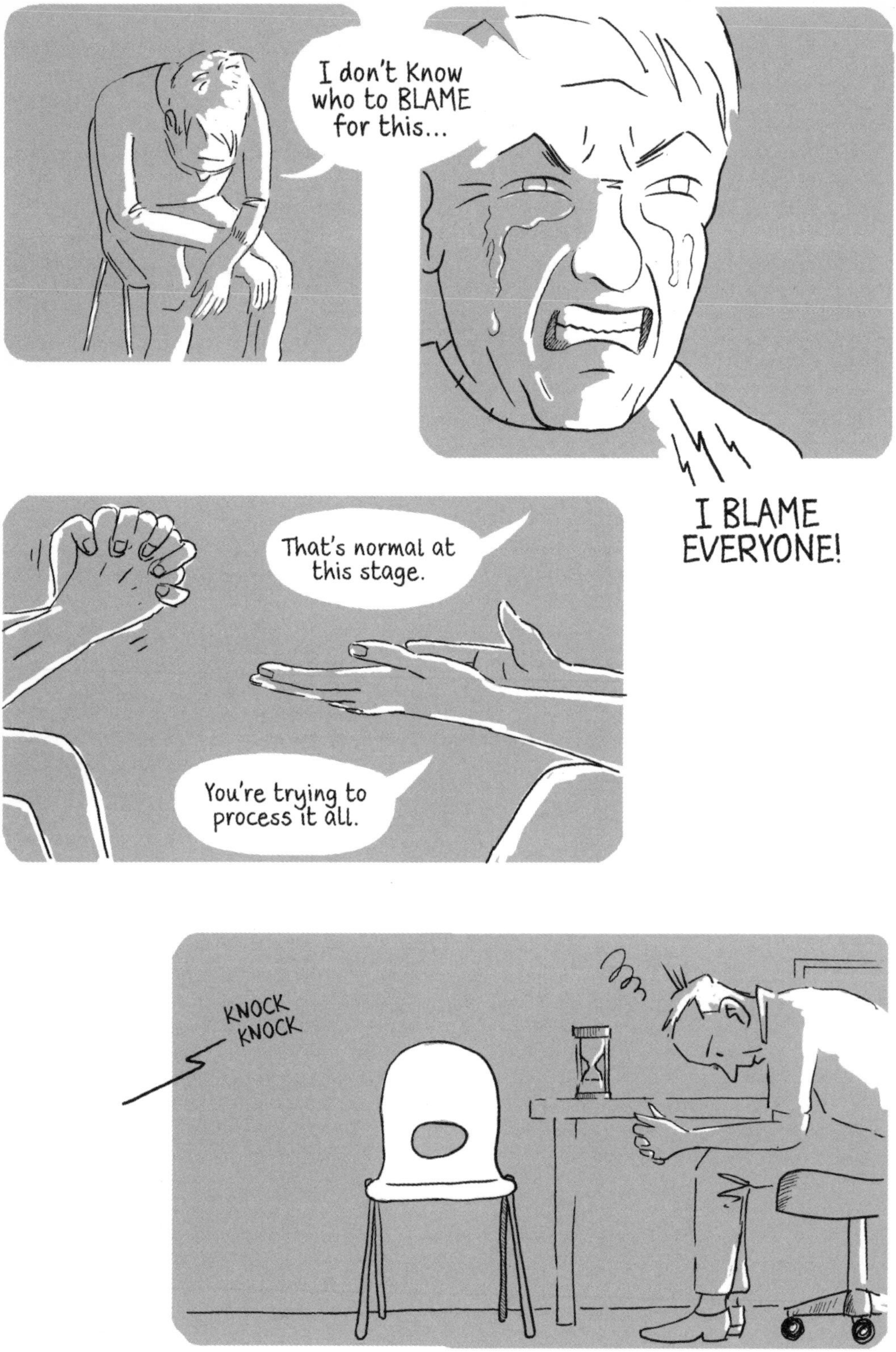
I don't Know who to BLAME for this...
I BLAME EVERYONE!
That's normal at this stage.
You're trying to process it all.
KNOCK KNOCK

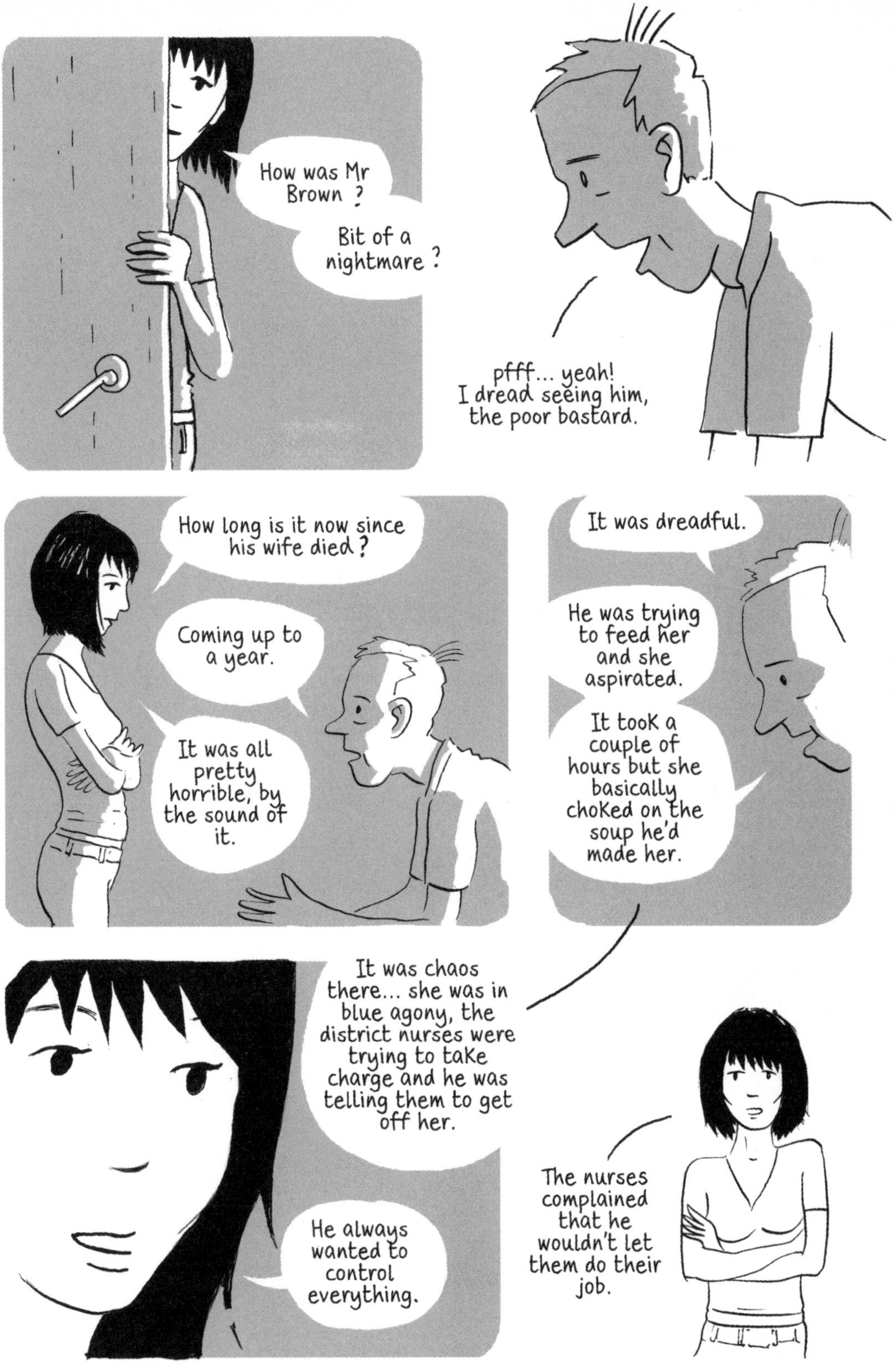
How was Mr Brown ?
Bit of a nightmare ?
pfff... yeah! I dread seeing him, the poor bastard.
How long is it now since his wife died ?
Coming up to a year.
It was all pretty horrible, by the sound of it.
It was dreadful.
He was trying to feed her and she aspirated.
It took a couple of hours but she basically choked on the soup he'd made her.
It was chaos there... she was in blue agony, the district nurses were trying to take charge and he was telling them to get off her.
He always wanted to control everything.
The nurses complained that he wouldn't let them do their job.

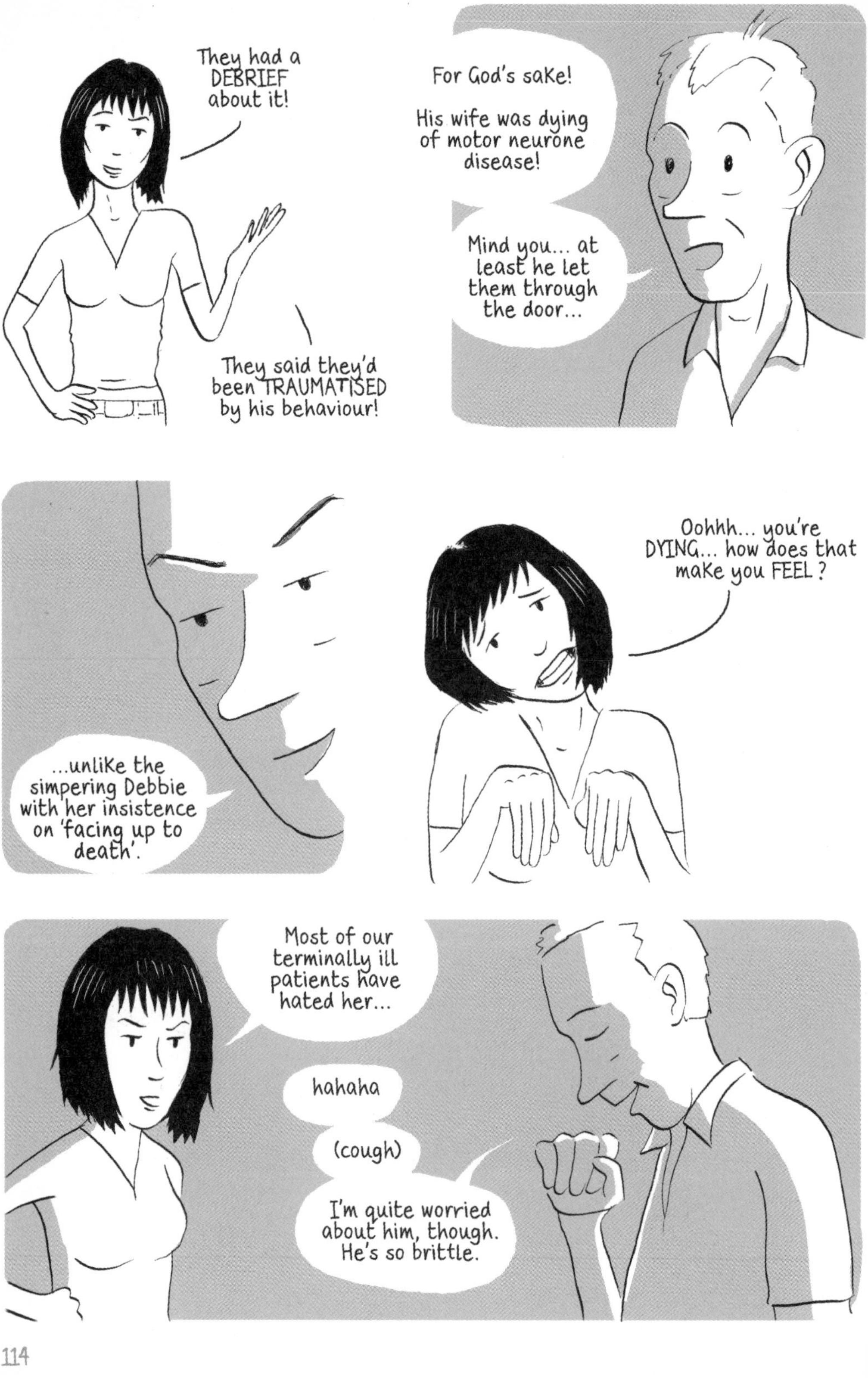
They had a DEBRIEF about it!
They said they'd been TRAUMATISED by his behaviour!
For God's sake!
His wife was dying of motor neurone disease!
Mind you... at least he let them through the door...
...unlike the simpering Debbie with her insistence on 'facing up to death'.
Oohhh... you're DYING... how does that make you FEEL ?
Most of our terminally ill patients have hated her...
hahaha
(cough)
I'm quite worried about him, though. He's so brittle.

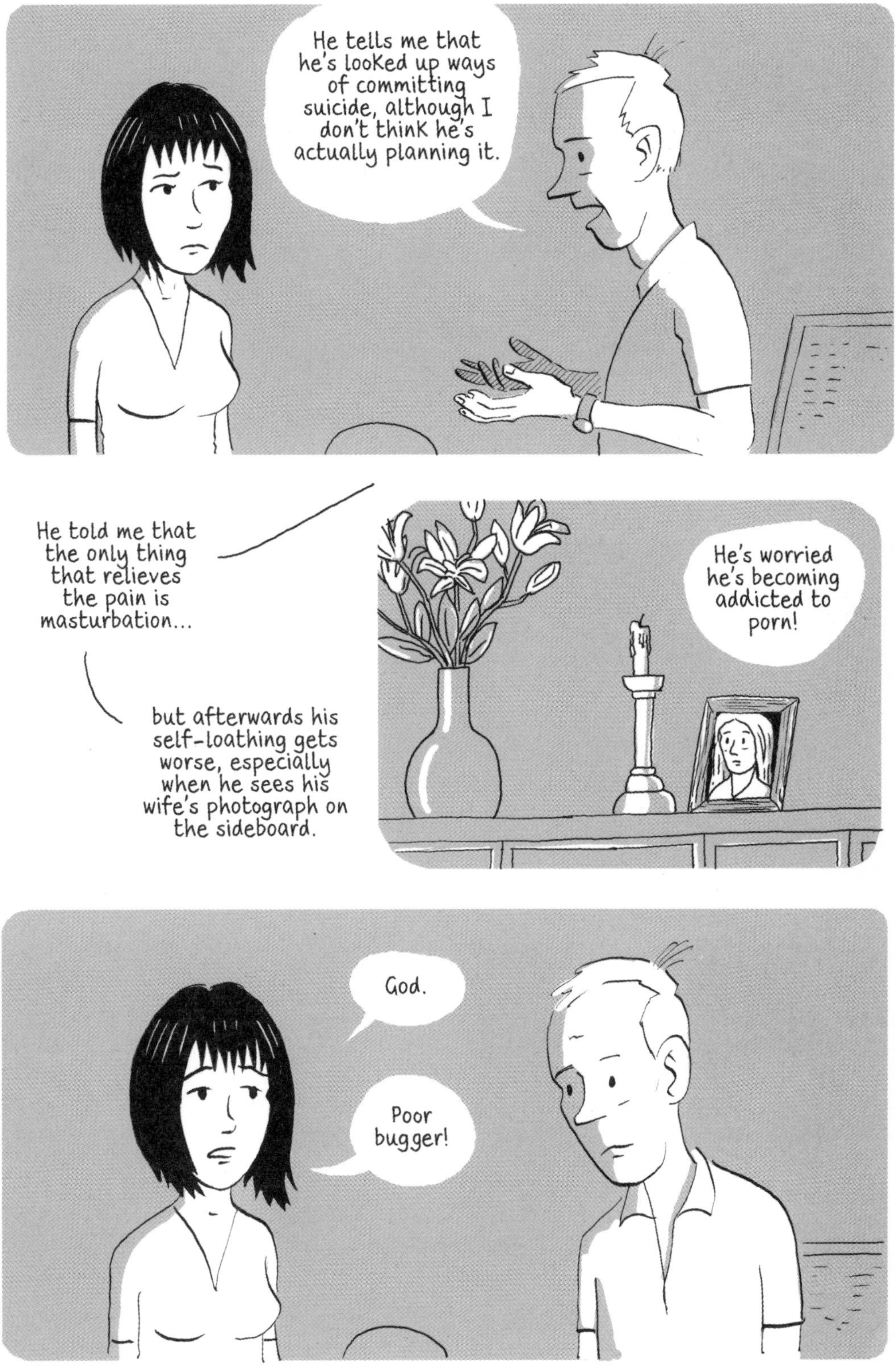
He tells me that he's looked up ways of committing suicide, although I don't think he's actually planning it.
He told me that the only thing that relieves the pain is masturbation...
but afterwards his self-loathing gets worse, especially when he sees his wife's photograph on the sideboard.
He's worried he's becoming addicted to porn!
God.
Poor bugger!

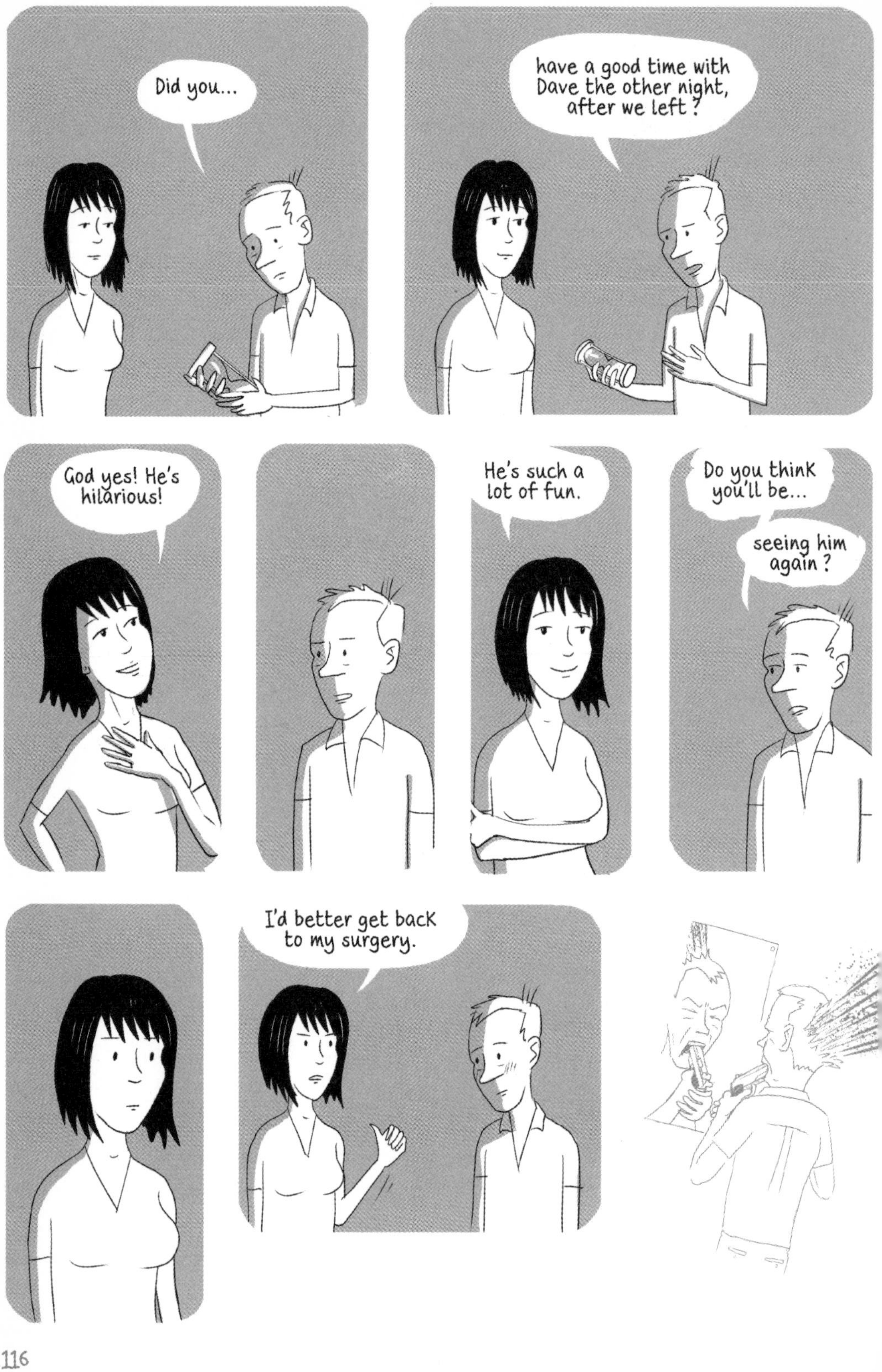
Did you...
have a good time with Dave the other night, after we left?
God yes! He's hilarious!
He's such a lot of fun.
Do you think you'll be...
seeing him again?
I'd better get back to my surgery.

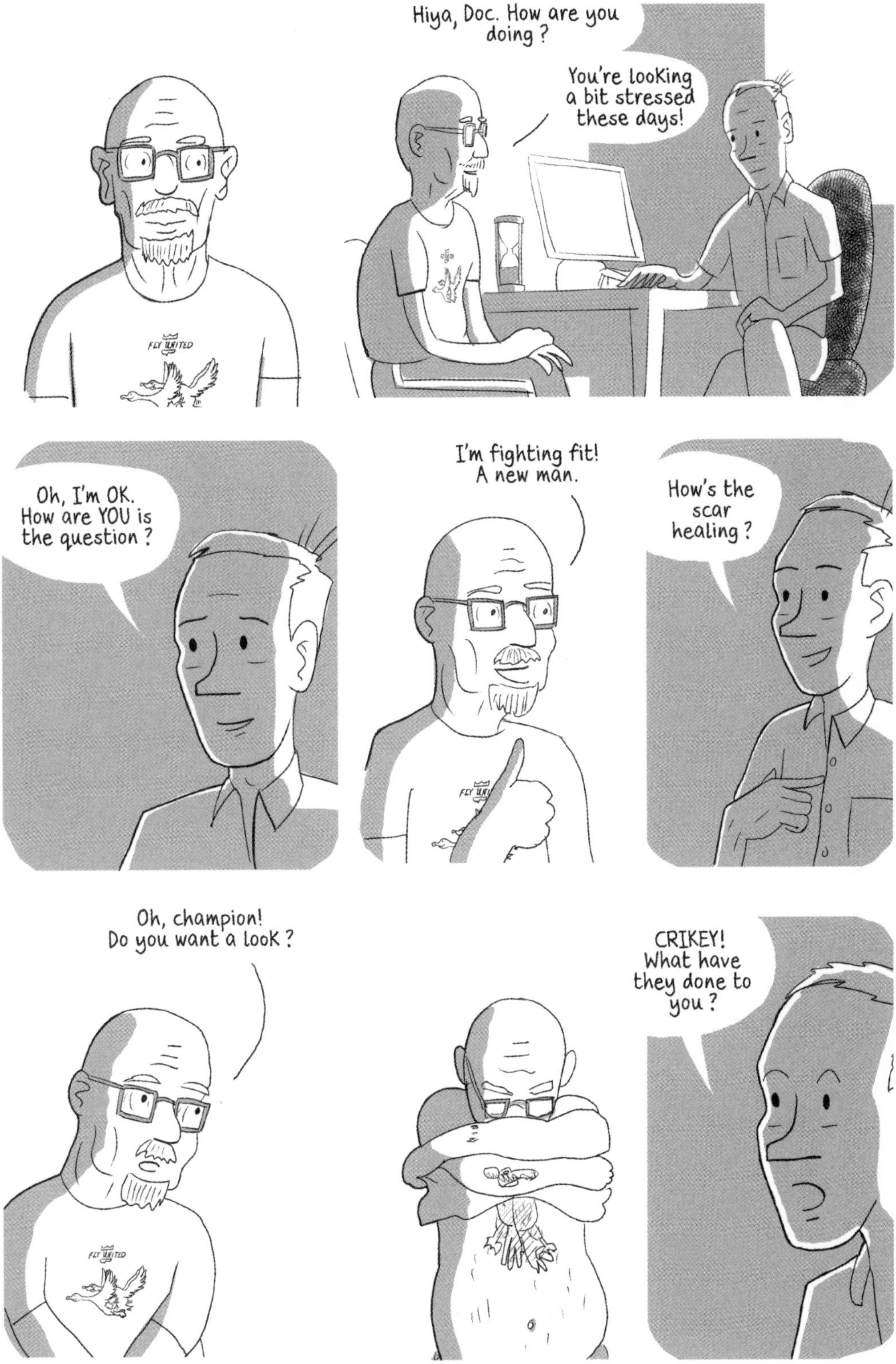
Hiya, Doc. How are you doing ?
You're looking a bit stressed these days!
FLY UNITED
Oh, I'm OK. How are YOU is the question ?
I'm fighting fit! A new man.
How's the scar healing ?
Oh, champion! Do you want a look ?
CRIKEY! What have they done to you ?

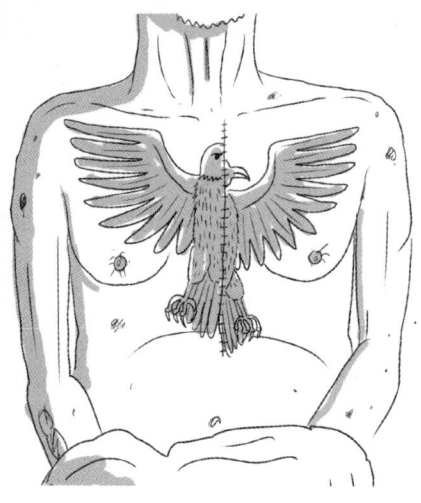

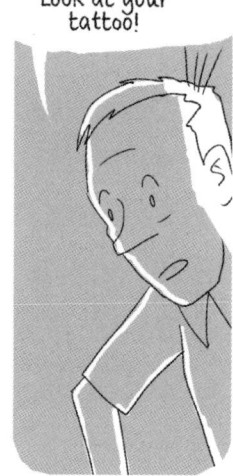

Look at your tattoo!

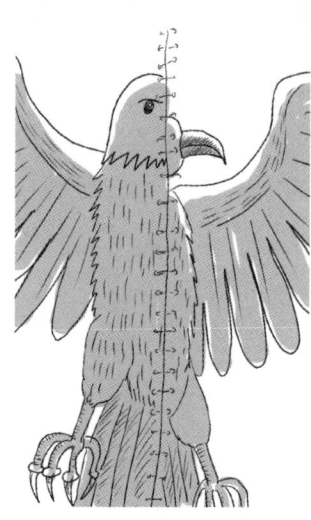

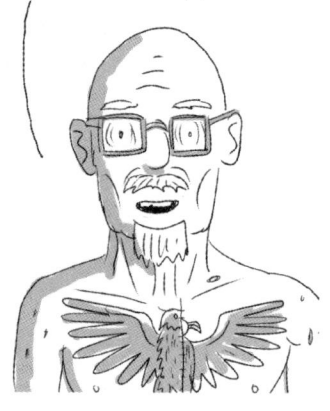

Heh heh. Looks like they got the medical student to sew me up!

That's bonkers!

The scar is the only bit of the operation that you can see!

You could sue them for that!

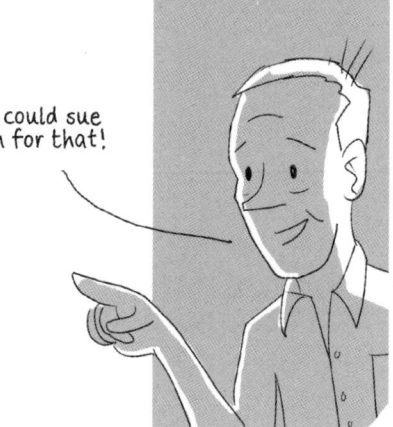

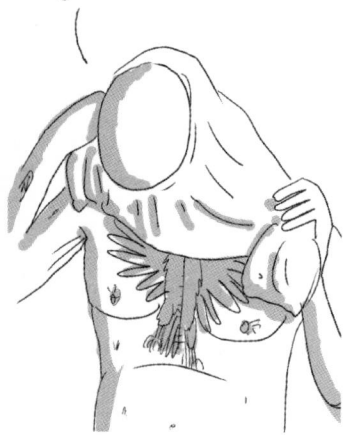

Why would I want to do that?

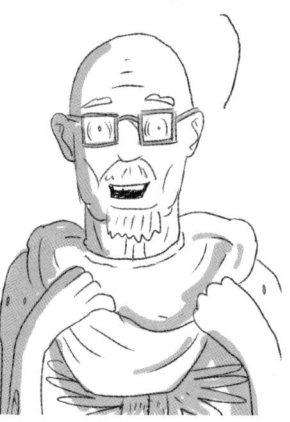

I'm seventy-five, I don't give a damn about how I look.

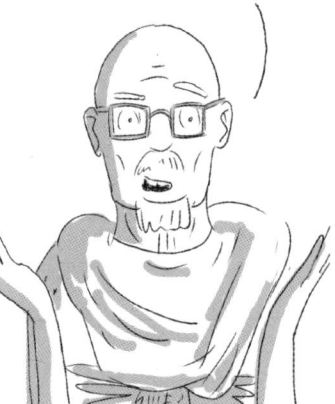

It didn't cost me anything and I've got a new lease of life!

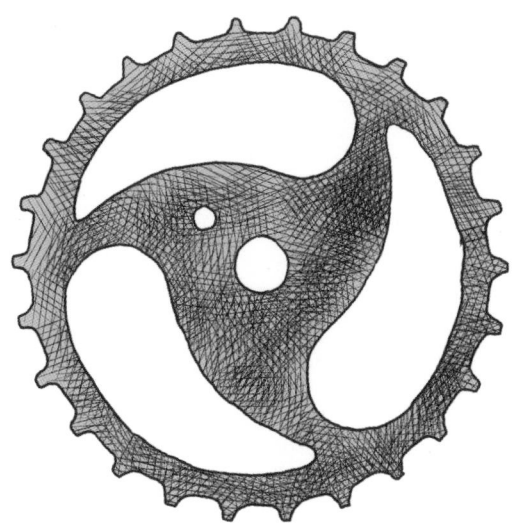

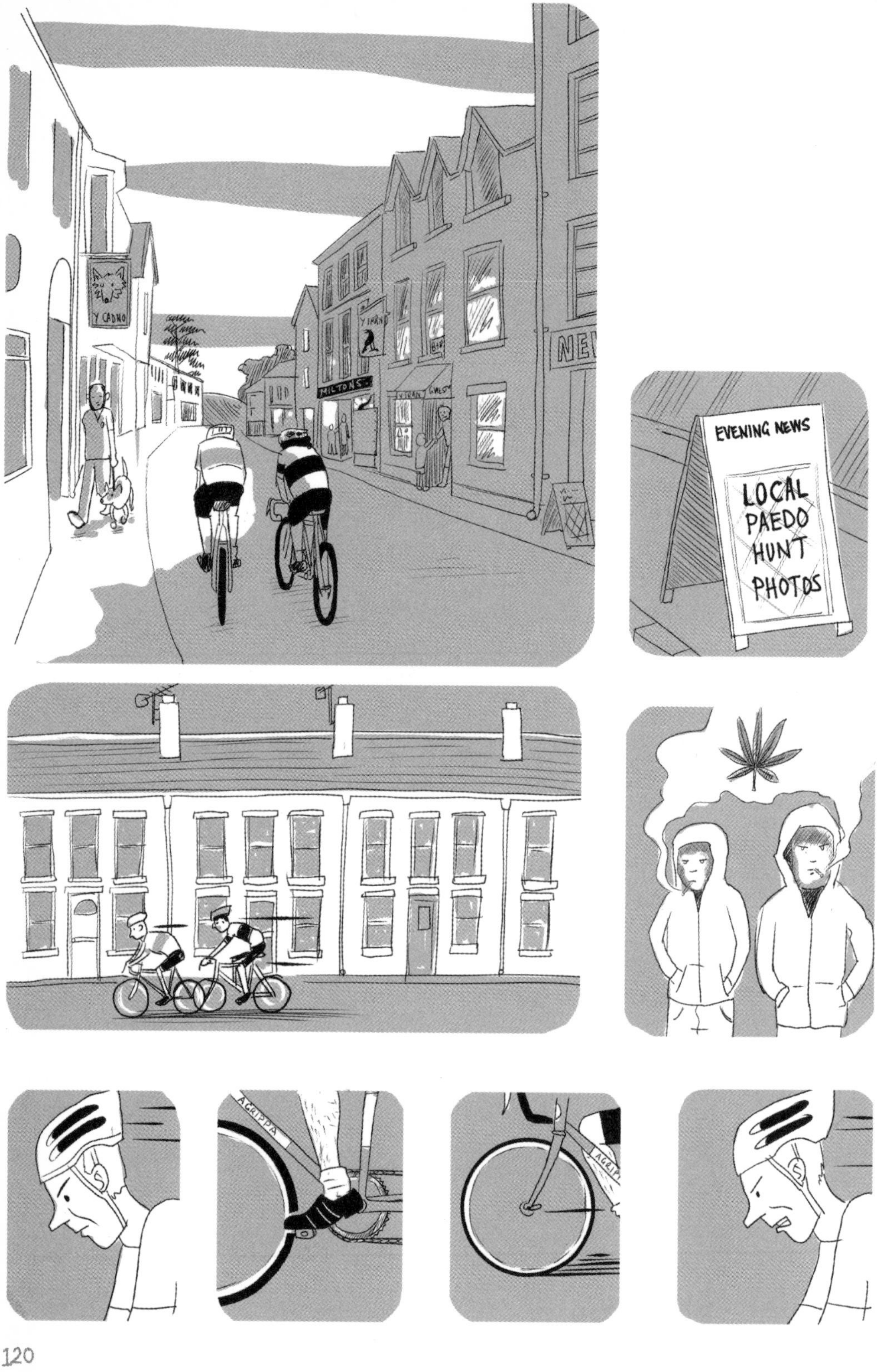
Y CADNO
MILTONS
EVENING NEWS
LOCAL PAEDO HUNT PHOTOS
AGRIPPA

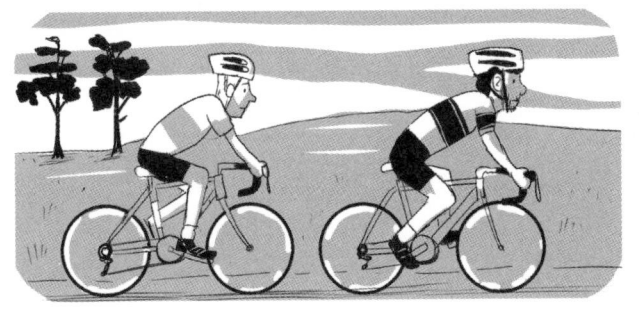

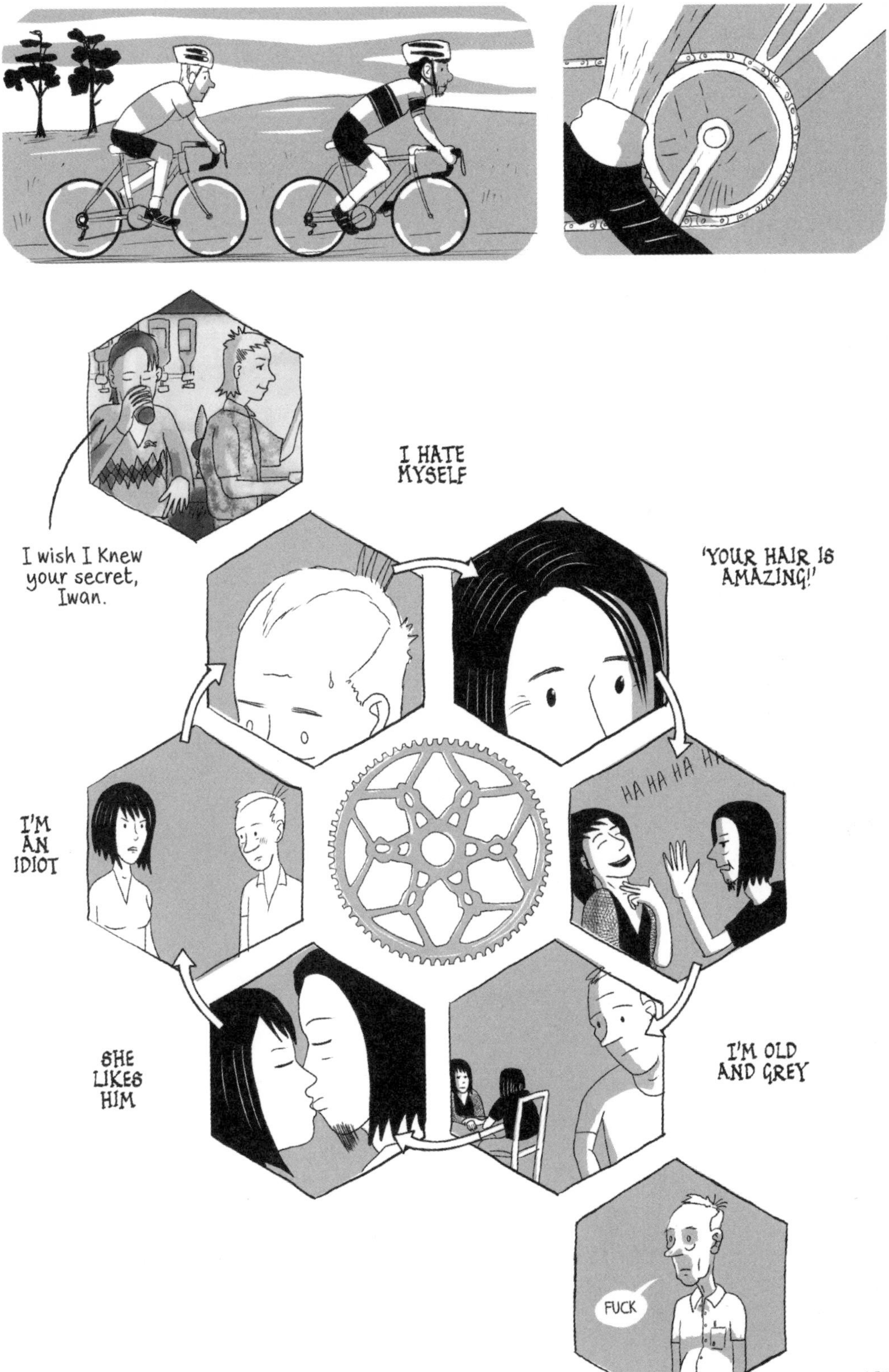

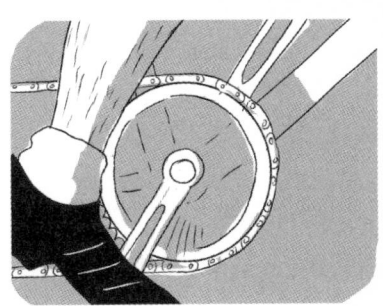

I wish I knew your secret, Iwan.

I HATE MYSELF

'YOUR HAIR IS AMAZING!'

I'M AN IDIOT

HA HA HA HA

I'M OLD AND GREY

SHE LIKES HIM

FUCK

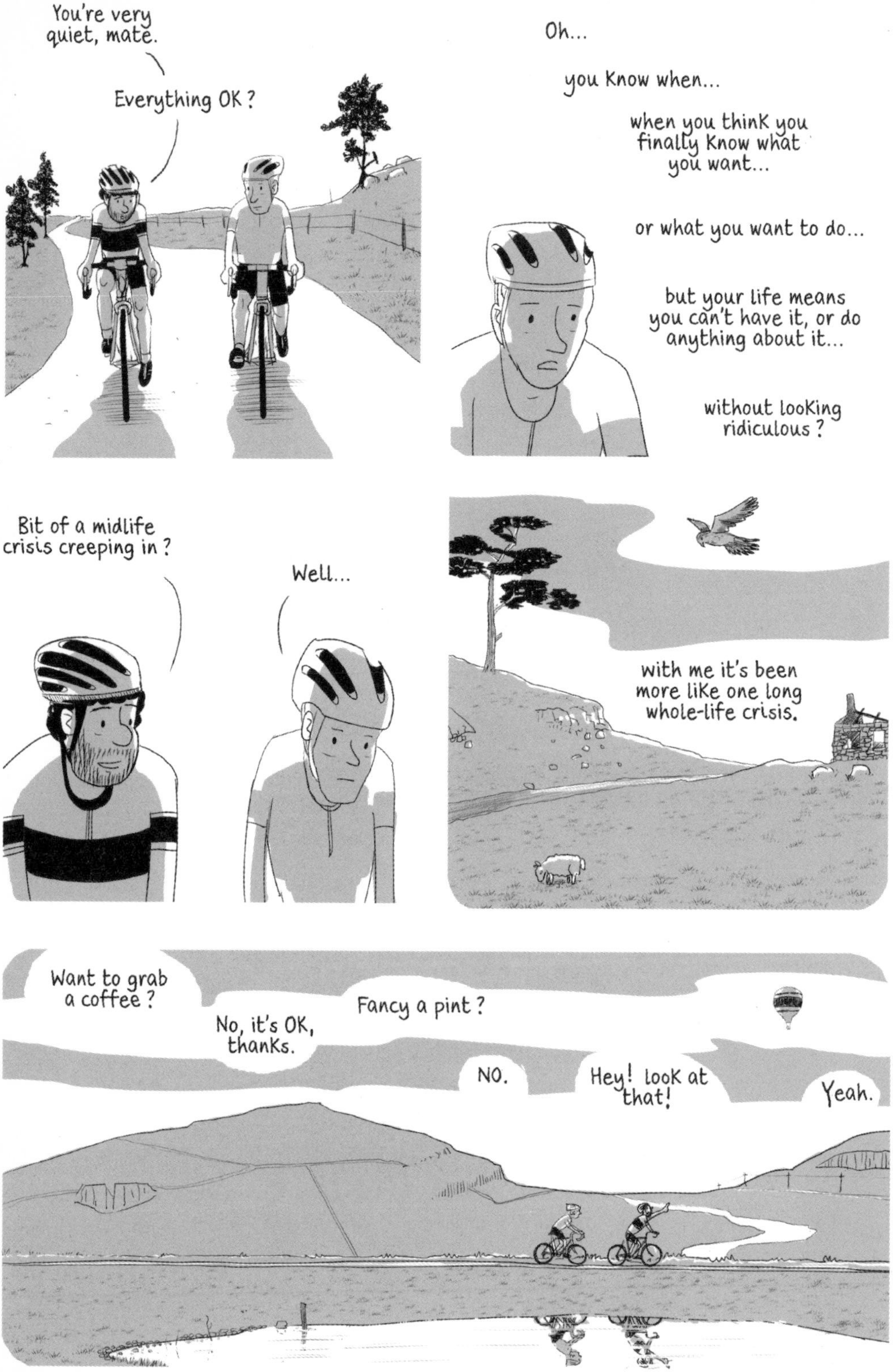
You're very quiet, mate.
Everything OK ?
Oh...
you know when...
when you think you finally know what you want...
or what you want to do...
but your life means you can't have it, or do anything about it...
without looking ridiculous ?
Bit of a midlife crisis creeping in ?
Well...
with me it's been more like one long whole-life crisis.
Want to grab a coffee ?
No, it's OK, thanks.
Fancy a pint ?
NO.
Hey! look at that!
Yeah.

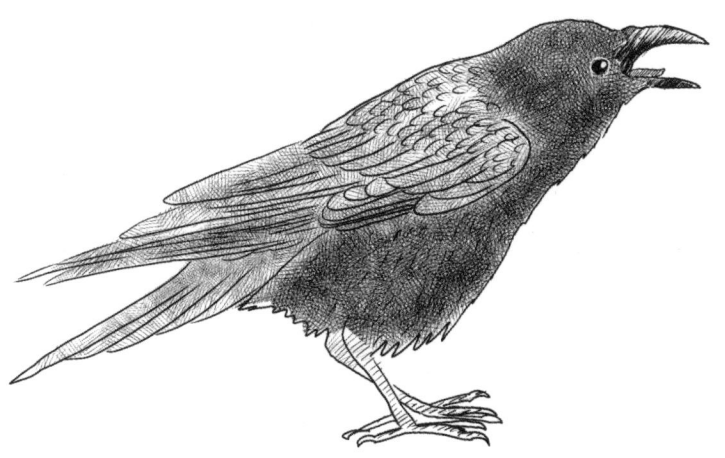

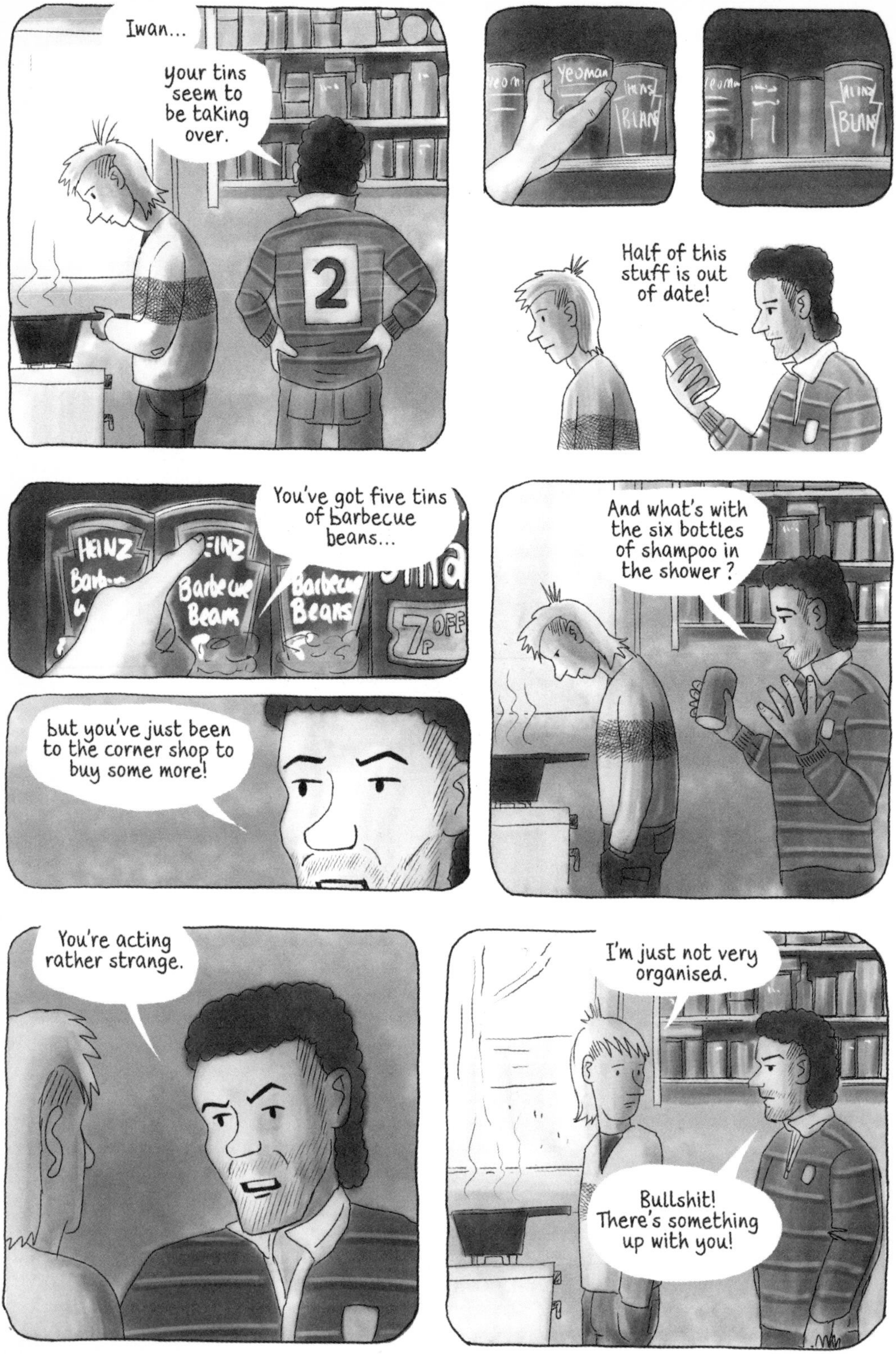
Iwan...
your tins seem to be taking over.
Yeoman
HEINZ BEANS
Half of this stuff is out of date!
HEINZ Barbecue Beans
You've got five tins of barbecue beans...
7p OFF
but you've just been to the corner shop to buy some more!
And what's with the six bottles of shampoo in the shower?
You're acting rather strange.
I'm just not very organised.
Bullshit! There's something up with you!

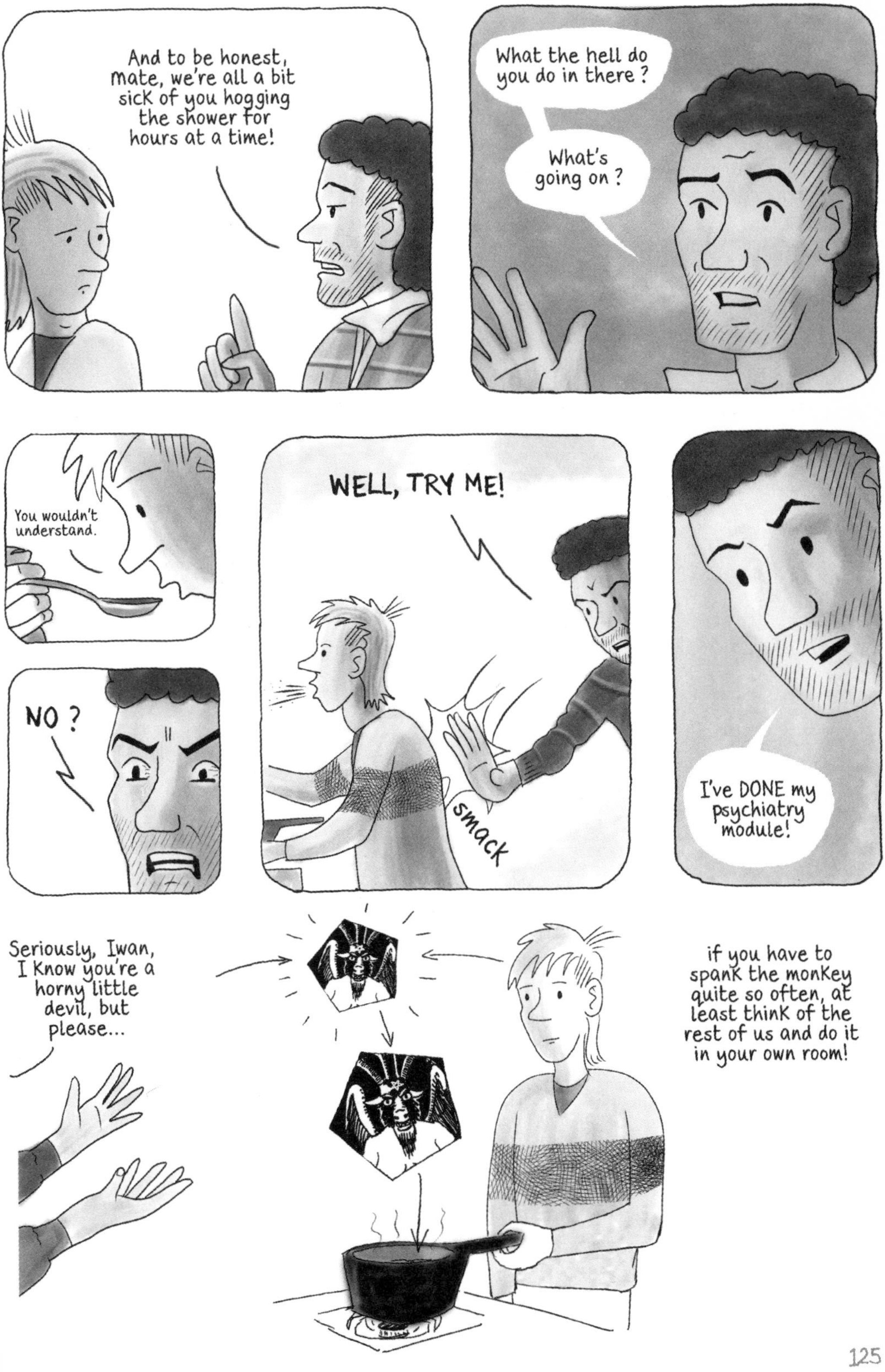
And to be honest, mate, we're all a bit sick of you hogging the shower for hours at a time!
What the hell do you do in there?
What's going on?
You wouldn't understand.
NO?
WELL, TRY ME!
smack
I've DONE my psychiatry module!
Seriously, Iwan, I know you're a horny little devil, but please...
if you have to spank the monkey quite so often, at least think of the rest of us and do it in your own room!

THE CHILLI IS CONTAMINATED
BY THE SABBATIC GOAT
BEGONE ALL DARKNESS AND EVIL
BLESS THIS FOOD WITH GOOD-NESS AND LIGHT.
BANG!
FUCKING HELL!

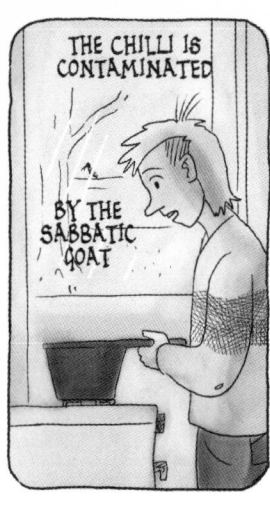

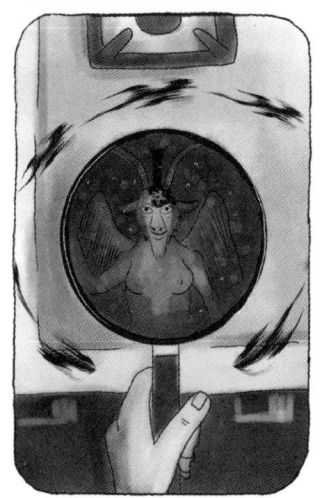

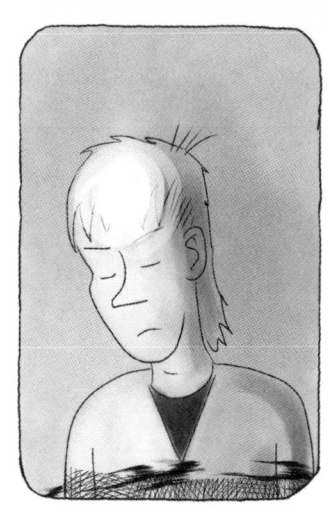

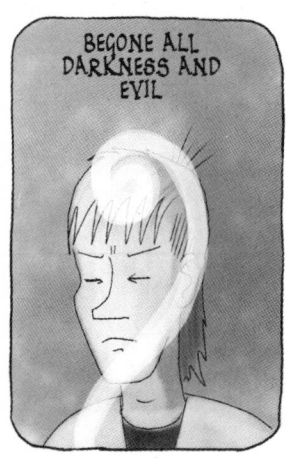

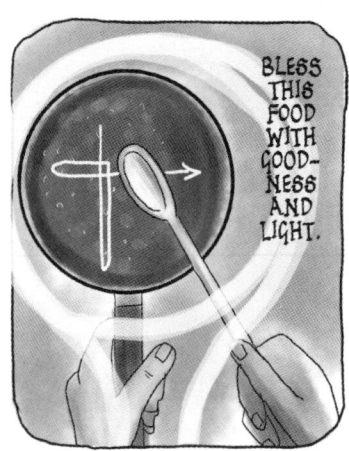

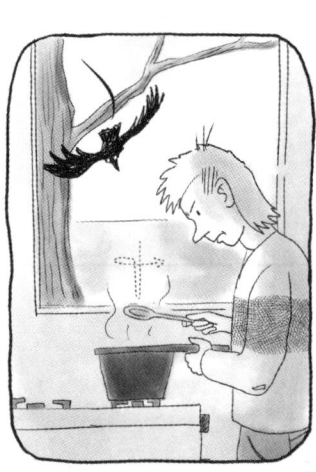

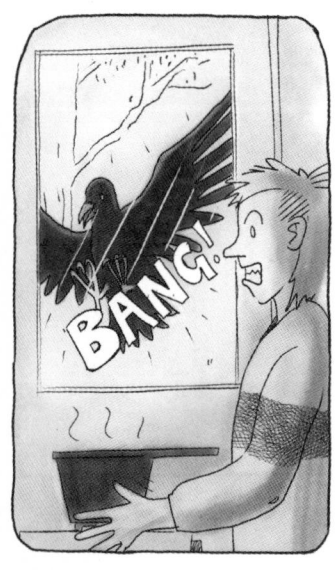

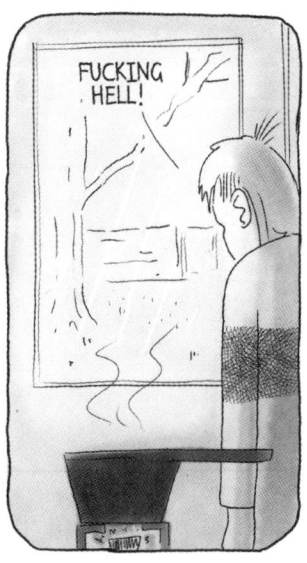

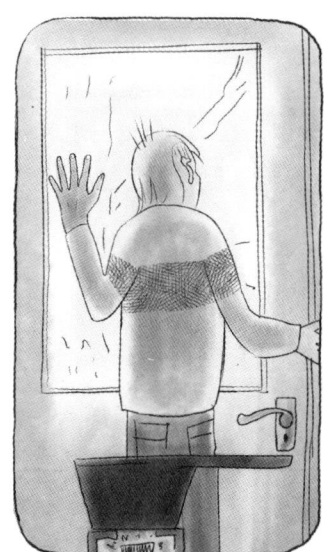

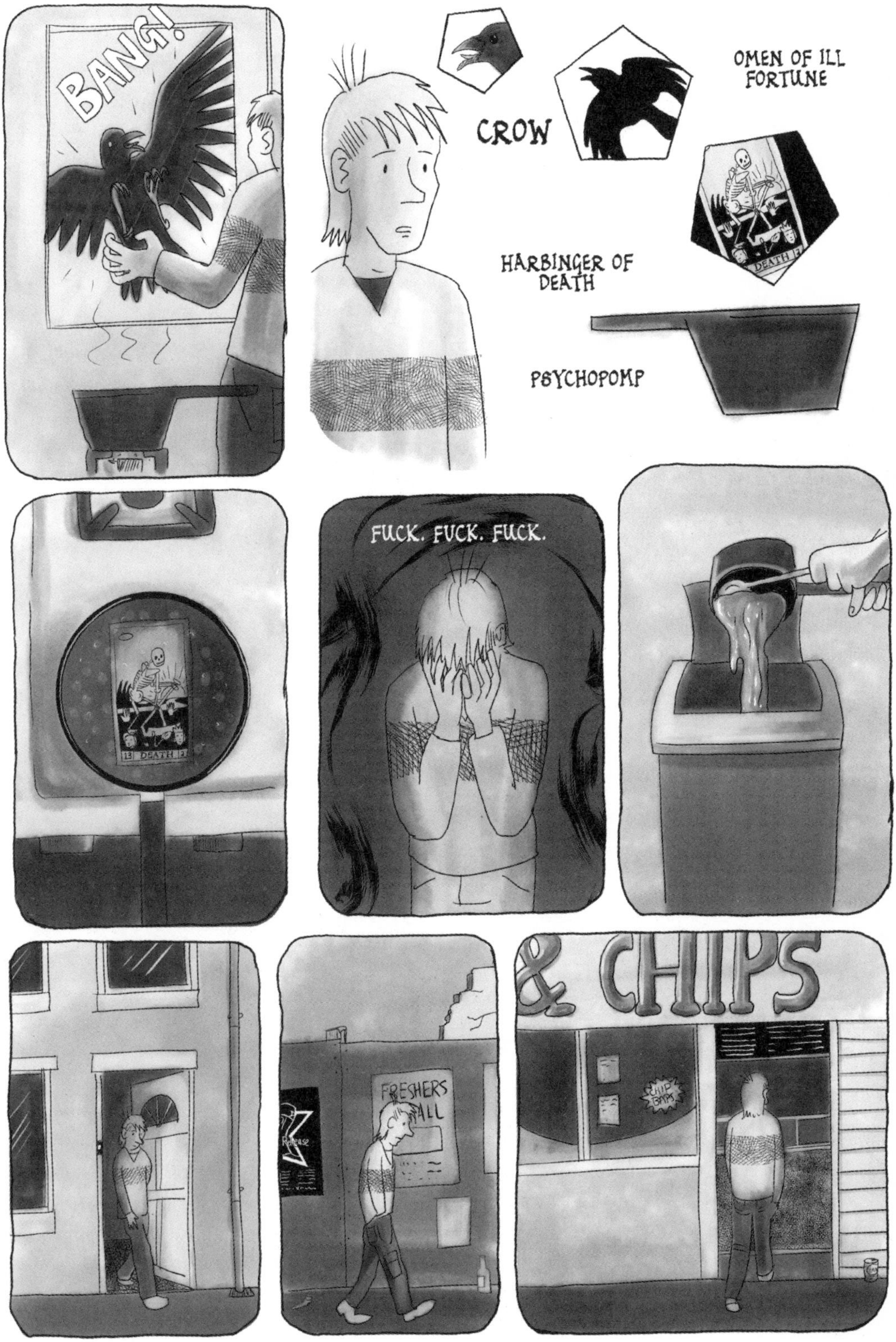
BANG!
CROW
OMEN OF ILL FORTUNE
HARBINGER OF DEATH
PSYCHOPOMP
DEATH
13 DEATH 13
FUCK. FUCK. FUCK.
FRESHERS BALL
Release
& CHIPS
CHIP BAPS

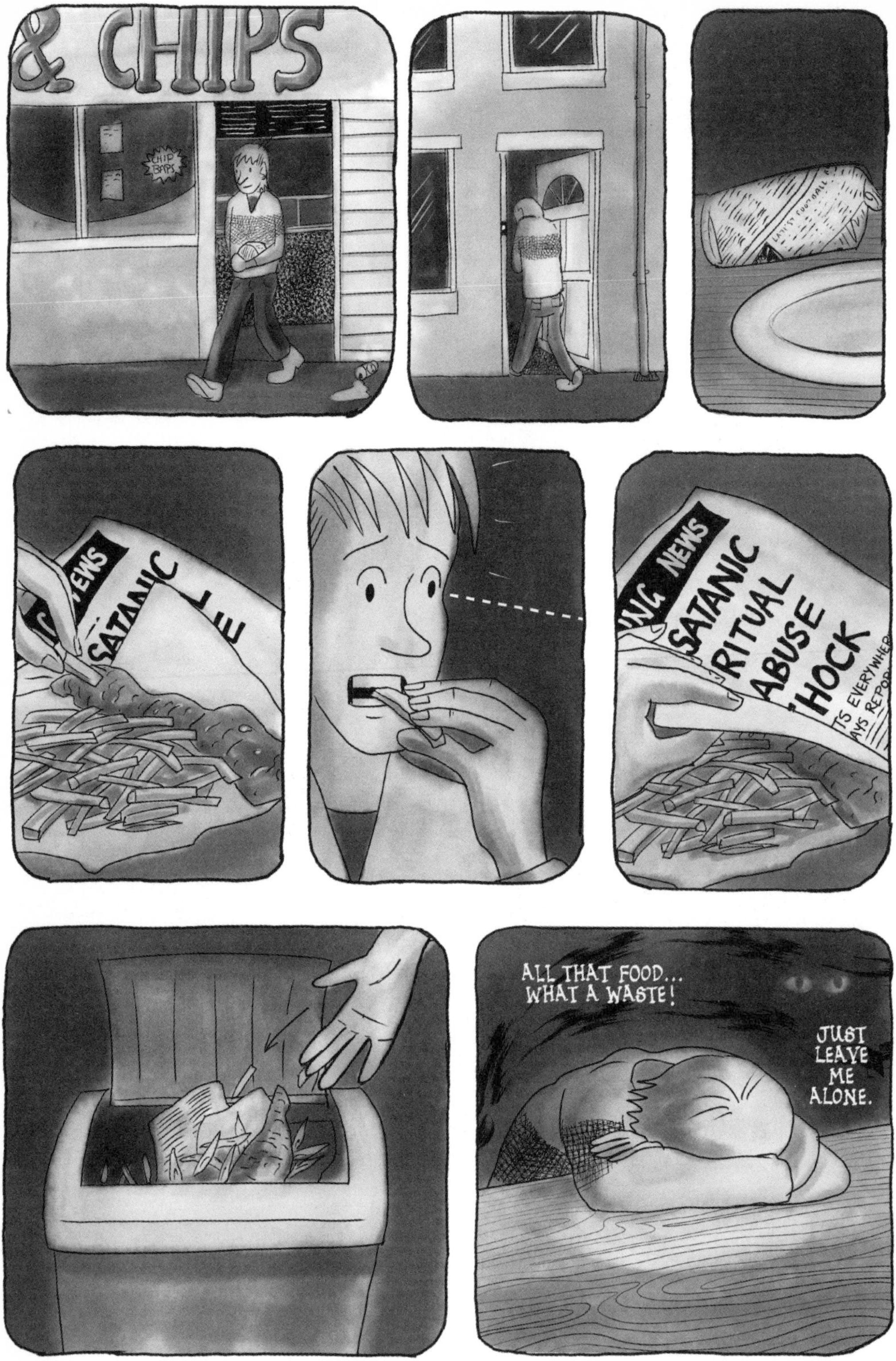
& CHIPS
CHIP BAPS
NEWS
SATANIC
SATANIC RITUAL ABUSE
ALL THAT FOOD... WHAT A WASTE!
JUST LEAVE ME ALONE.

FLEGMAT
SANGVIN
JALLANC
COLERIC

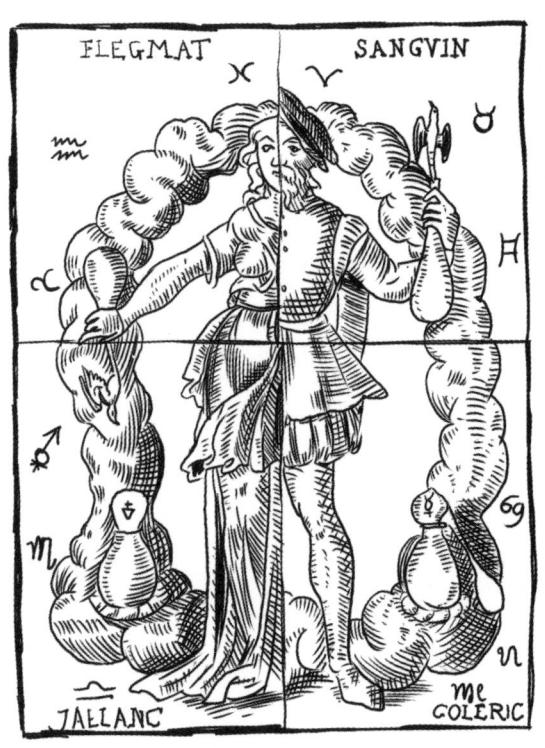

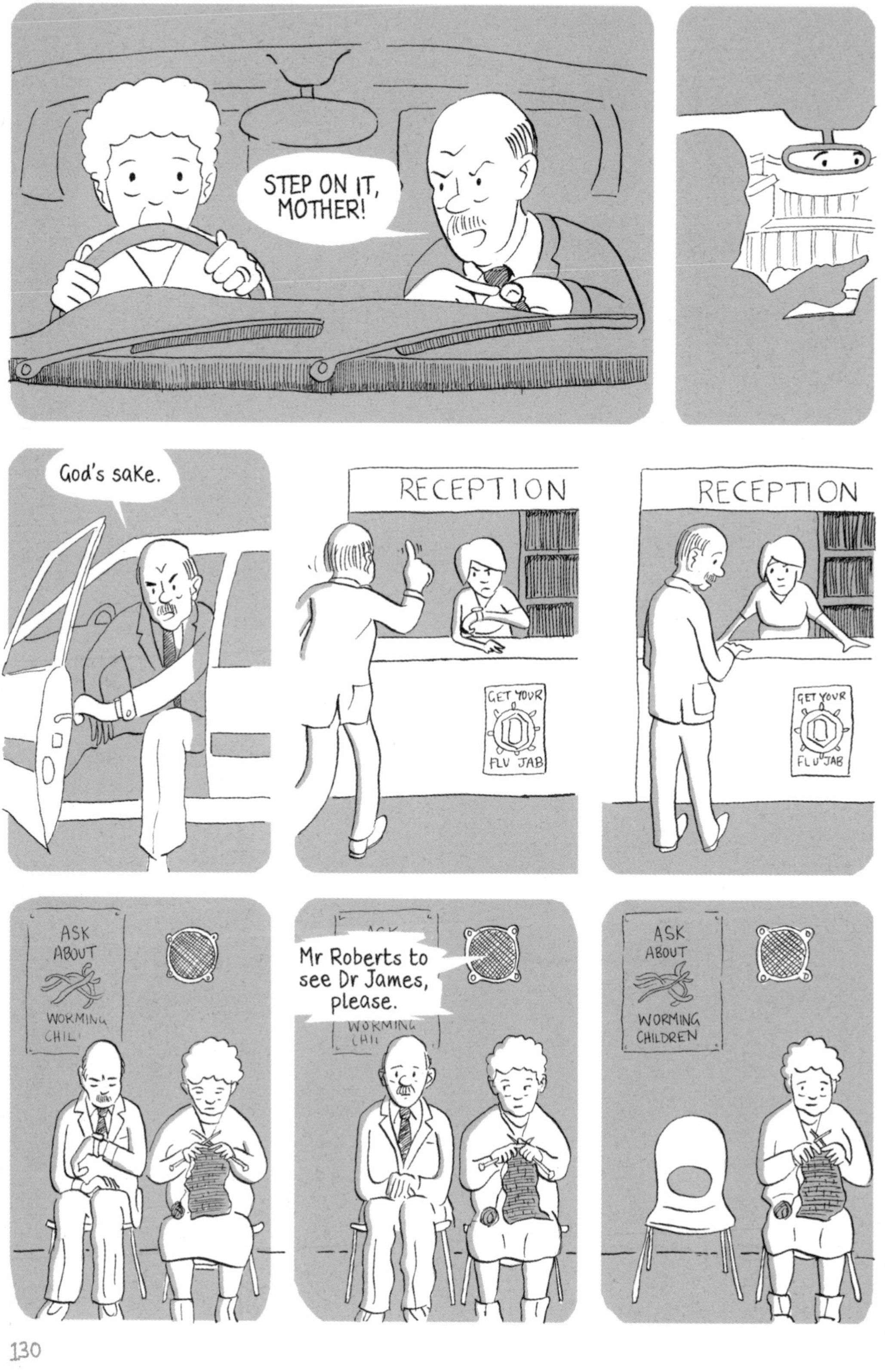
STEP ON IT, MOTHER!
God's sake.
RECEPTION
GET YOUR FLU JAB
RECEPTION
GET YOUR FLU JAB
ASK ABOUT WORMING
Mr Roberts to see Dr James, please.
ASK ABOUT WORMING CHILDREN

What can I do for you, Mr Roberts?
Thanks for seeing me, Iwan.
These headaches are getting worse.
Hmmm... This has been going on for some time now...
I think we should get a scan and refer you to a neurologist.
We'll need to do some blood tests first.
How's Mrs Roberts?
TAP TAP TAP
Zack Mills to see Dr James, please.

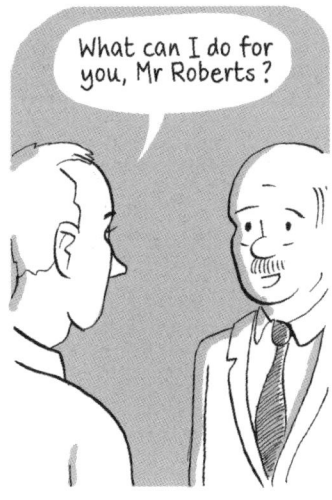

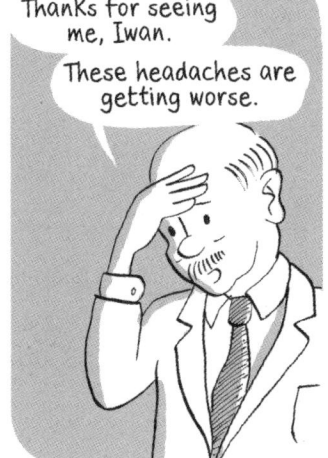

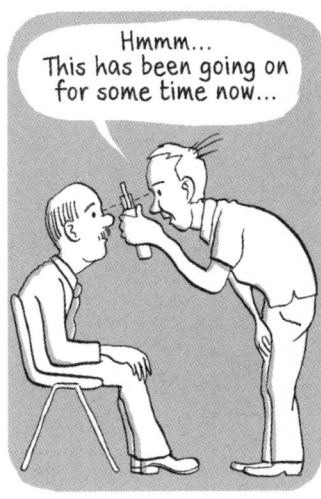

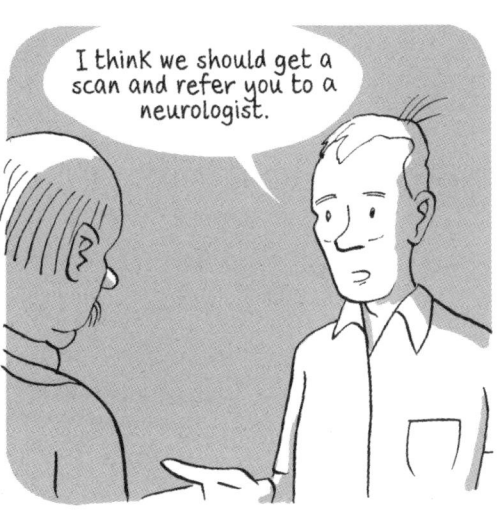

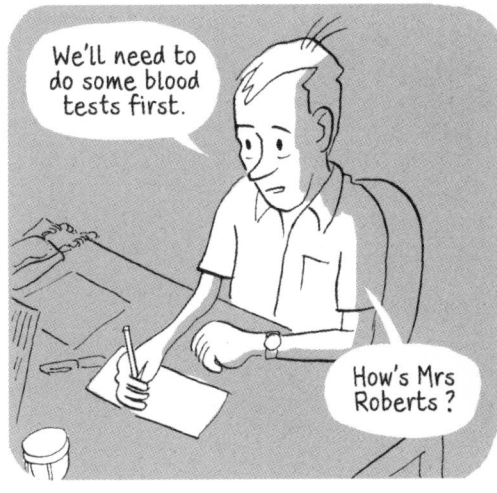

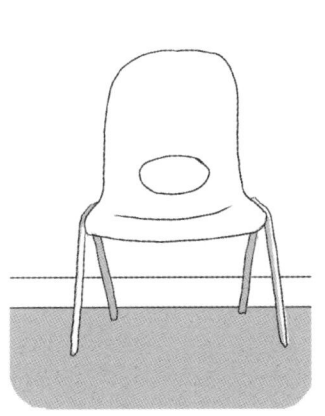

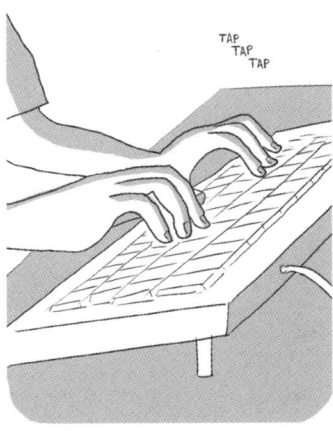

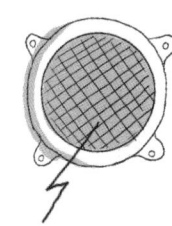

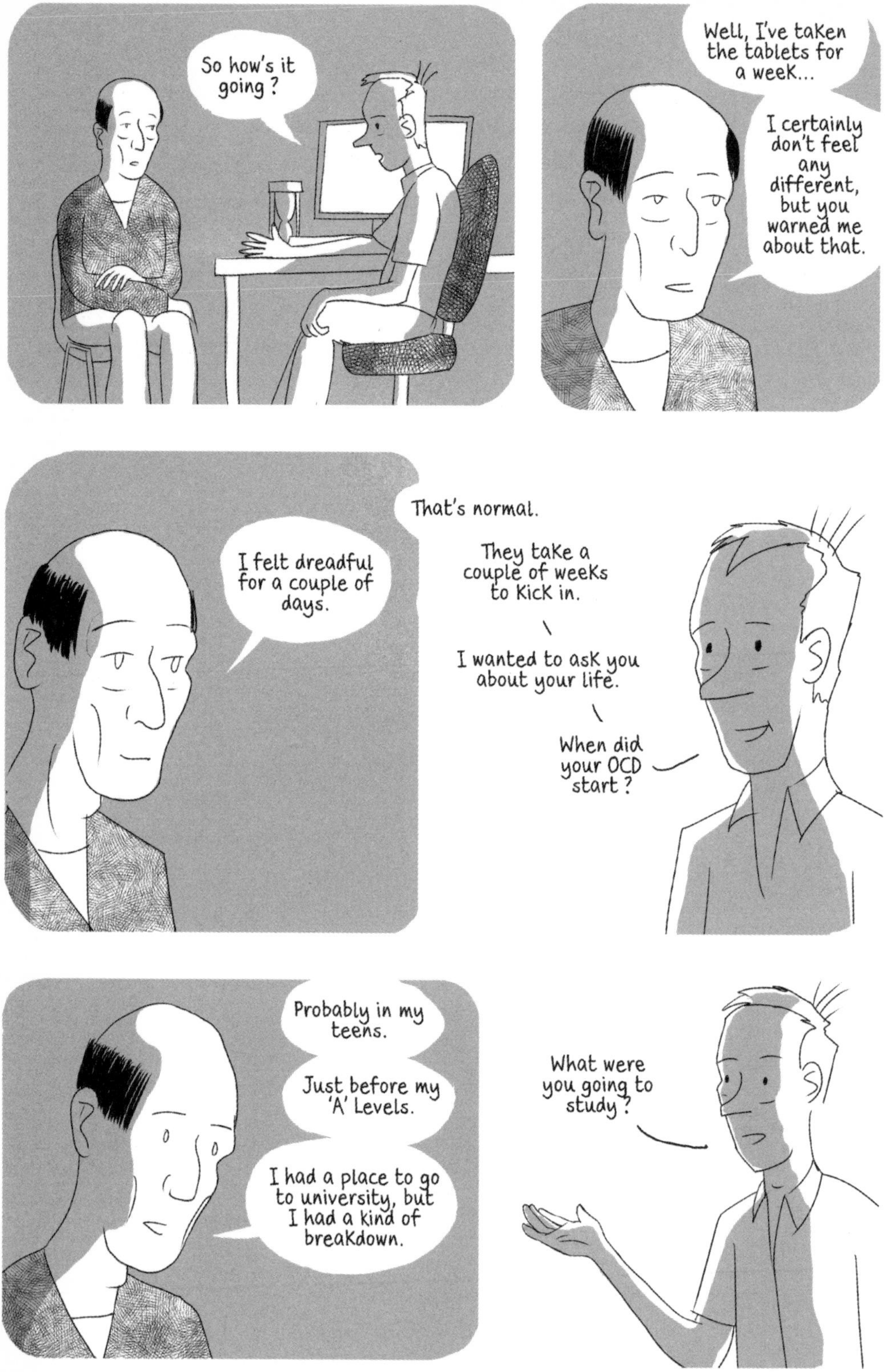
So how's it going?
Well, I've taken the tablets for a week...
I certainly don't feel any different, but you warned me about that.
I felt dreadful for a couple of days.
That's normal.
They take a couple of weeks to kick in.
I wanted to ask you about your life.
When did your OCD start?
Probably in my teens.
Just before my 'A' Levels.
I had a place to go to university, but I had a kind of breakdown.
What were you going to study?

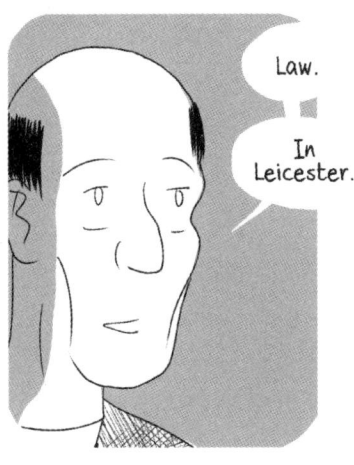

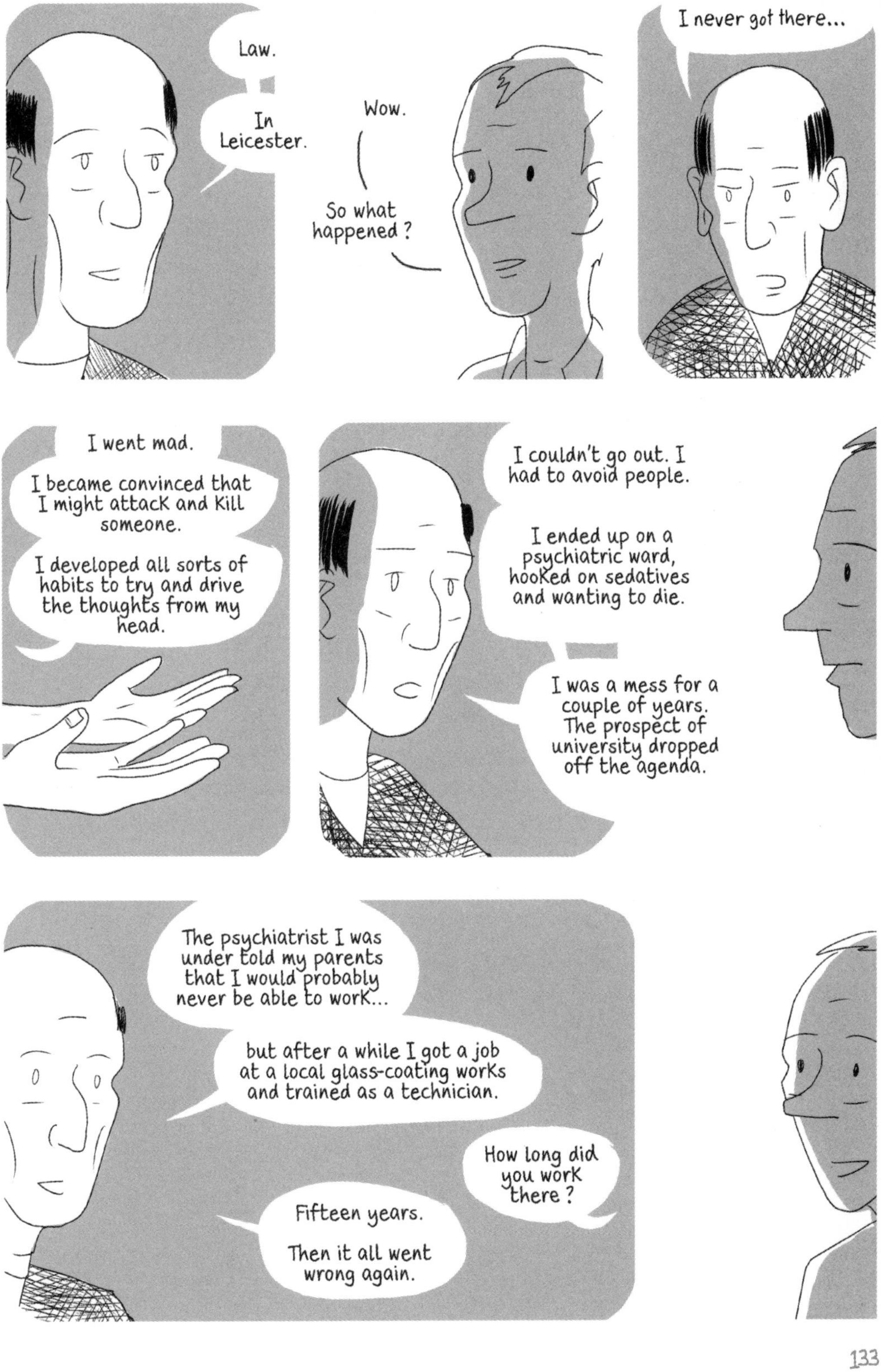

Law.

In Leicester.

Wow.

So what happened?

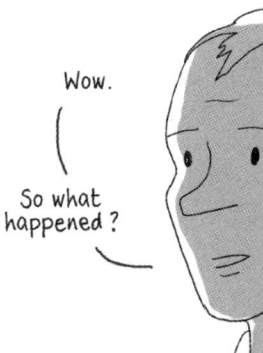

I never got there...

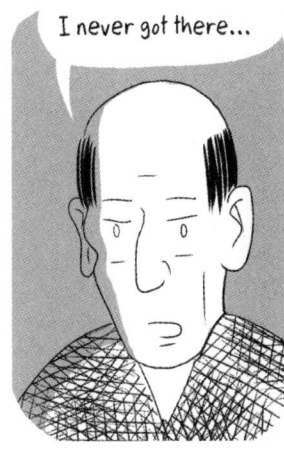

I went mad.

I became convinced that I might attack and kill someone.

I developed all sorts of habits to try and drive the thoughts from my head.

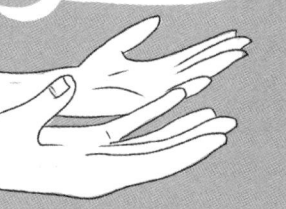

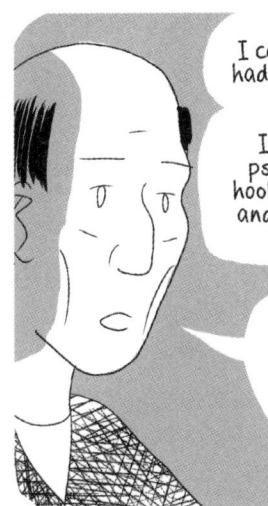

I couldn't go out. I had to avoid people.

I ended up on a psychiatric ward, hooked on sedatives and wanting to die.

I was a mess for a couple of years. The prospect of university dropped off the agenda.

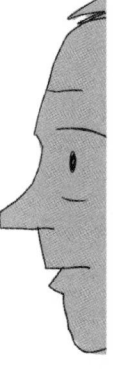

The psychiatrist I was under told my parents that I would probably never be able to work...

but after a while I got a job at a local glass-coating works and trained as a technician.

How long did you work there?

Fifteen years.

Then it all went wrong again.

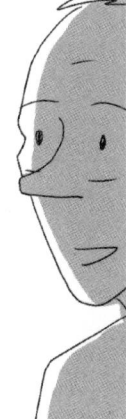

133

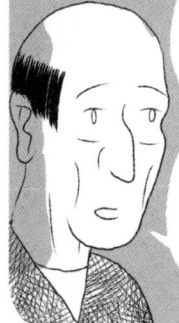

I started to associate certain parts of the coating process with bad luck.

I couldn't do my job properly, so I lost it.

Then I started drinking and didn't stop for a couple of years.

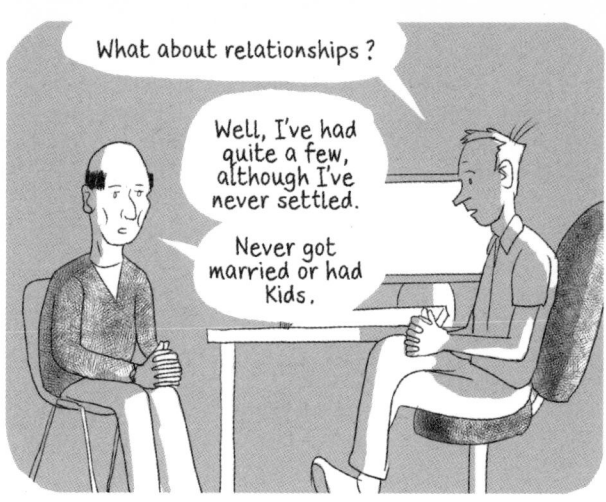

What about relationships?

Well, I've had quite a few, although I've never settled.

Never got married or had kids.

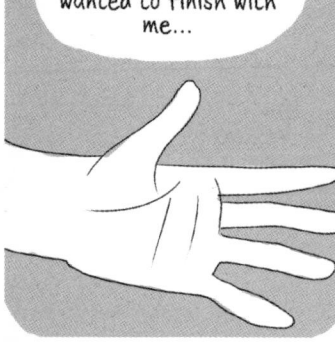

I either finished them because things didn't 'feel right' to me...

or I would constantly worry that the girl wanted to finish with me...

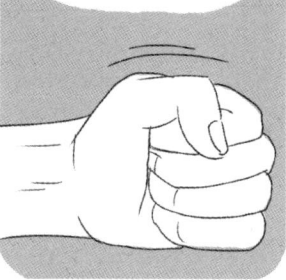

and end up driving her away.

Either way I'd screw it up, and the more I screwed up the more I hated myself.

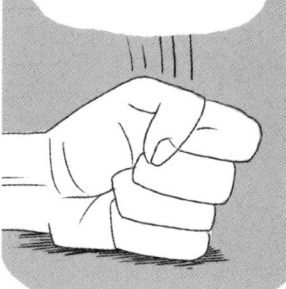

The more I hated myself, the more complex the obsessions got, and I became convinced that I was responsible for all kinds of calamities.

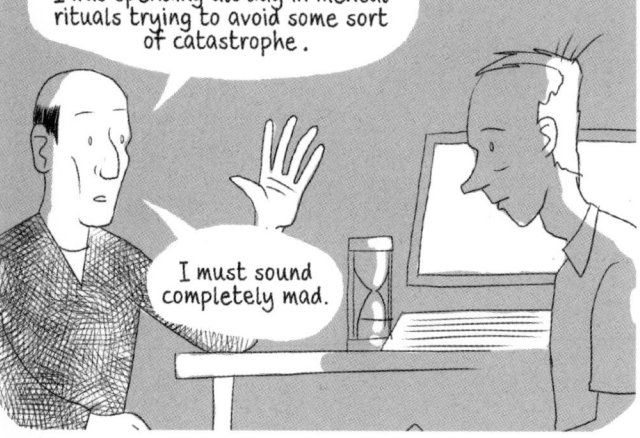

I was spending all day in mental rituals trying to avoid some sort of catastrophe.

I must sound completely mad.

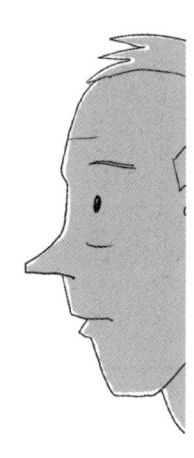

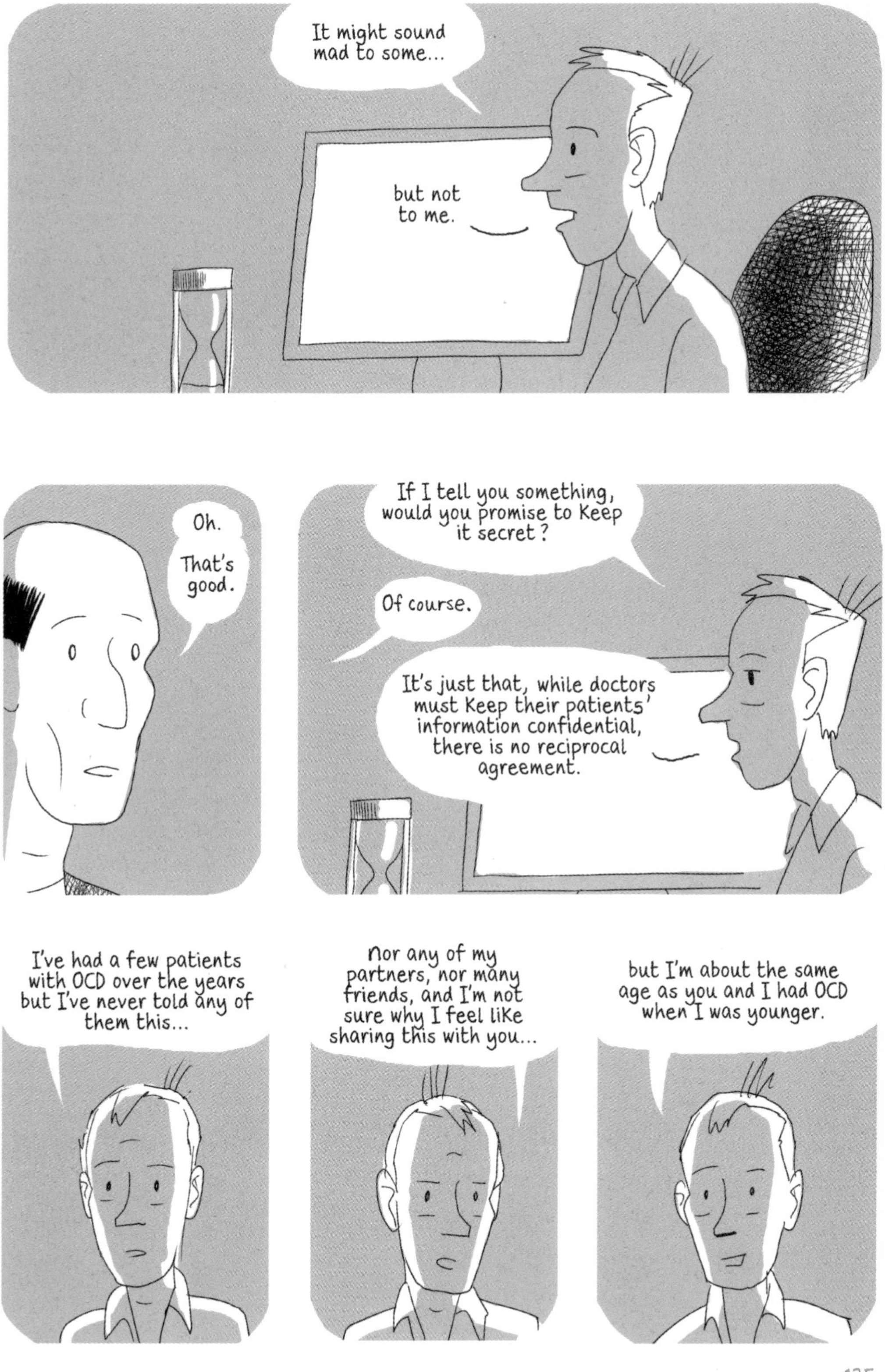
It might sound mad to some...
but not to me.
Oh.
That's good.
If I tell you something, would you promise to keep it secret?
Of course.
It's just that, while doctors must keep their patients' information confidential, there is no reciprocal agreement.
I've had a few patients with OCD over the years but I've never told any of them this...
Nor any of my partners, nor many friends, and I'm not sure why I feel like sharing this with you...
but I'm about the same age as you and I had OCD when I was younger.

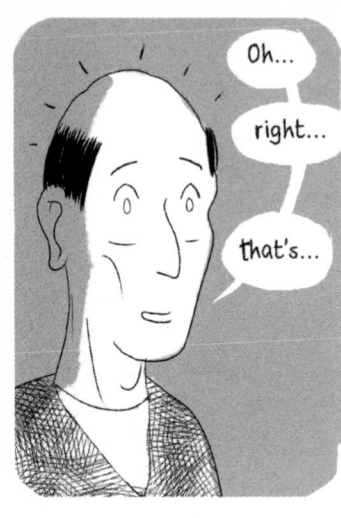

Oh...

right...

that's...

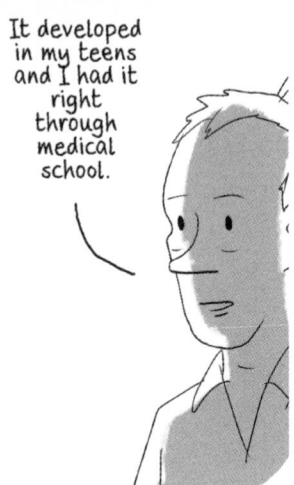

It developed in my teens and I had it right through medical school.

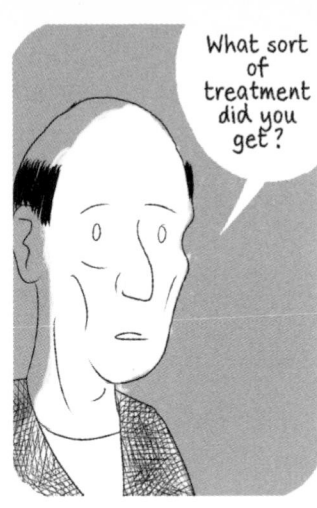

What sort of treatment did you get?

None.

I hid it.

It was hellish.

I thought I was insane.

I just tried to act as normally as I could.

It wasn't until years later that I sought help.

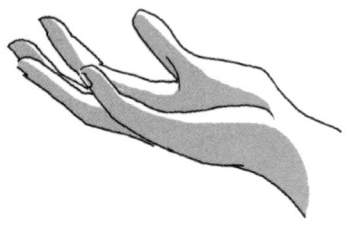

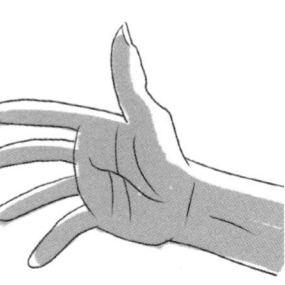

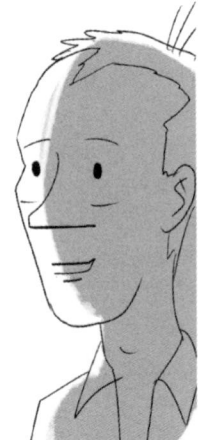

Oh, and I drank very heavily...

but that wasn't unusual at medical school.

Did you know what was wrong with you?

I was terrified. I thought I was schizophrenic at first.

Then I did some reading in the medical library and it all fitted with OCD.

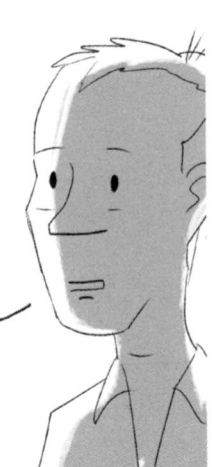

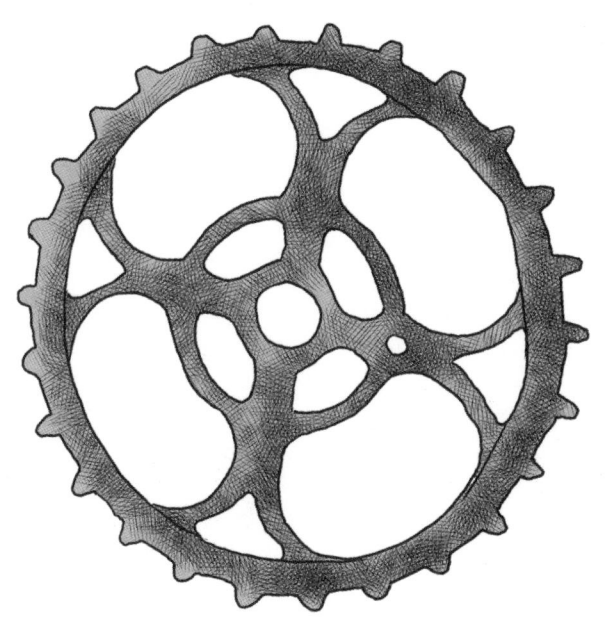

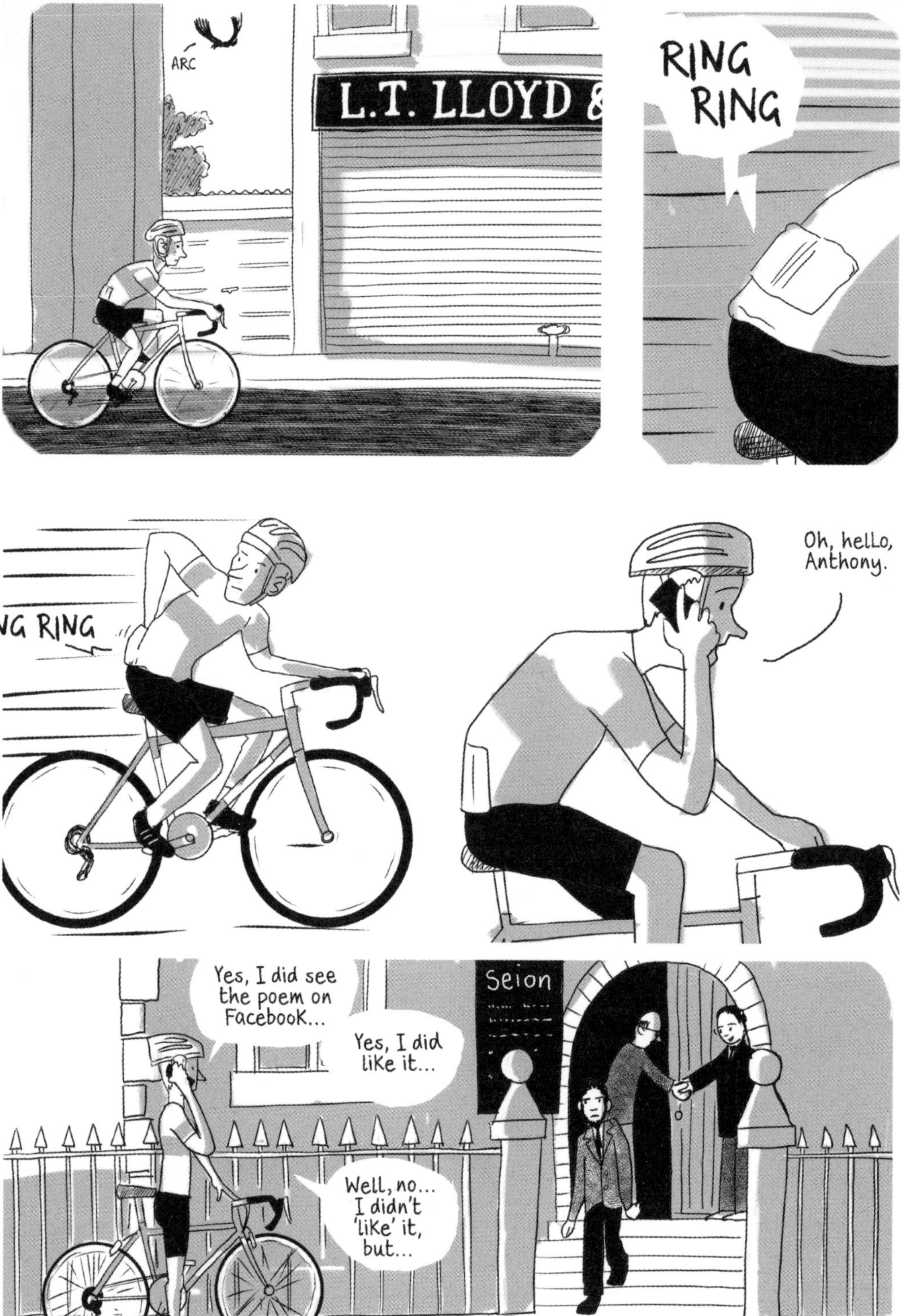
ARC
L.T. LLOYD &
RING RING
RING RING
Oh, hello, Anthony.
Yes, I did see the poem on Facebook...
Yes, I did like it...
Seion
Well, no... I didn't 'like' it, but...

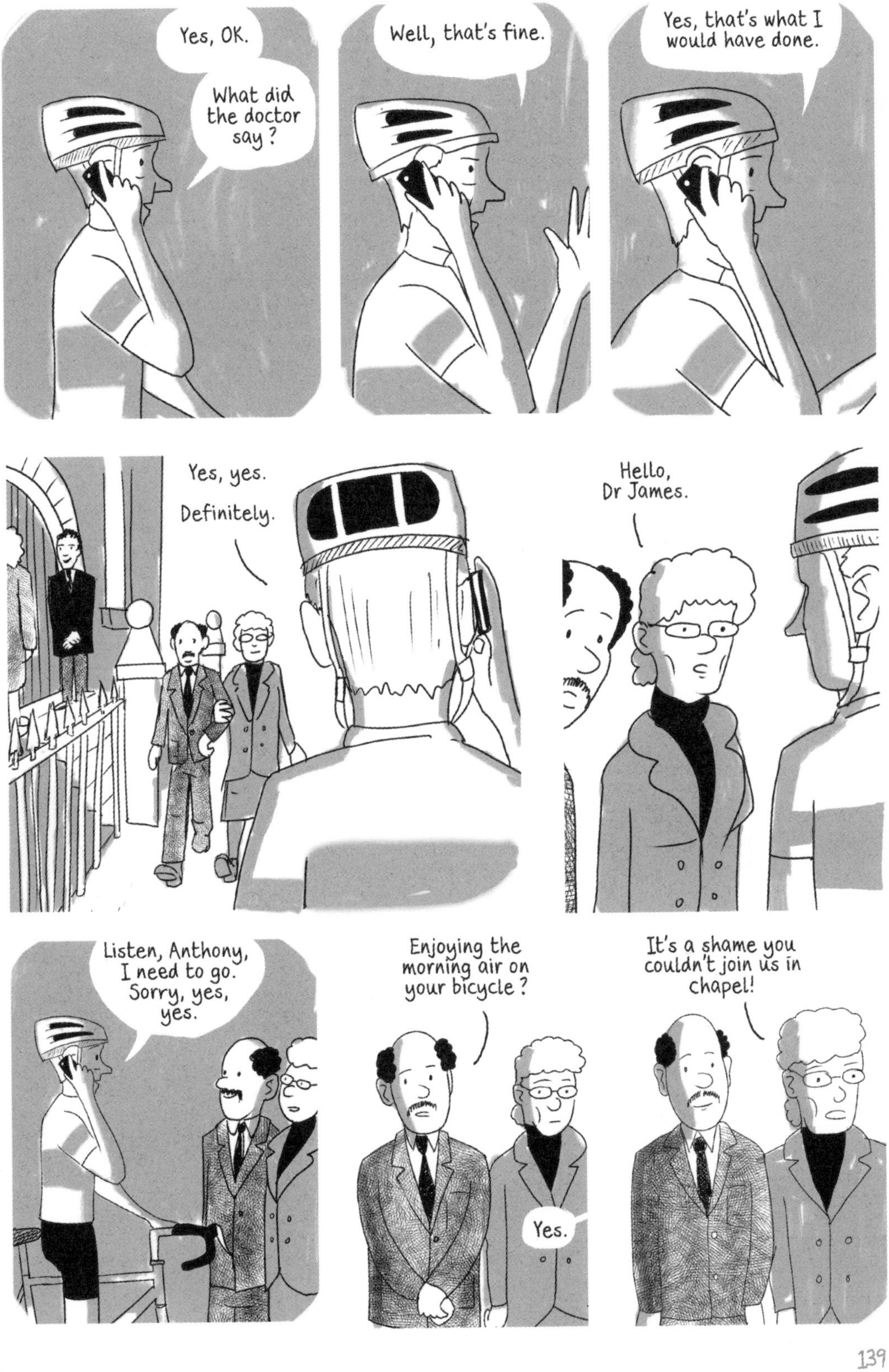
Yes, OK.
What did the doctor say?
Well, that's fine.
Yes, that's what I would have done.
Yes, yes.
Definitely.
Hello, Dr James.
Listen, Anthony, I need to go. Sorry, yes, yes.
Enjoying the morning air on your bicycle?
Yes.
It's a shame you couldn't join us in chapel!

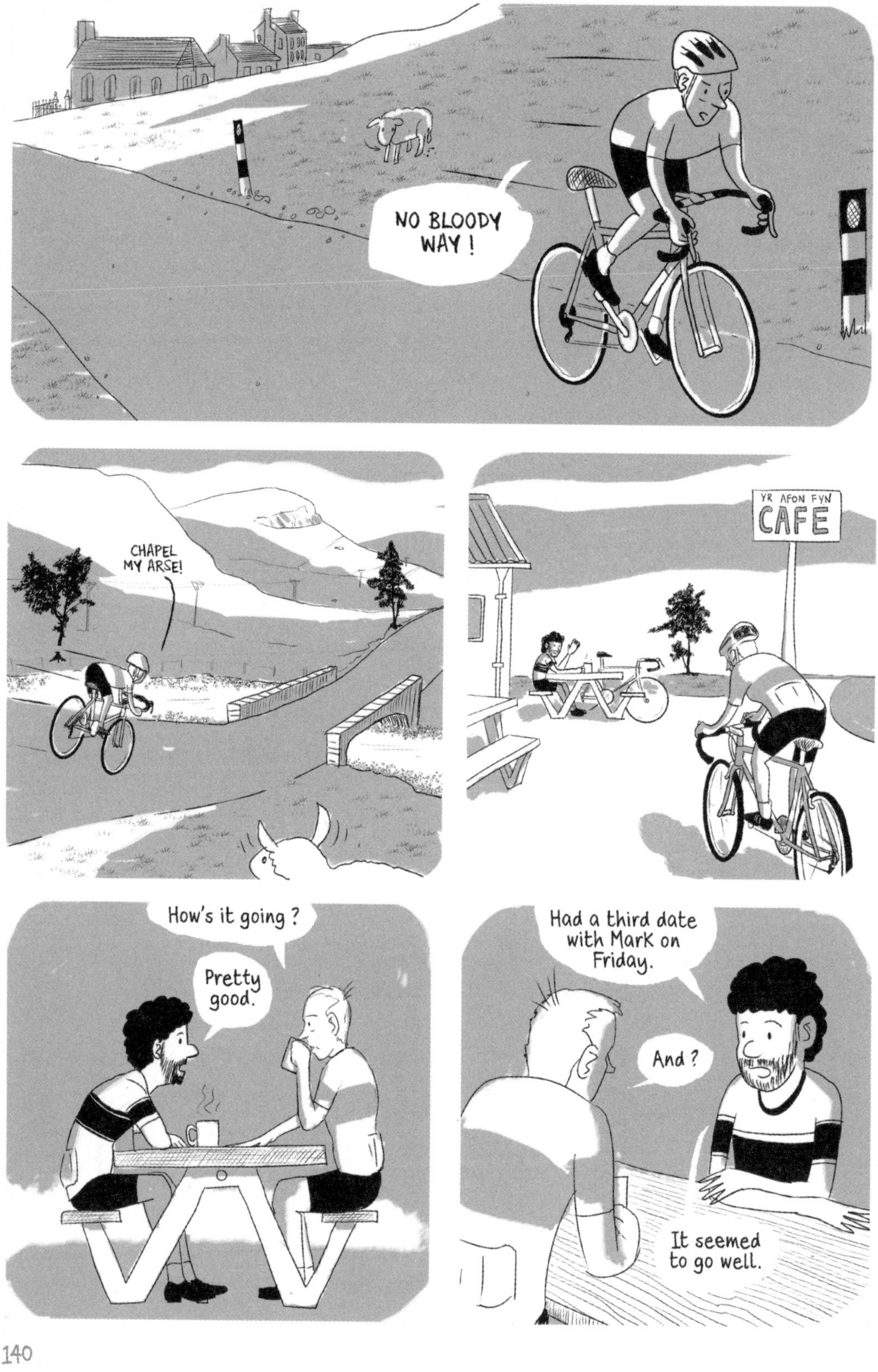
NO BLOODY WAY!
CHAPEL MY ARSE!
YR AFON FYN
CAFE
How's it going?
Pretty good.
Had a third date with Mark on Friday.
And?
It seemed to go well.

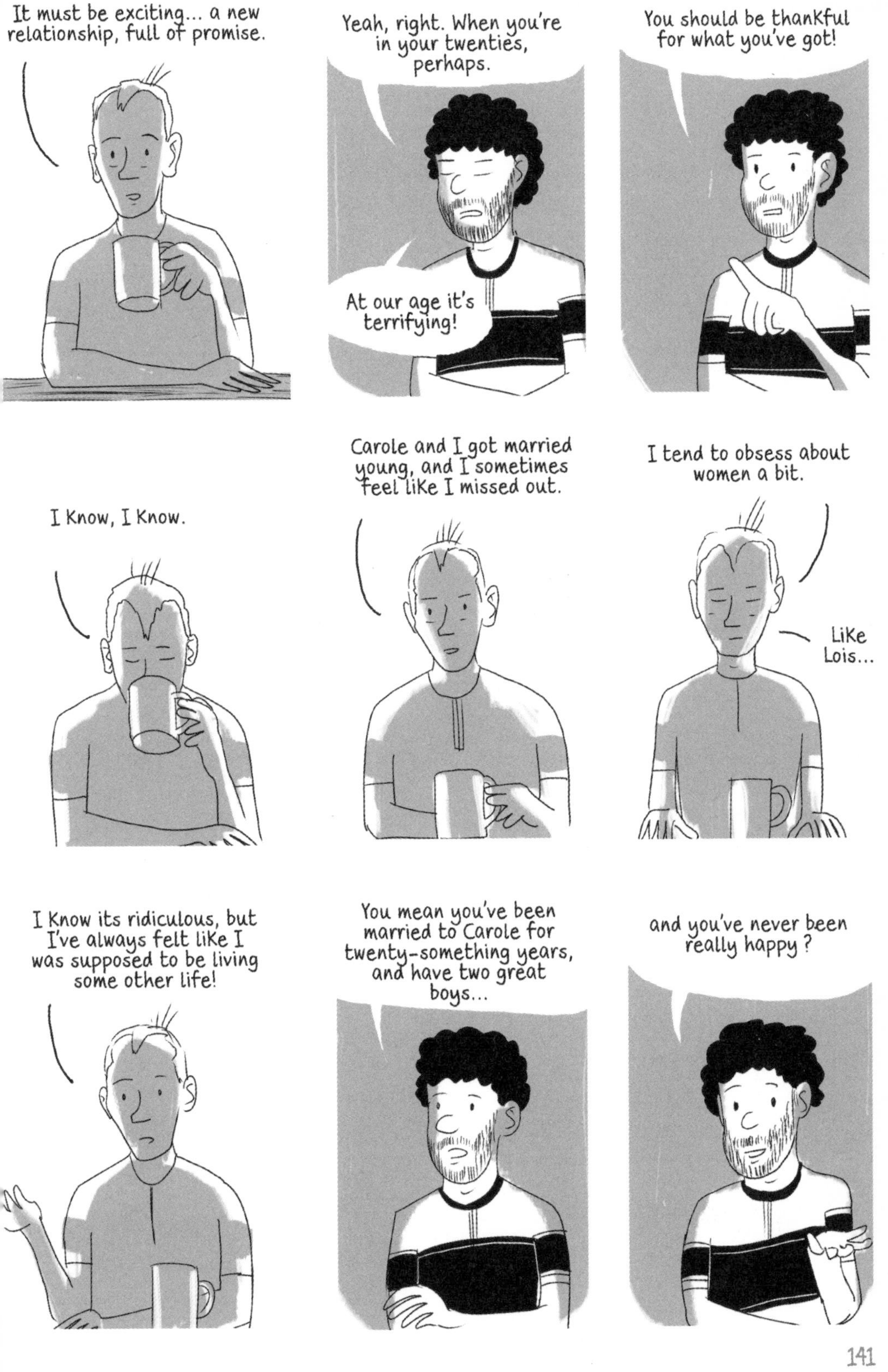
It must be exciting... a new relationship, full of promise.
Yeah, right. When you're in your twenties, perhaps.
At our age it's terrifying!
You should be thankful for what you've got!
I Know, I Know.
Carole and I got married young, and I sometimes feel liKe I missed out.
I tend to obsess about women a bit.
LiKe Lois...
I Know its ridiculous, but I've always felt liKe I was supposed to be living some other life!
You mean you've been married to Carole for twenty-something years, and have two great boys...
and you've never been really happy ?

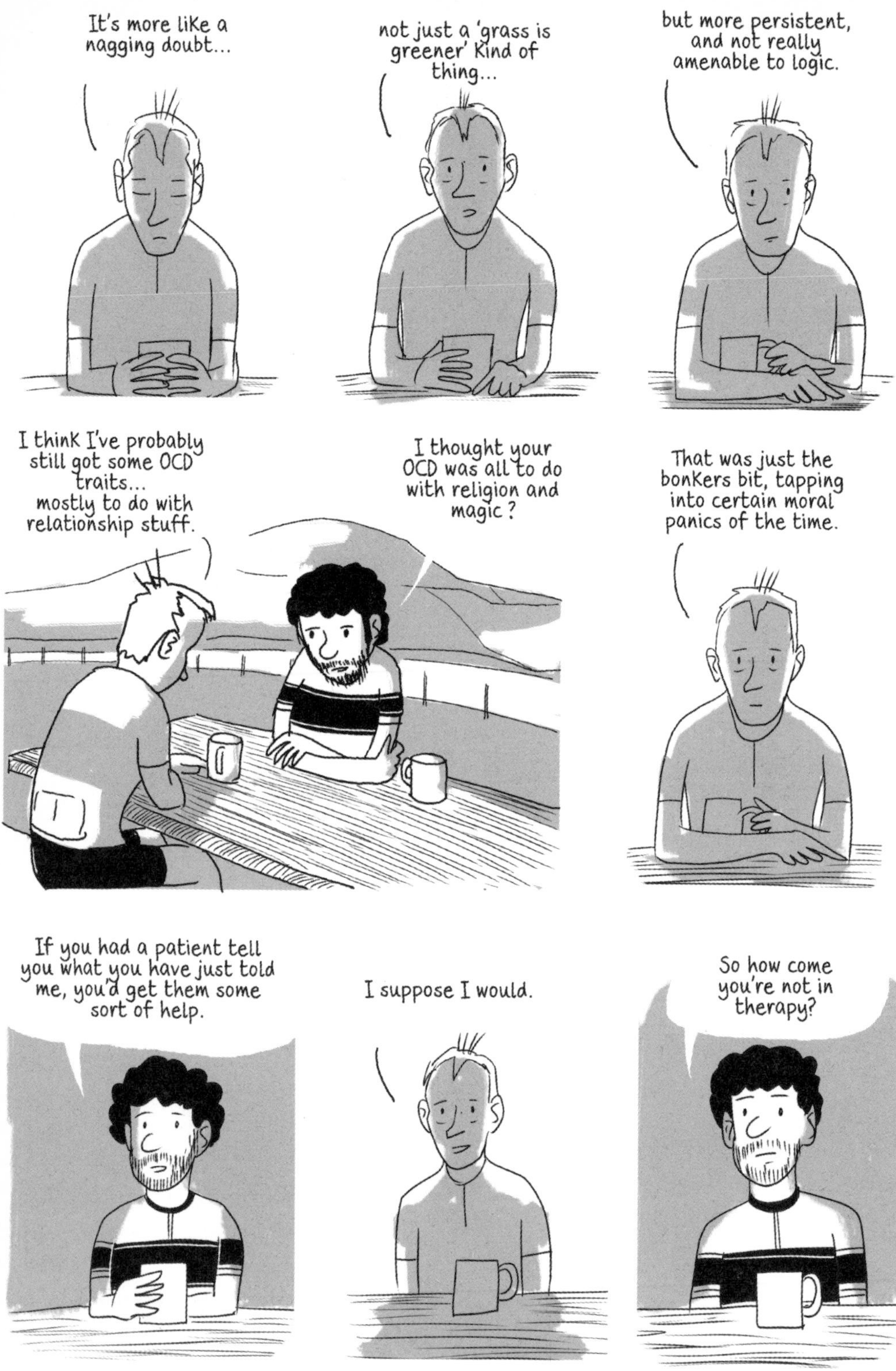
It's more like a nagging doubt...
not just a 'grass is greener' kind of thing...
but more persistent, and not really amenable to logic.
I think I've probably still got some OCD traits... mostly to do with relationship stuff.
I thought your OCD was all to do with religion and magic?
That was just the bonkers bit, tapping into certain moral panics of the time.
If you had a patient tell you what you have just told me, you'd get them some sort of help.
I suppose I would.
So how come you're not in therapy?

INRI

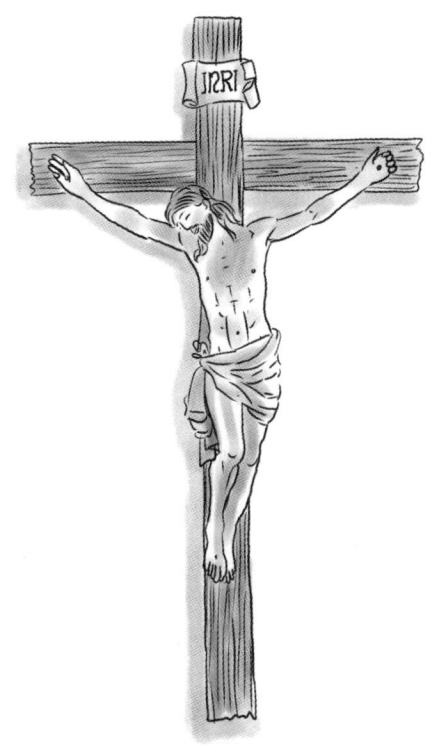

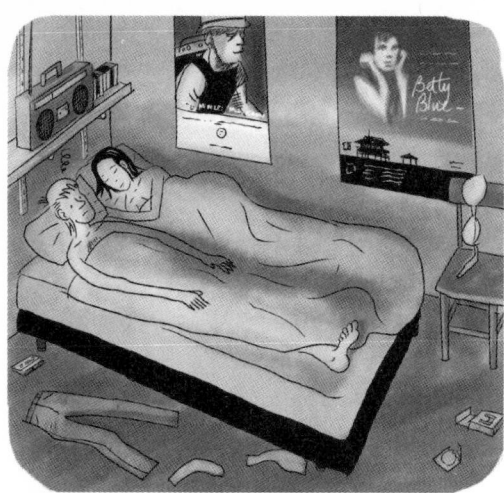

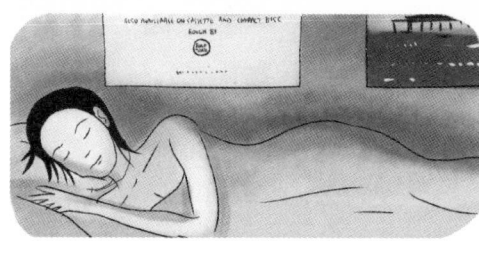

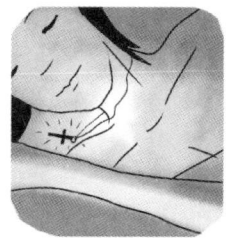

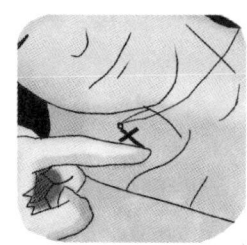

YAWWN

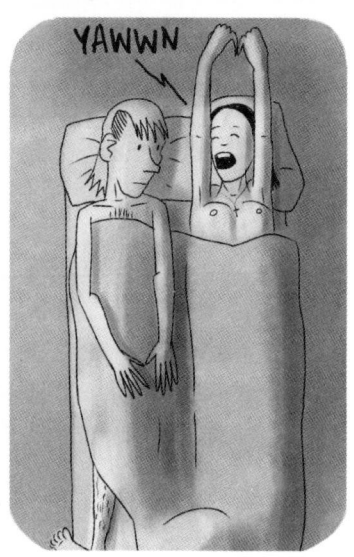

Carole, I think I might go out this morning.

Mmm? Where to?

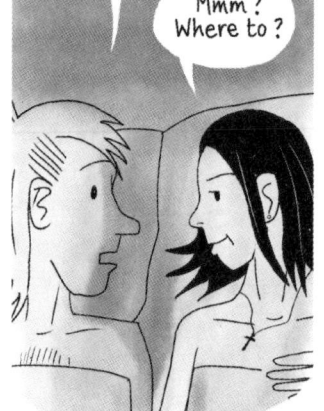

I need to go to the Med School library.

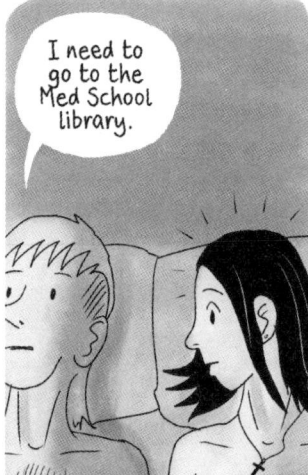

In the six months we've been going out I've NEVER known you go to the library!

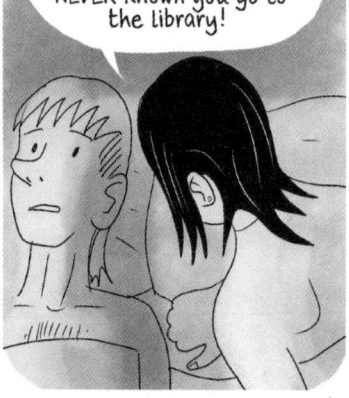

Let alone on a Sunday morning!

Where are you really going?

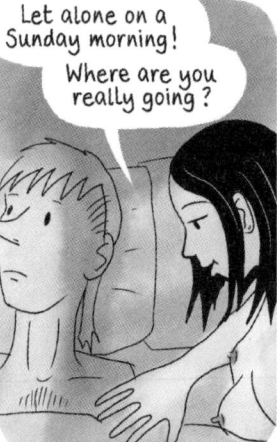

I'm going to the LIBRARY!

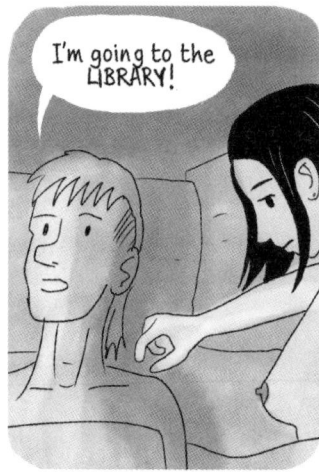

144

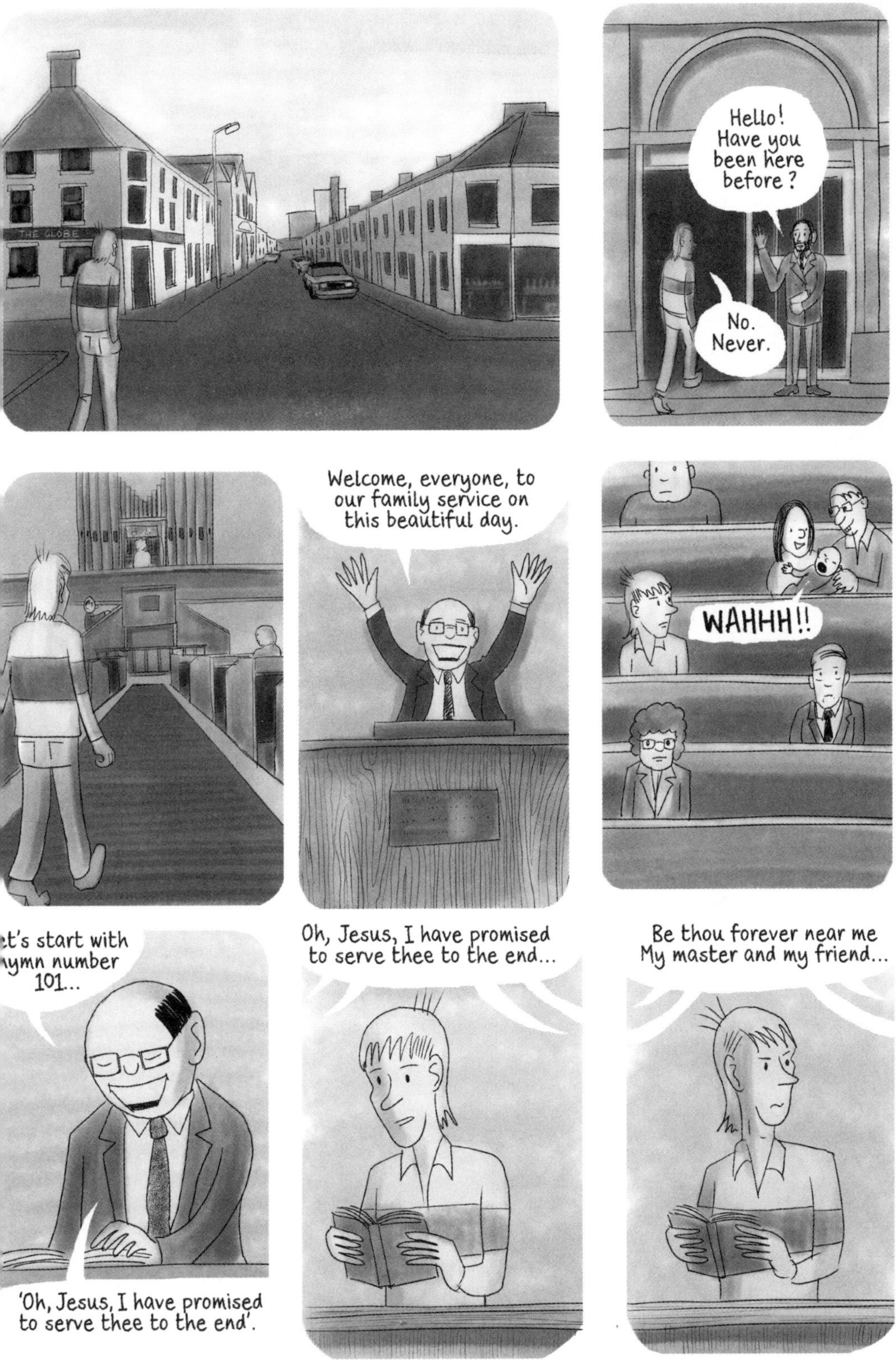

THE GLOBE
Hello! Have you been here before?
No. Never.
Welcome, everyone, to our family service on this beautiful day.
WAHHH!!
t's start with
ymn number
101...
'Oh, Jesus, I have promised to serve thee to the end'.
Oh, Jesus, I have promised to serve thee to the end...
Be thou forever near me My master and my friend...

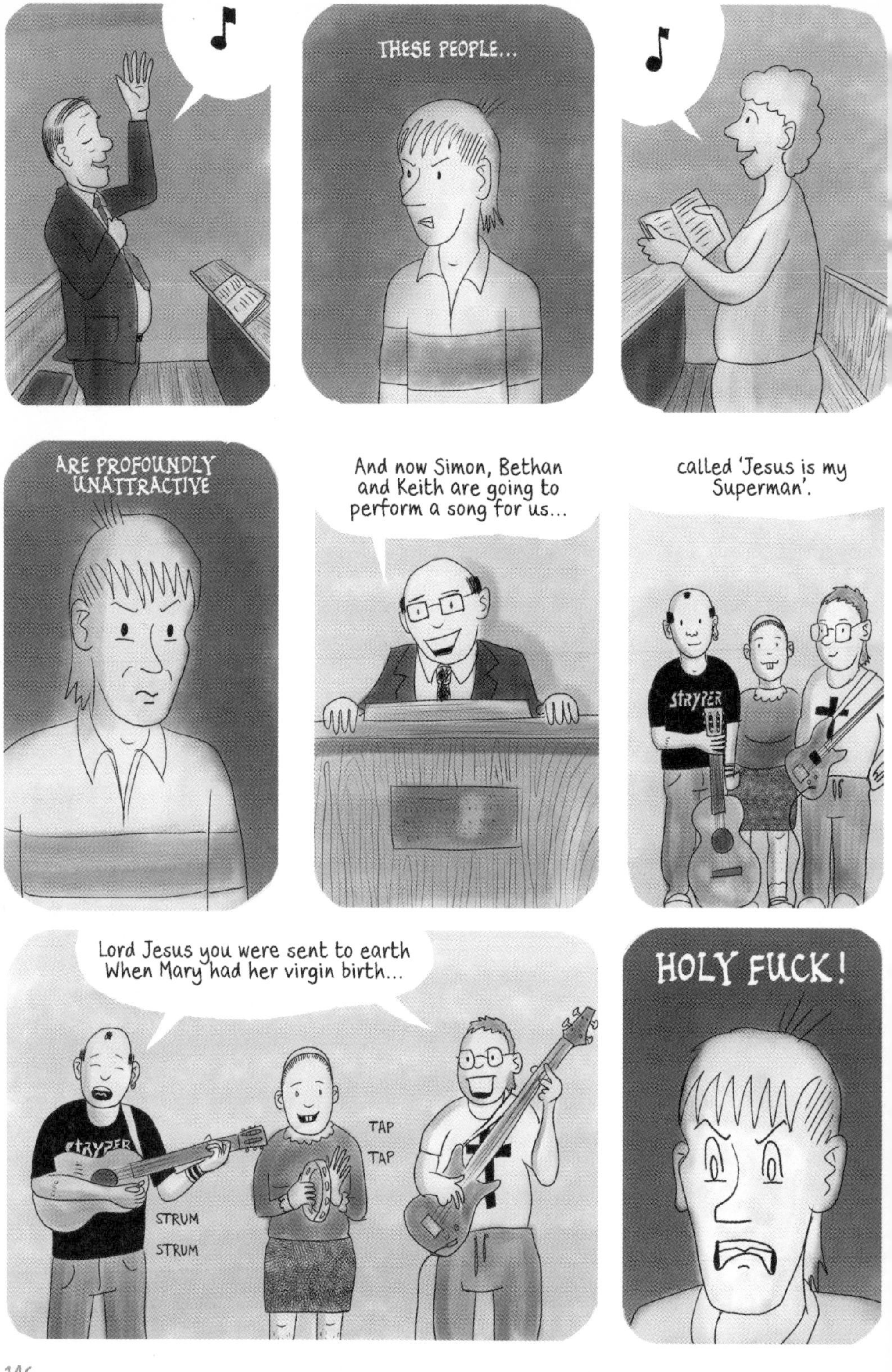
THESE PEOPLE...
ARE PROFOUNDLY UNATTRACTIVE
And now Simon, Bethan and Keith are going to perform a song for us...
called 'Jesus is my Superman'.
STRYPER
Lord Jesus you were sent to earth When Mary had her virgin birth...
STRYPER
STRUM
STRUM
TAP
TAP
HOLY FUCK!

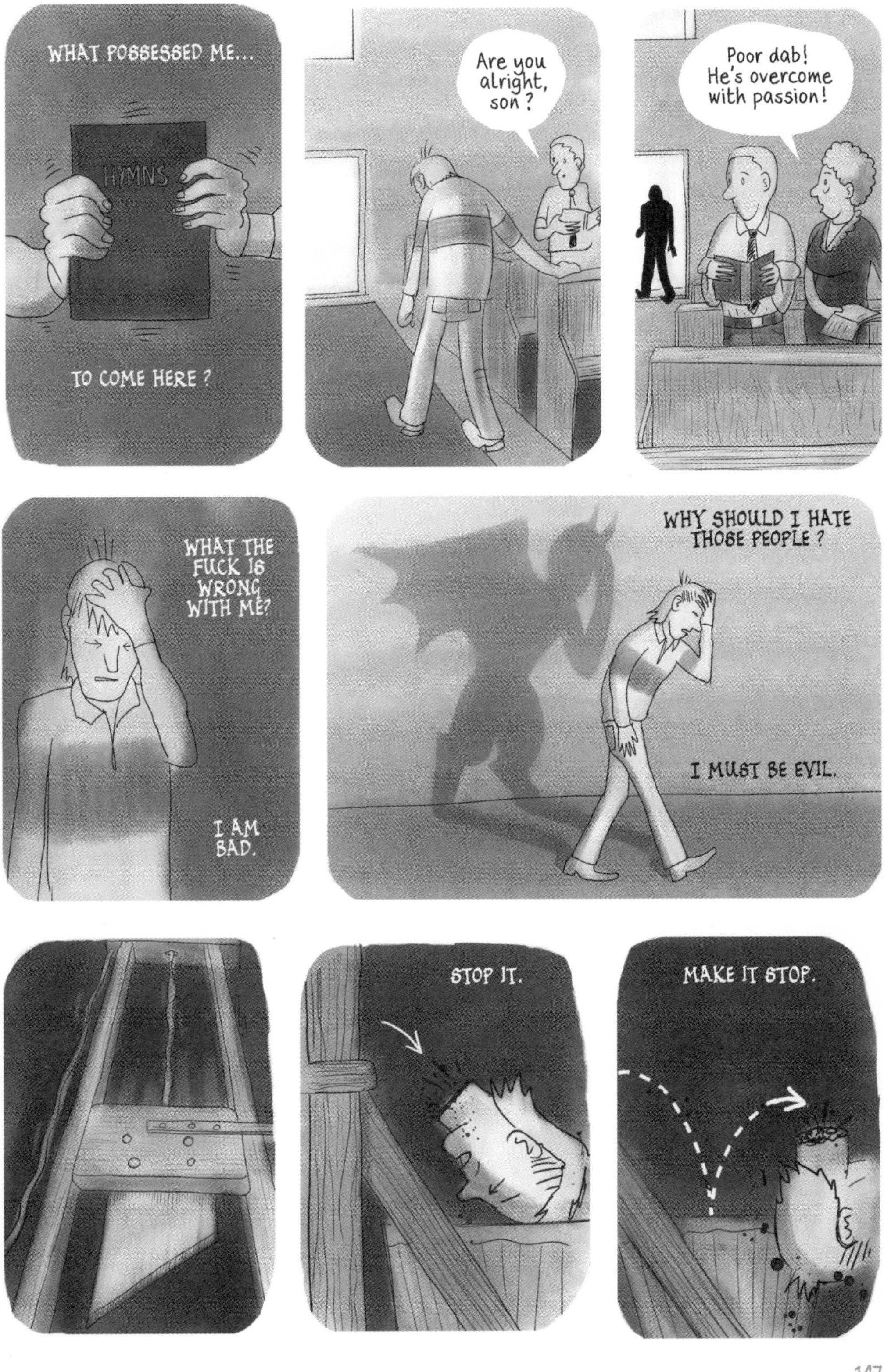
WHAT POSSESSED ME...
HYMNS
TO COME HERE ?
Are you alright, son ?
Poor dab! He's overcome with passion!
WHAT THE FUCK IS WRONG WITH ME?
I AM BAD.
WHY SHOULD I HATE THOSE PEOPLE ?
I MUST BE EVIL.
STOP IT.
MAKE IT STOP.

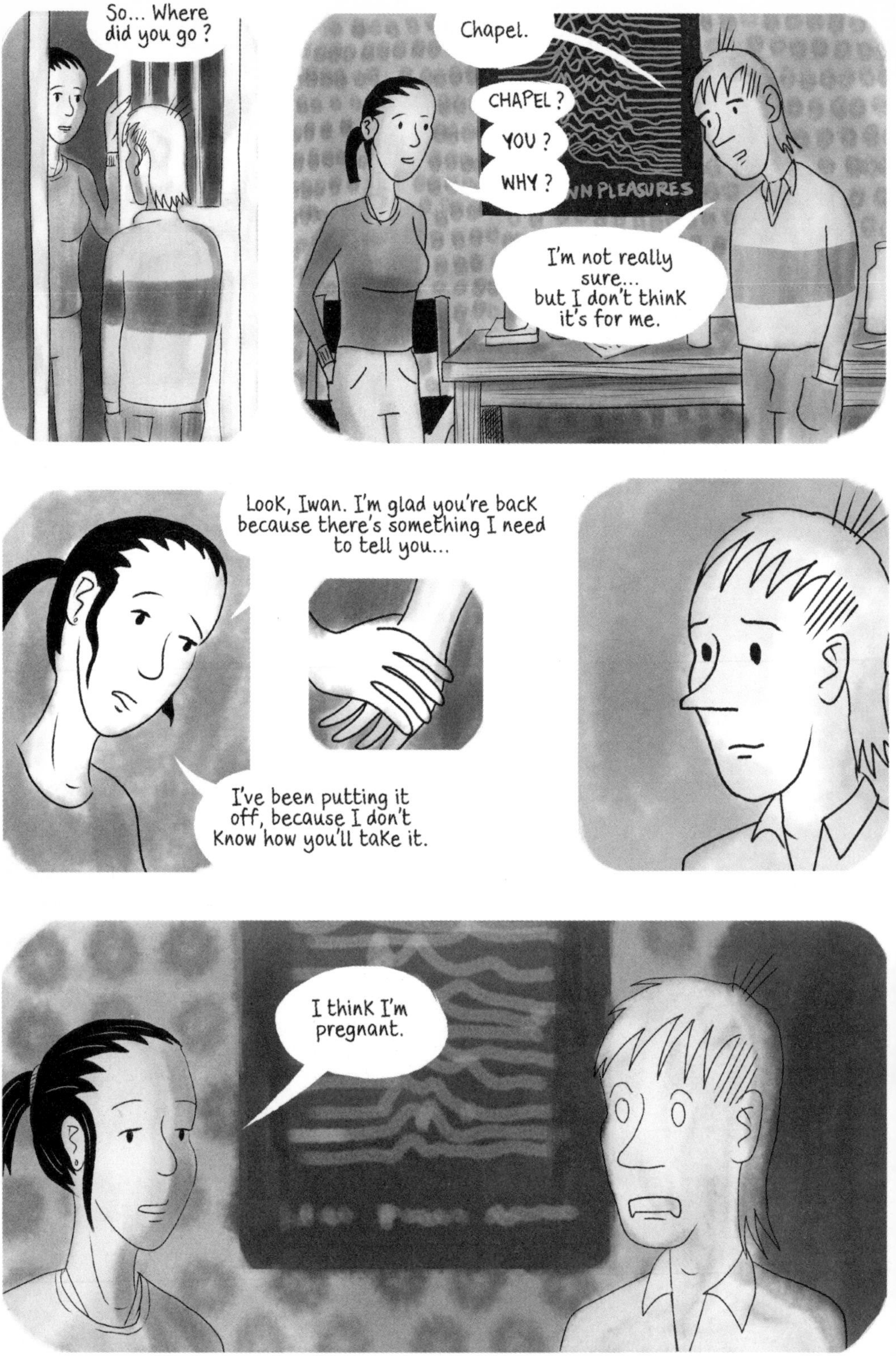
So... Where did you go ?
Chapel.
CHAPEL ?
YOU ?
WHY ?
WN PLEASURES
I'm not really sure... but I don't think it's for me.
Look, Iwan. I'm glad you're back because there's something I need to tell you...
I've been putting it off, because I don't know how you'll take it.
I think I'm pregnant.

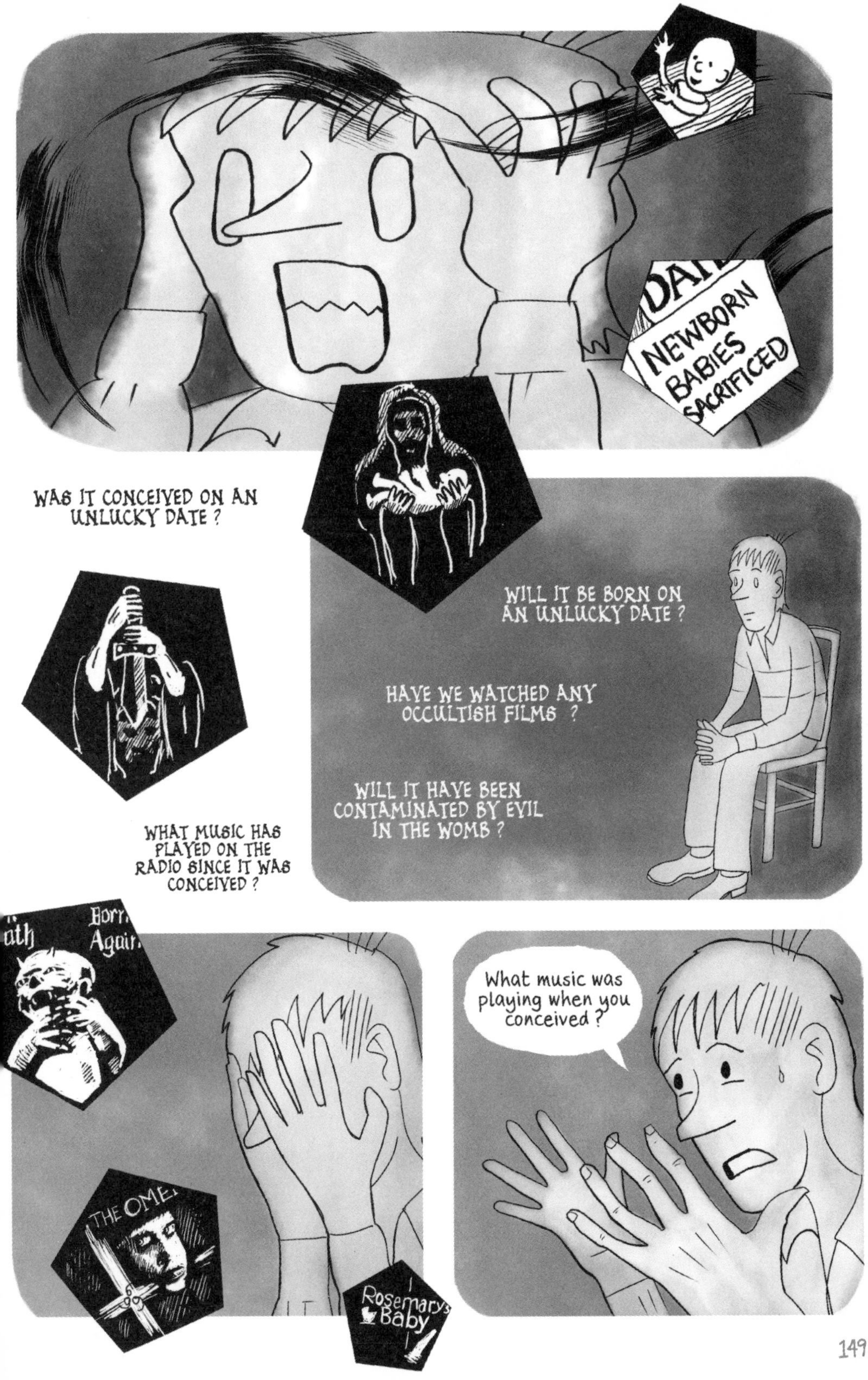
NEWBORN BABIES SACRIFICED
WAS IT CONCEIVED ON AN UNLUCKY DATE ?
WILL IT BE BORN ON AN UNLUCKY DATE ?
HAVE WE WATCHED ANY OCCULTISH FILMS ?
WILL IT HAVE BEEN CONTAMINATED BY EVIL IN THE WOMB ?
WHAT MUSIC HAS PLAYED ON THE RADIO SINCE IT WAS CONCEIVED ?
Rosemarys Baby
What music was playing when you conceived ?

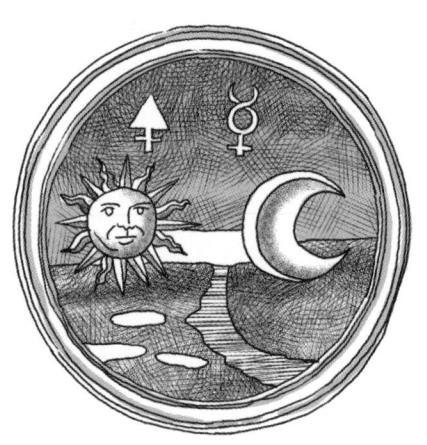

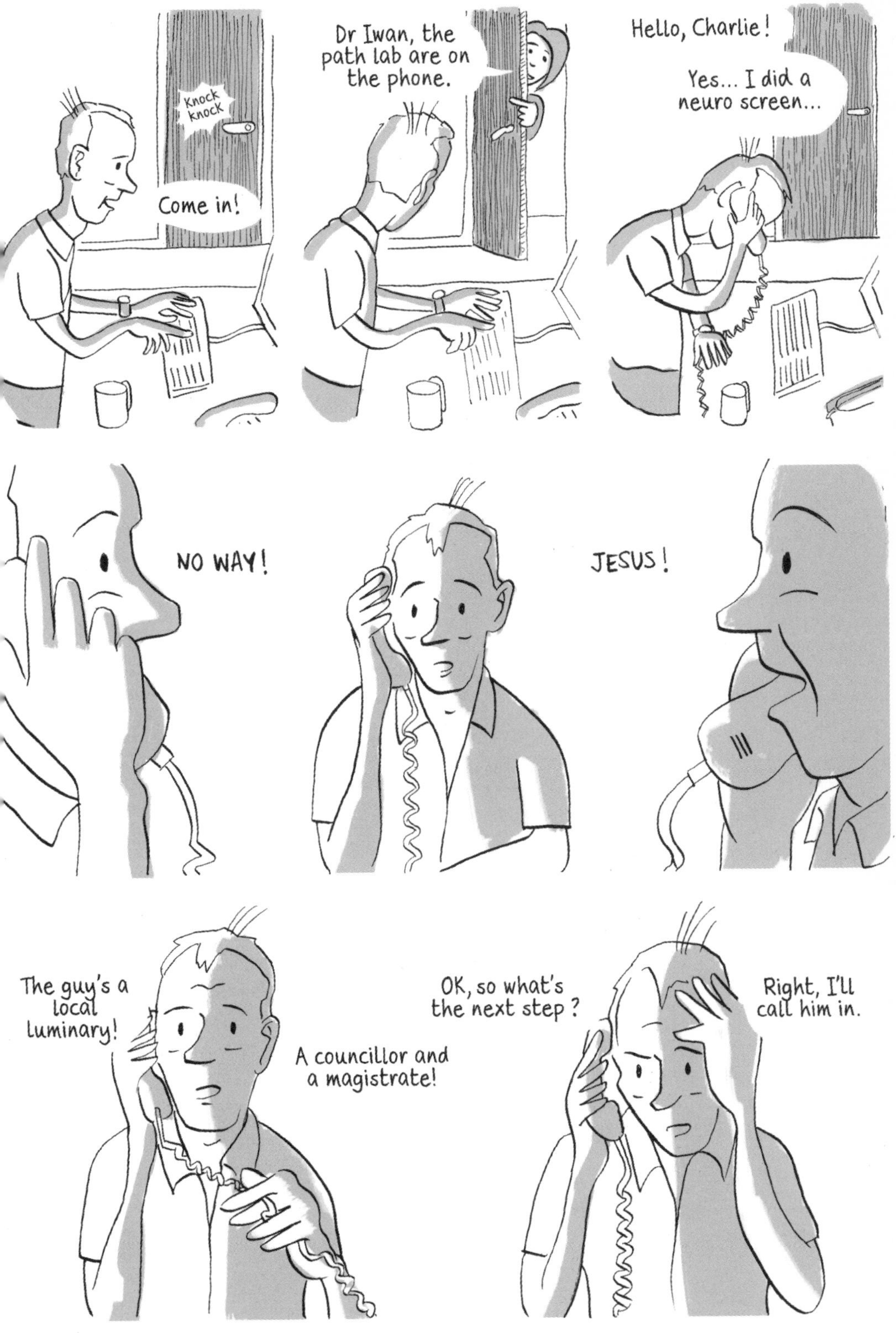
Knock knock
Come in!
Dr Iwan, the path lab are on the phone.
Hello, Charlie!
Yes... I did a neuro screen...
NO WAY!
JESUS!
The guy's a local luminary!
A councillor and a magistrate!
OK, so what's the next step?
Right, I'll call him in.

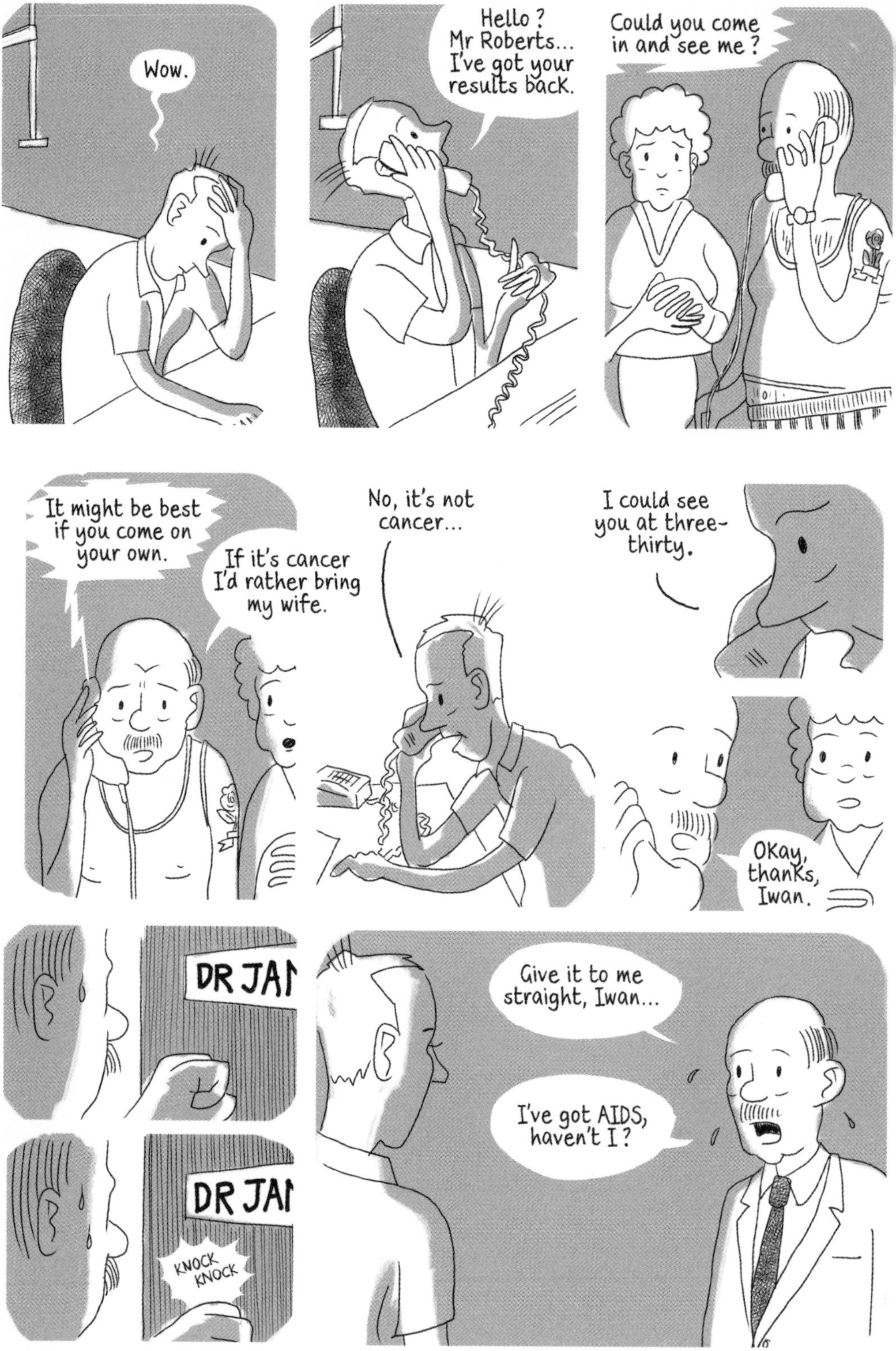
Wow.
Hello ? Mr Roberts... I've got your results back.
Could you come in and see me ?
It might be best if you come on your own.
If it's cancer I'd rather bring my wife.
No, it's not cancer...
I could see you at three-thirty.
OKay, thanks, Iwan.
DR JA
DR JA
KNOCK KNOCK
Give it to me straight, Iwan...
I've got AIDS, haven't I ?

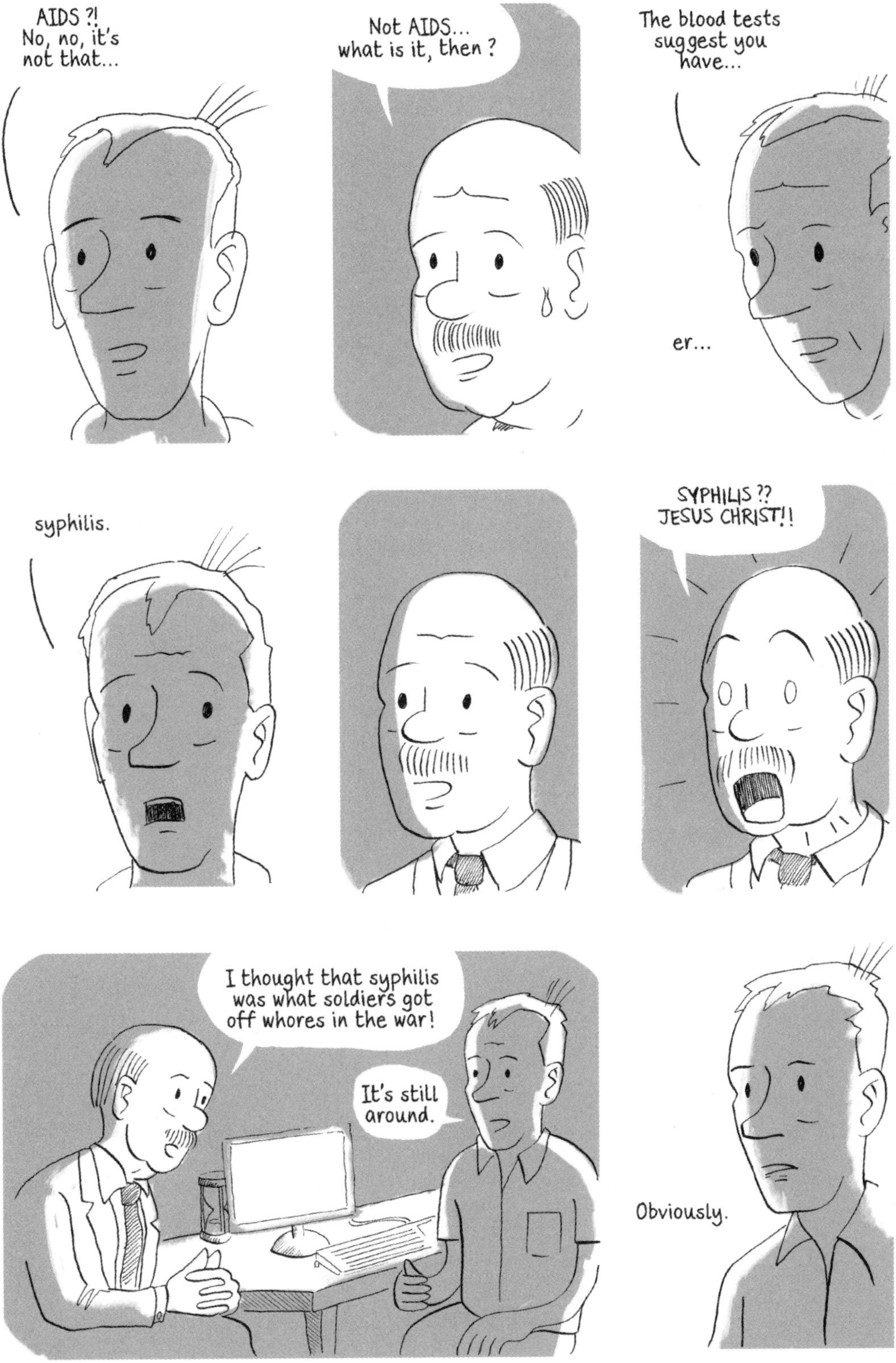
AIDS ?! No, no, it's not that...
Not AIDS... what is it, then ?
The blood tests suggest you have...
er...
syphilis.
SYPHILIS ?? JESUS CHRIST!!
I thought that syphilis was what soldiers got off whores in the war!
It's still around.
Obviously.

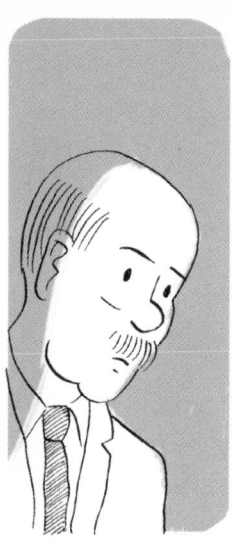
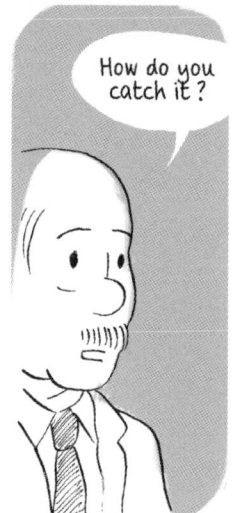

How do you catch it?

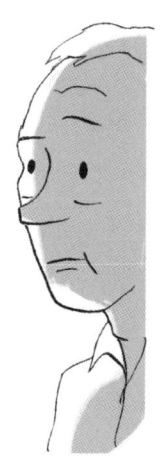
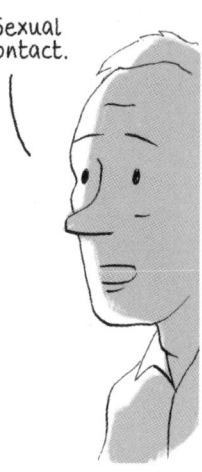

Sexual contact.

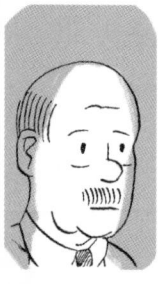
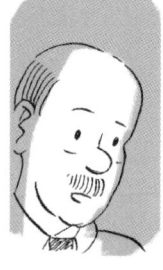
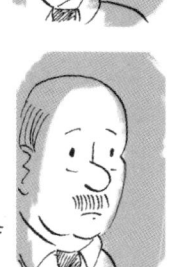

KOF

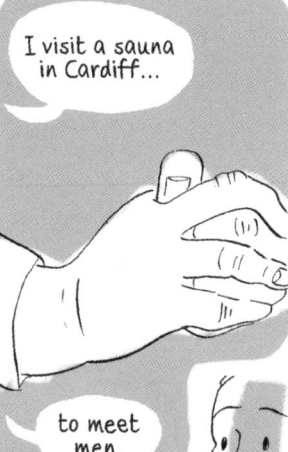

I visit a sauna in Cardiff...

to meet men.

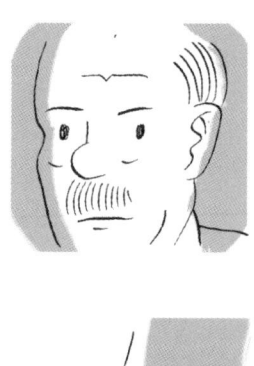
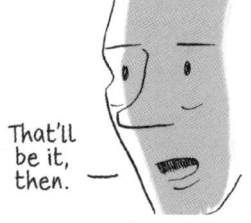

That'll be it, then.

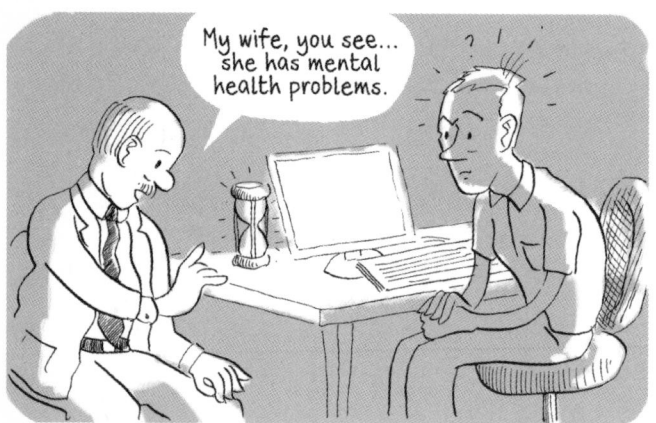

My wife, you see... she has mental health problems.

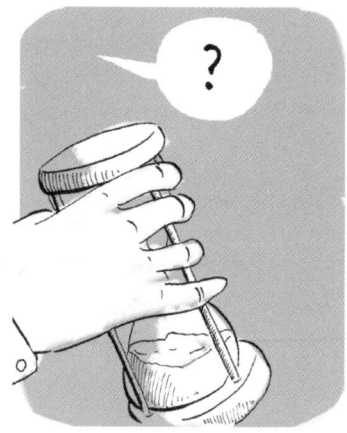

?

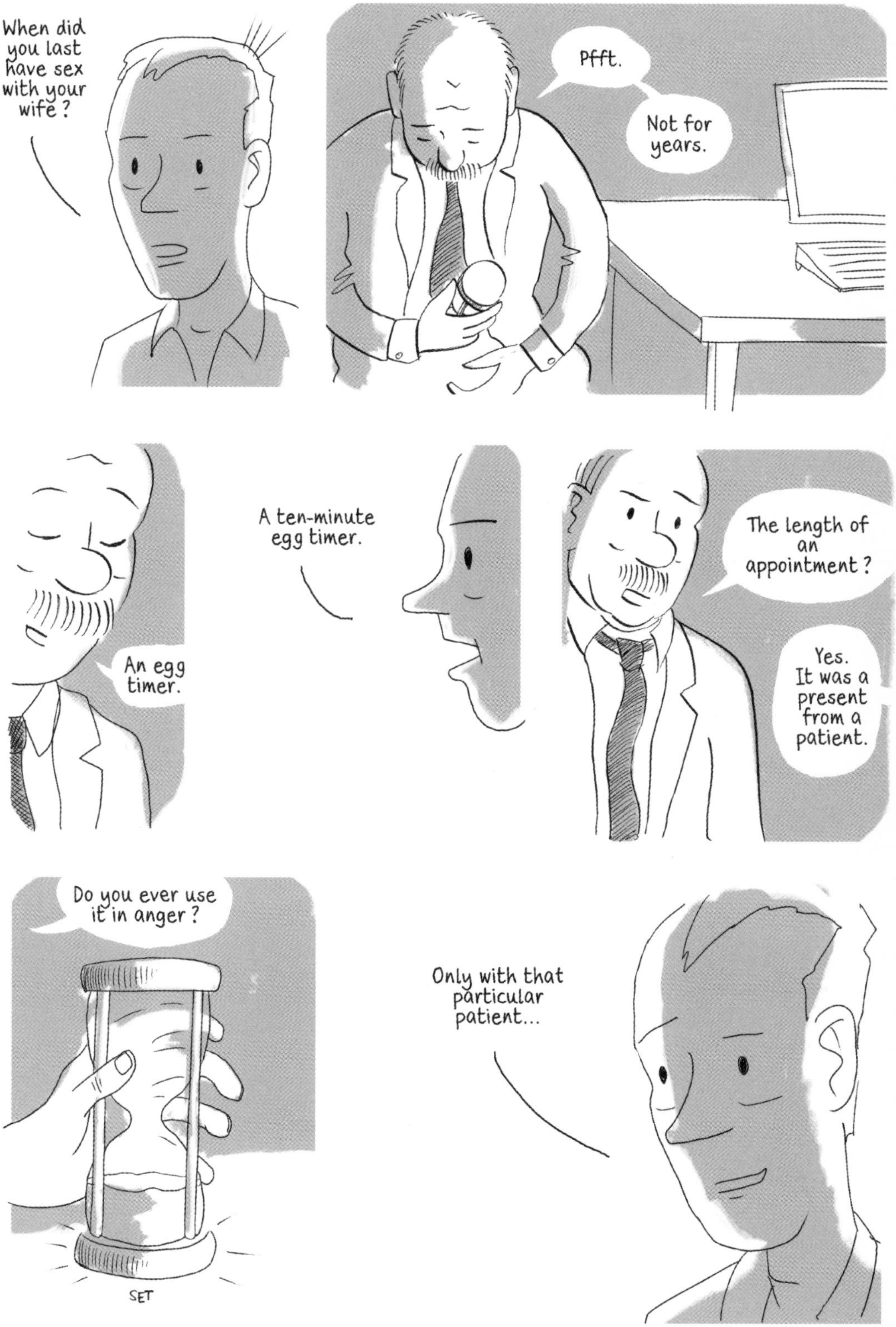

When did you last have sex with your wife ?
Pfft.
Not for years.
An egg timer.
A ten-minute egg timer.
The length of an appointment ?
Yes. It was a present from a patient.
Do you ever use it in anger ?
SET
Only with that particular patient...

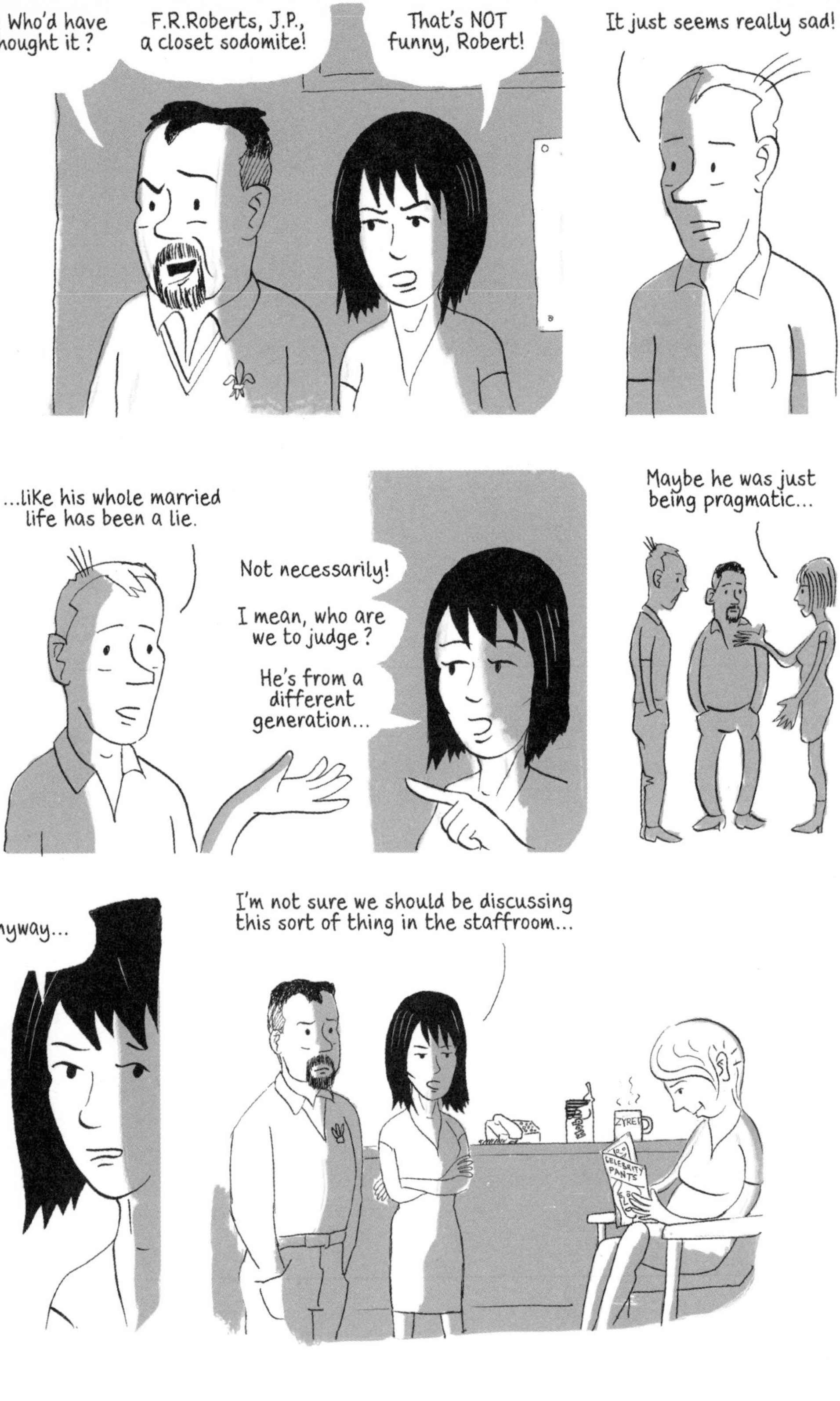
Ha! Who'd have thought it?
F.R.Roberts, J.P., a closet sodomite!
That's NOT funny, Robert!
It just seems really sad!
...like his whole married life has been a lie.
Not necessarily!
I mean, who are we to judge?
He's from a different generation...
Maybe he was just being pragmatic...
Anyway...
I'm not sure we should be discussing this sort of thing in the staffroom...
CELEBRITY PANTS
ZYRET

Shit! What's he want now?
ANEURIN COTTER TO SEE DOCTOR JAMES, PLEASE.
KNOCK KNOCK
Come in!
Hi. Have a seat.
What can I do for you?

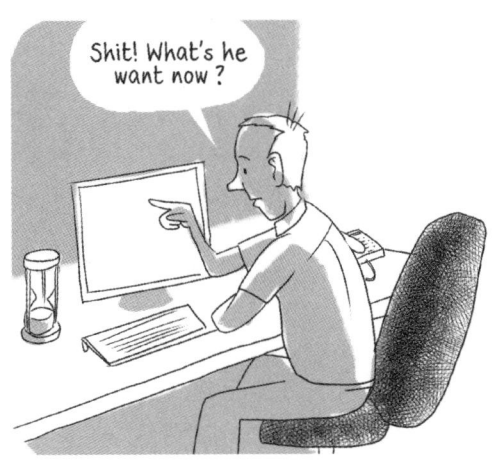

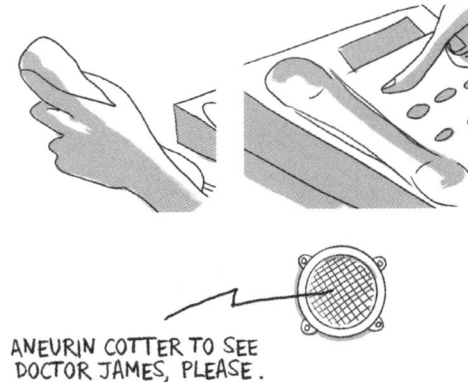

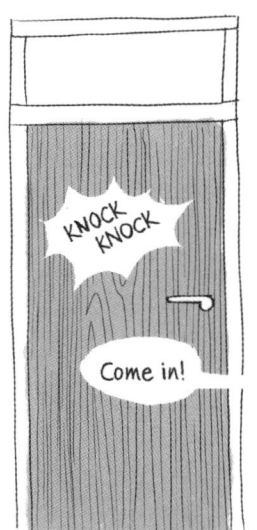

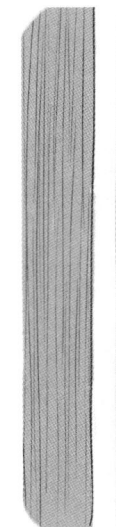

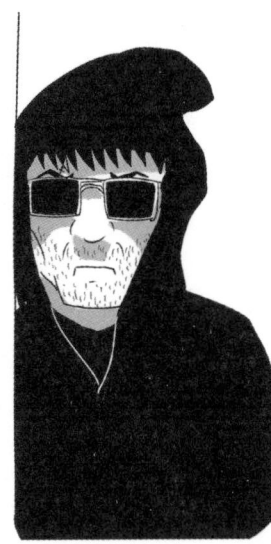

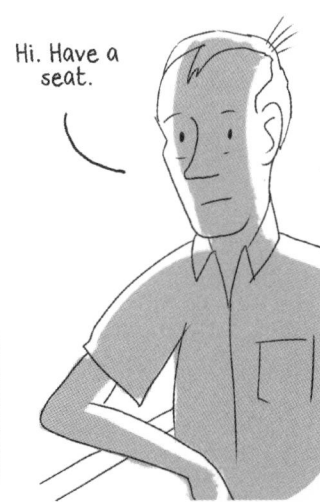

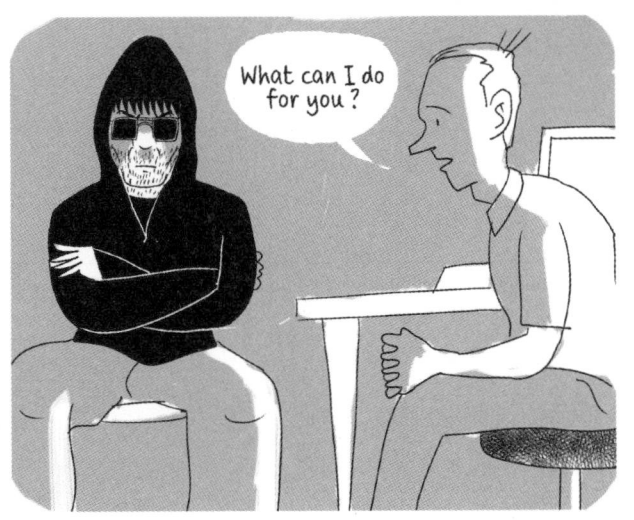

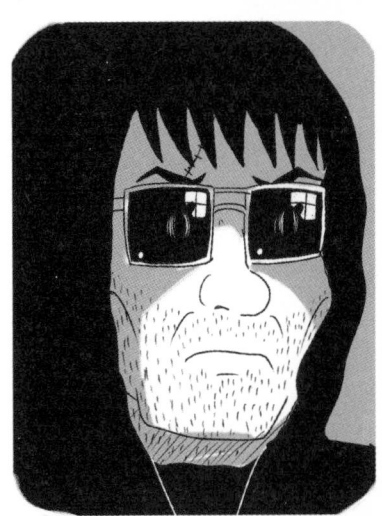

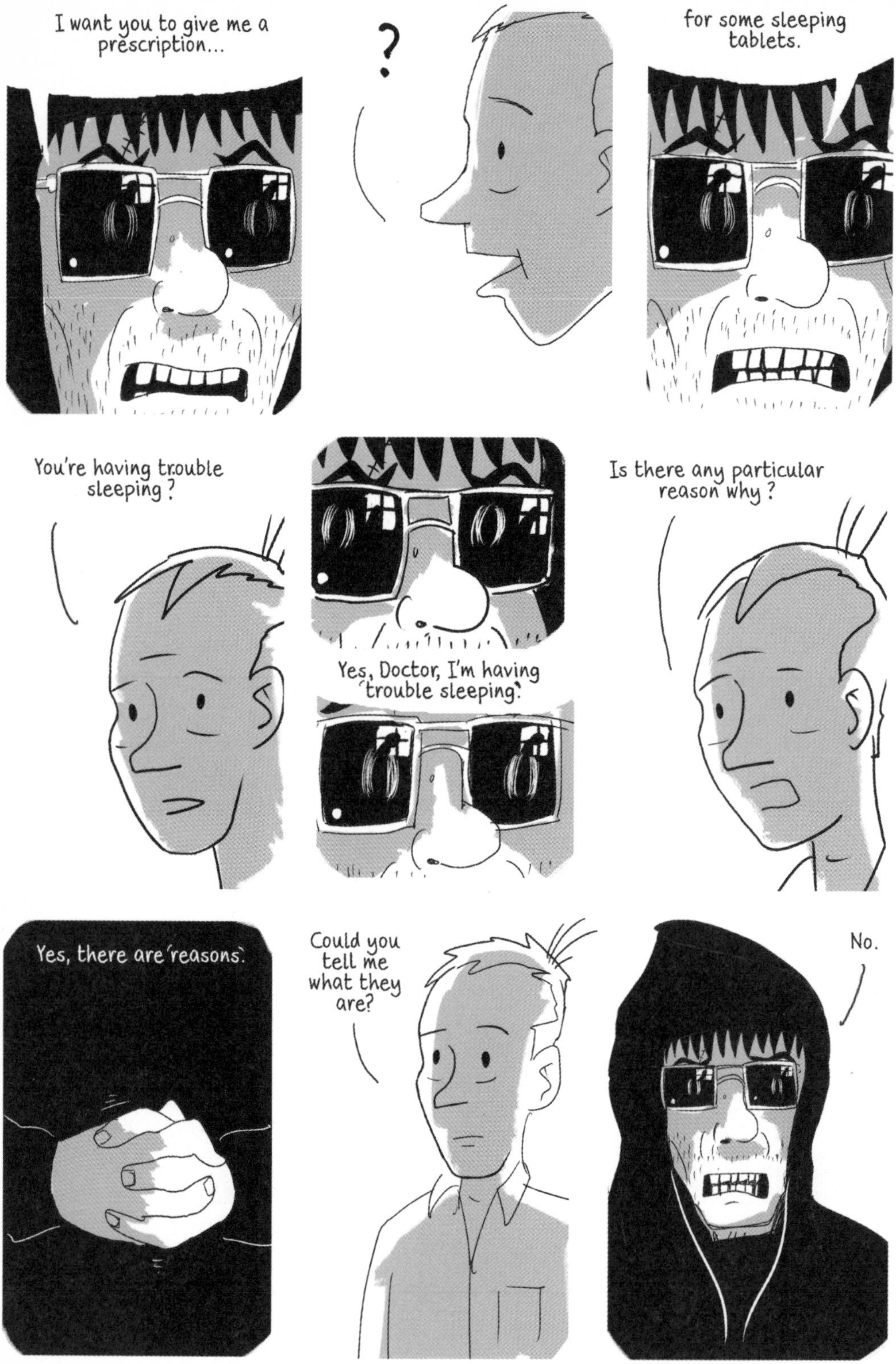
I want you to give me a prescription...
?
for some sleeping tablets.
You're having trouble sleeping?
Yes, Doctor, I'm having 'trouble sleeping'.
Is there any particular reason why?
Yes, there are 'reasons'.
Could you tell me what they are?
No.

Is your mood okay?
I just want the tablets.
I've had them before but your Nazi receptionists wouldn't let me have them without seeing you.
Well, we don't like to just hand them out.
We like to try and discover the underlying reason for poor sleep.
Any 'underlying reasons' are none of your business, Doctor, and beyond your capacity to solve.
Well, why don't you try discussing them?
It may be that I can...
Oh, forget it. You're not listening to me!
SIGH
TAP TAP TAP

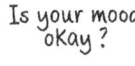

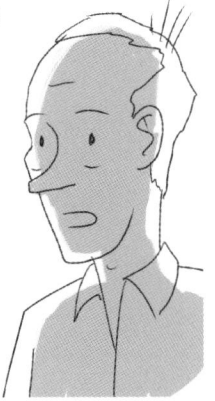

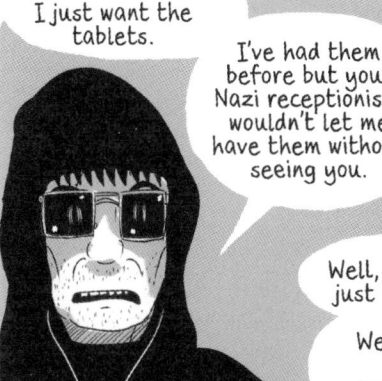

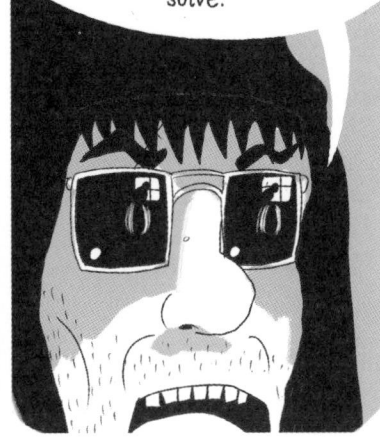

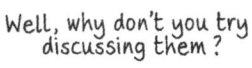

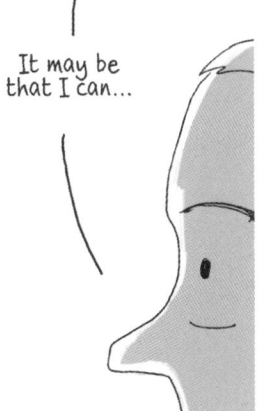

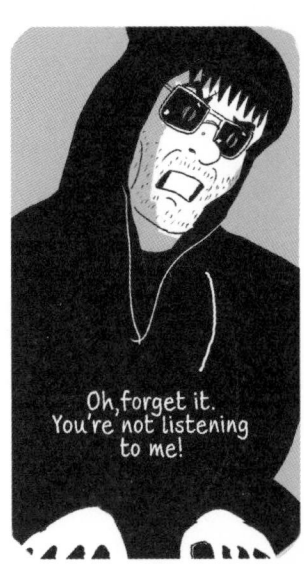

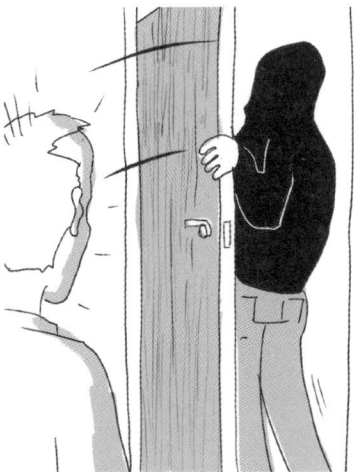

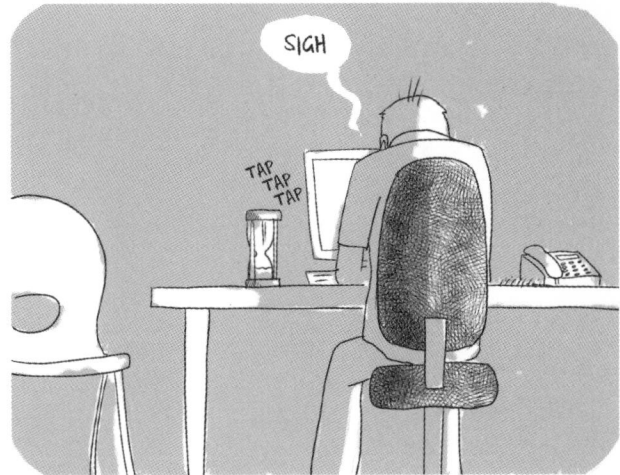

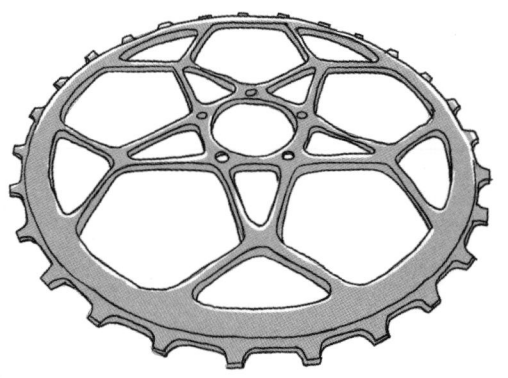

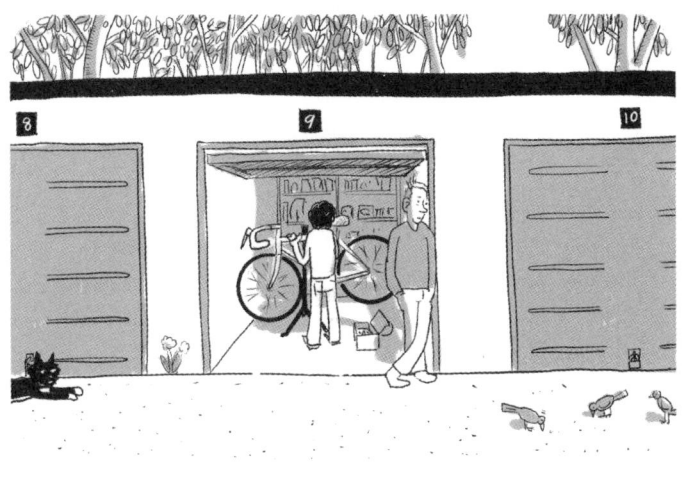

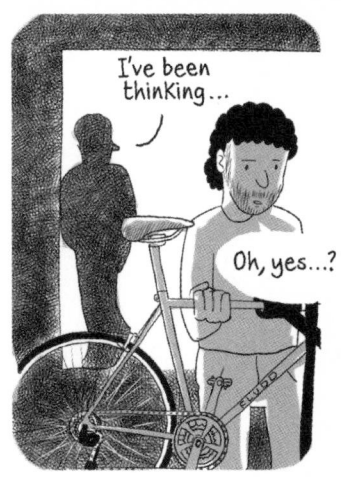

I've been thinking...

Oh, yes...?

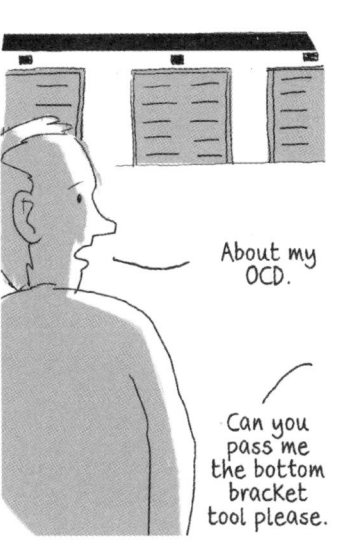

About my OCD.

Can you pass me the bottom bracket tool please.

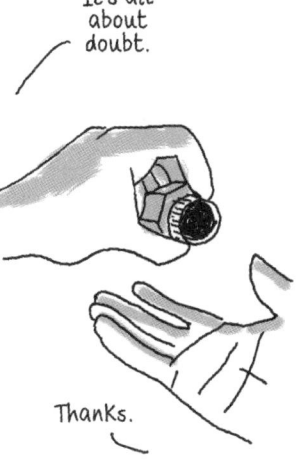

It's all about doubt.

Thanks.

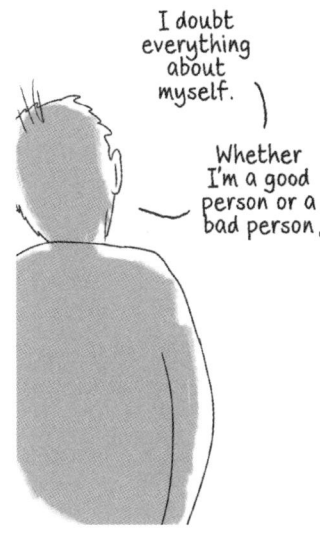

I doubt everything about myself.

Whether I'm a good person or a bad person.

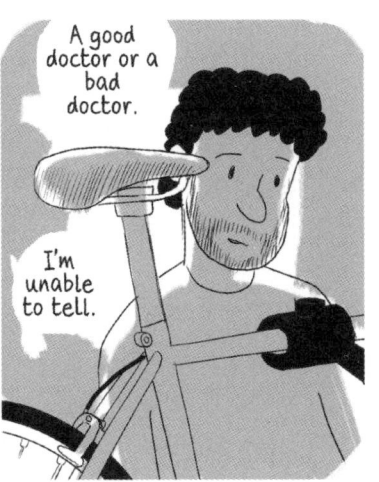

A good doctor or a bad doctor.

I'm unable to tell.

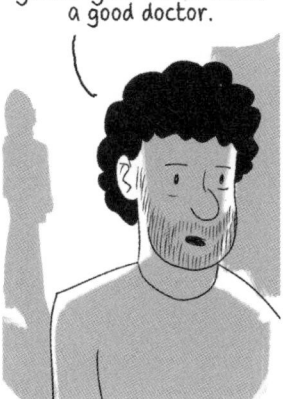

You're nice to patients, you do your best. You're a good doctor.

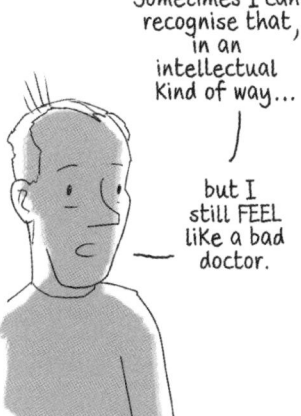

Sometimes I can recognise that, in an intellectual kind of way...

but I still FEEL like a bad doctor.

161

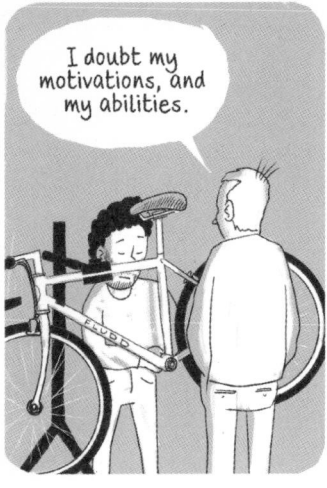

I doubt my motivations, and my abilities.

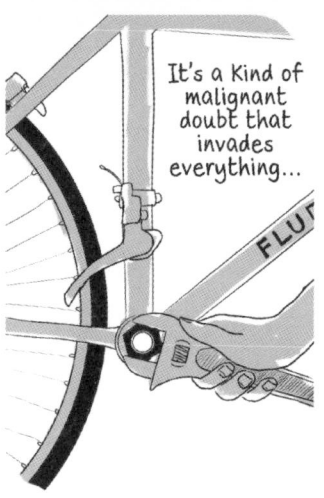

It's a kind of malignant doubt that invades everything...

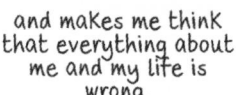
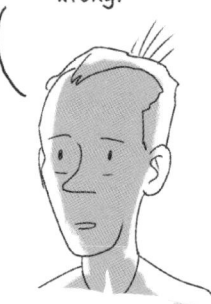

and makes me think that everything about me and my life is wrong.

Like what I told you about my marriage.

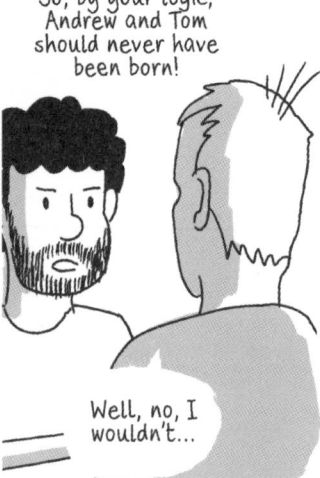

So, by your logic, Andrew and Tom should never have been born!

Well, no, I wouldn't...

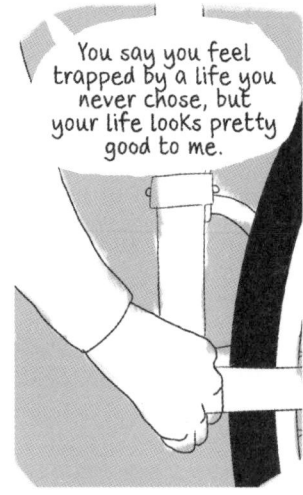

You say you feel trapped by a life you never chose, but your life looks pretty good to me.

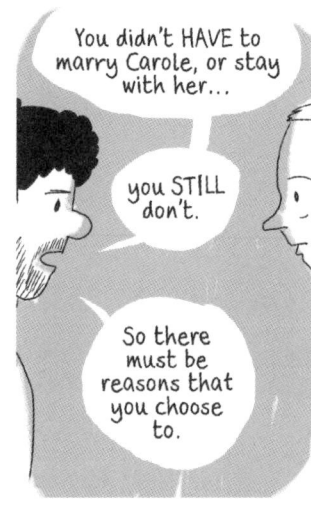

You didn't HAVE to marry Carole, or stay with her...

you STILL don't.

So there must be reasons that you choose to.

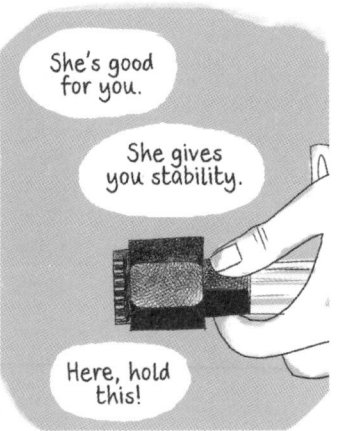

She's good for you.

She gives you stability.

Here, hold this!

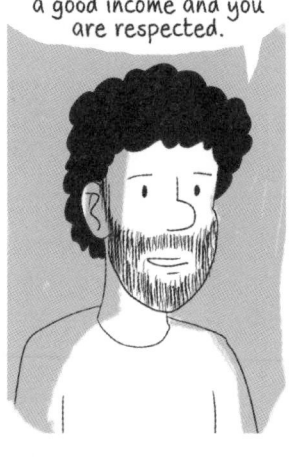

You've got a good job and a good income and you are respected.

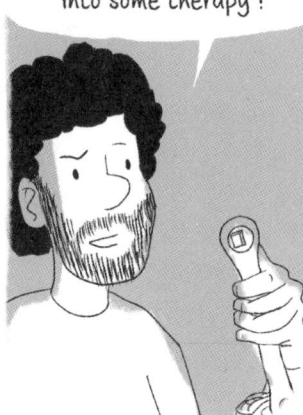

Like I said, you should probably get yourself into some therapy!

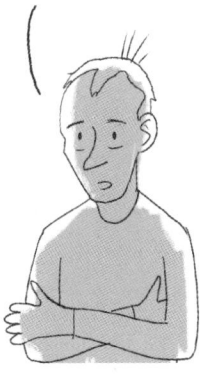

Yeah.

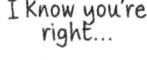

I know you're right...

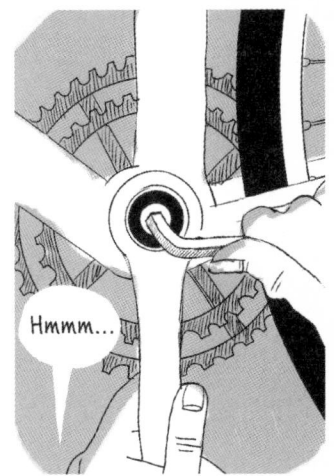

Hmmm...

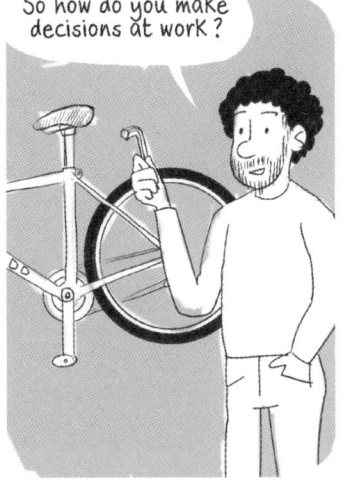

So how do you make decisions at work?

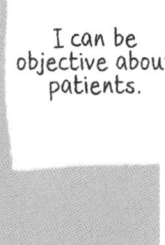

The doubt is only about myself.

I can be objective about patients.

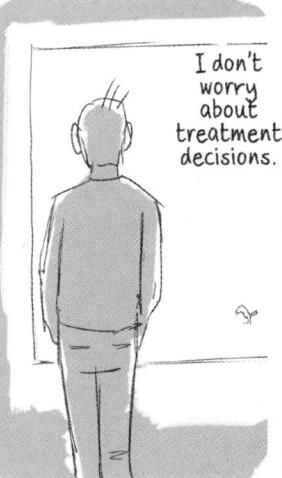

I don't worry about treatment decisions.

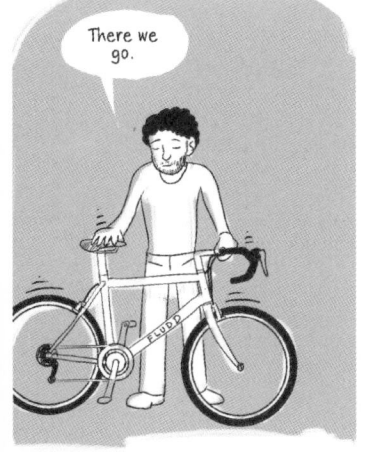

There we go.

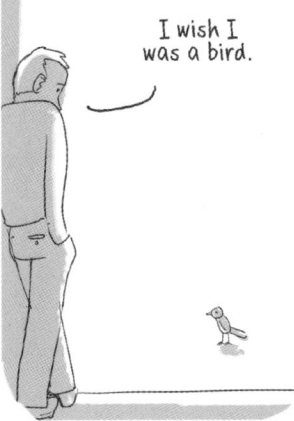

I wish I was a bird.

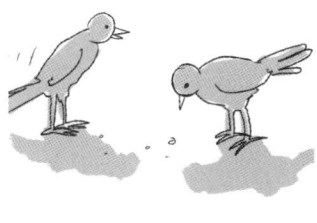

Wouldn't want to live in a freezing fucking hedge, mind.

163

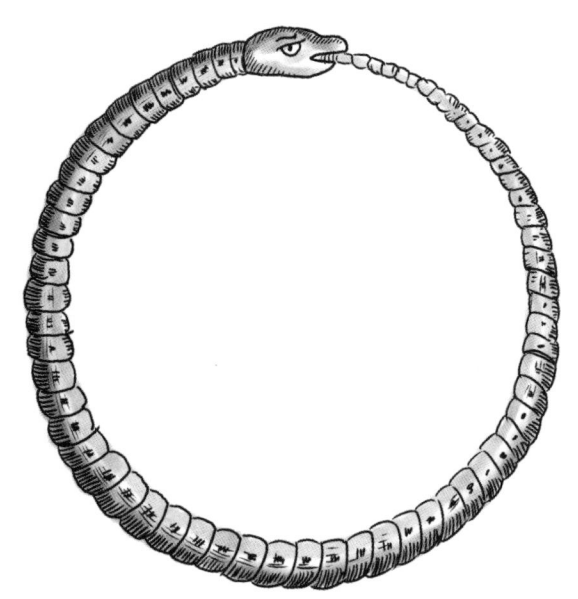

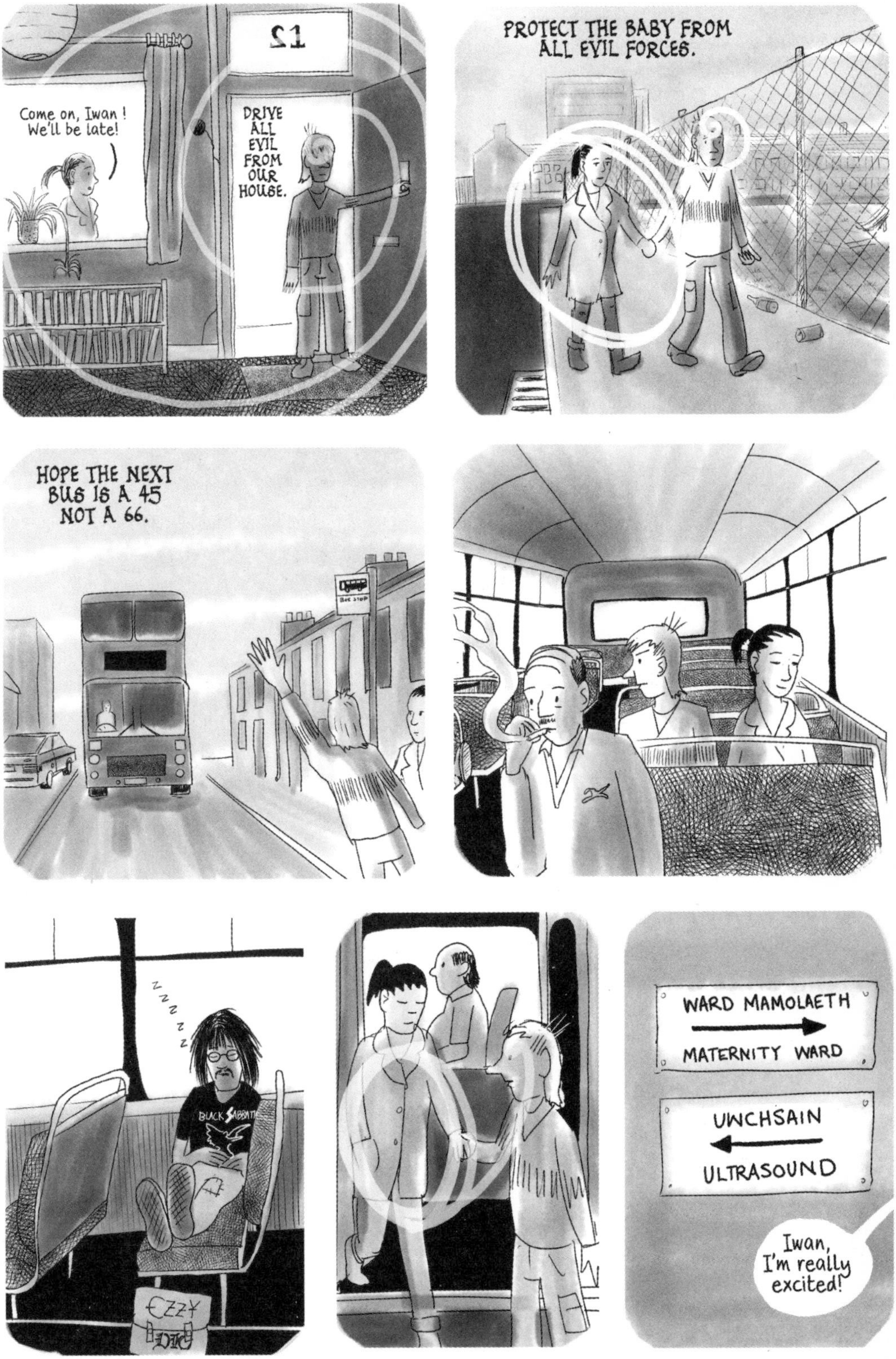

12
Come on, Iwan! We'll be late!
DRIVE ALL EVIL FROM OUR HOUSE.
PROTECT THE BABY FROM ALL EVIL FORCES.
HOPE THE NEXT BUS IS A 45 NOT A 66.
BUS STOP
BLACK SABBATH
OZZY
WARD MAMOLAETH
MATERNITY WARD
UWCHSAIN
ULTRASOUND
Iwan, I'm really excited!

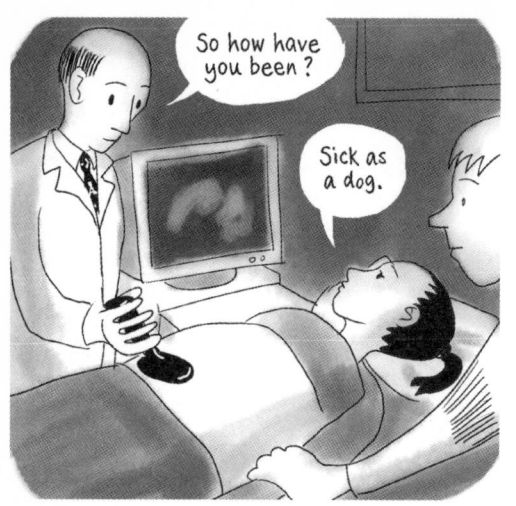

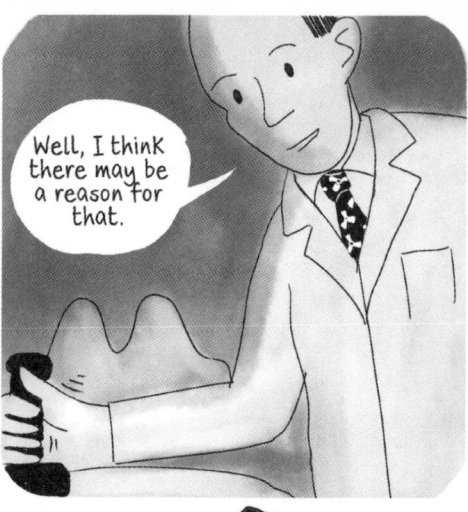

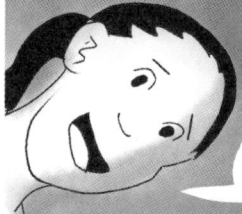

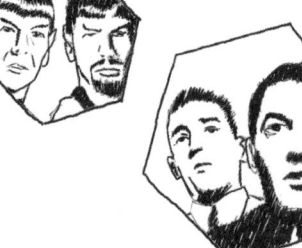

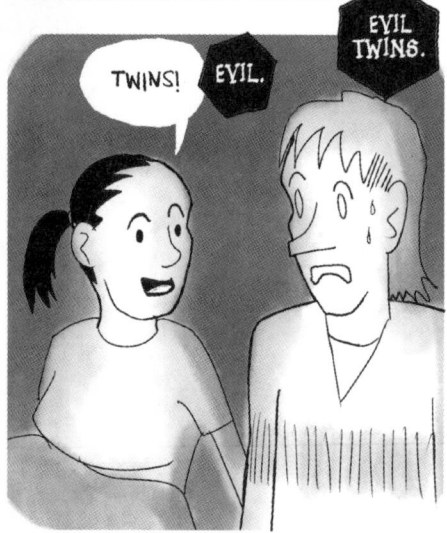

So how have you been?
Sick as a dog.
Well, I think there may be a reason for that.
There are two of them in there.
DOUBLE PROTECTION
DOUBLE THE COST
2
You mean I'm having twins?
Oh, my God! Iwan!
TWINS!
EVIL.
EVIL TWINS.
RONNIE AND REGGIE
ROMULUS AND REMUS
AHURA MAZDA AND ANGRA MAINYU
SUPERMAN AND BIZARRO
OH, GOD. I'M NOT SURE I CAN COPE WITH THIS.

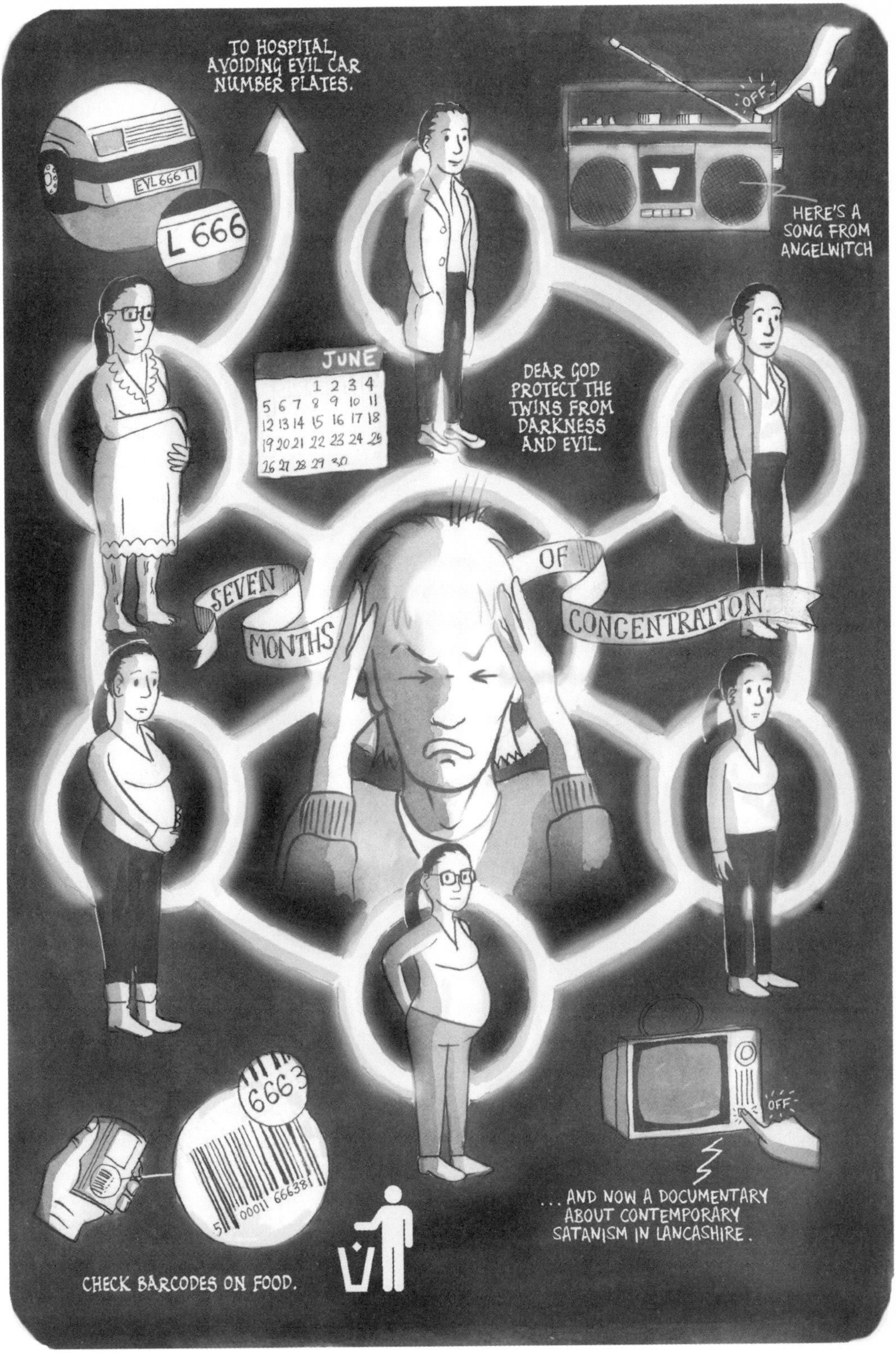
TO HOSPITAL, AVOIDING EVIL CAR NUMBER PLATES.
EVL 666 T
L 666
OFF
HERE'S A SONG FROM ANGELWITCH
JUNE
1 2 3 4
5 6 7 8 9 10 11
12 13 14 15 16 17 18
19 20 21 22 23 24 25
26 27 28 29 30
DEAR GOD PROTECT THE TWINS FROM DARKNESS AND EVIL.
SEVEN MONTHS OF CONCENTRATION
6663
5 00011 66638
OFF
...AND NOW A DOCUMENTARY ABOUT CONTEMPORARY SATANISM IN LANCASHIRE.
CHECK BARCODES ON FOOD.

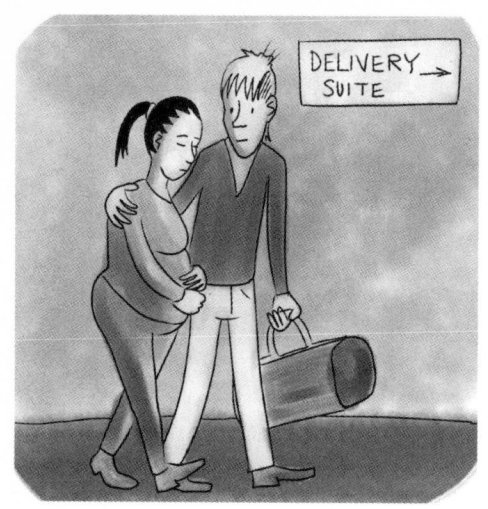

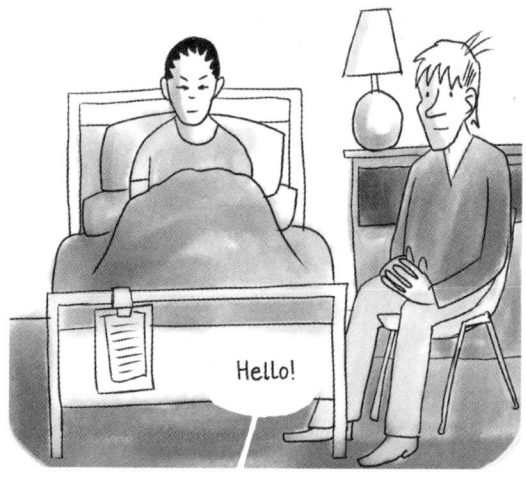

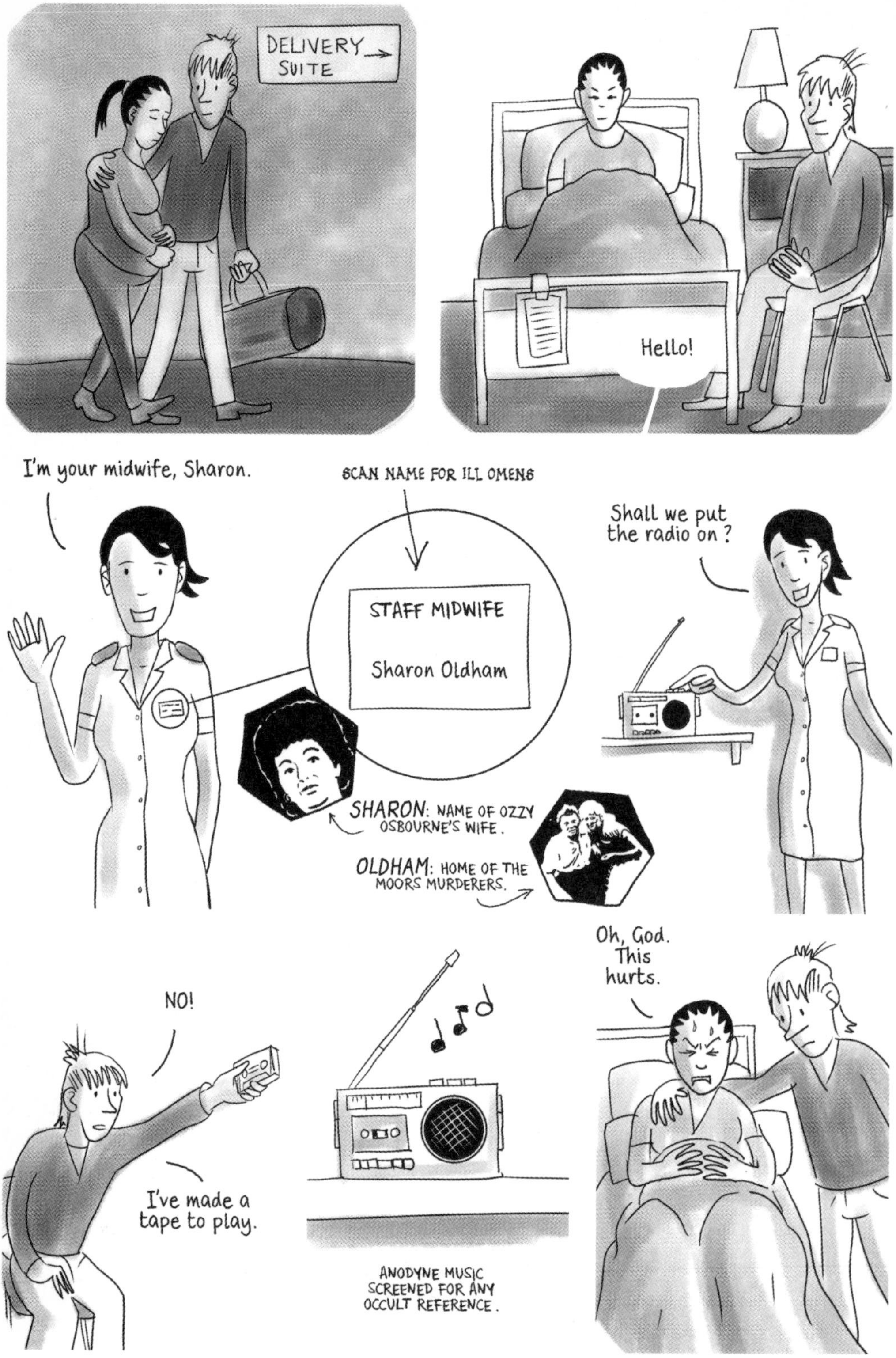
DELIVERY SUITE
Hello!
I'm your midwife, Sharon.
SCAN NAME FOR ILL OMENS
STAFF MIDWIFE
Sharon Oldham
SHARON: NAME OF OZZY OSBOURNE'S WIFE.
OLDHAM: HOME OF THE MOORS MURDERERS.
Shall we put the radio on?
NO!
I've made a tape to play.
ANODYNE MUSIC SCREENED FOR ANY OCCULT REFERENCE.
Oh, God. This hurts.

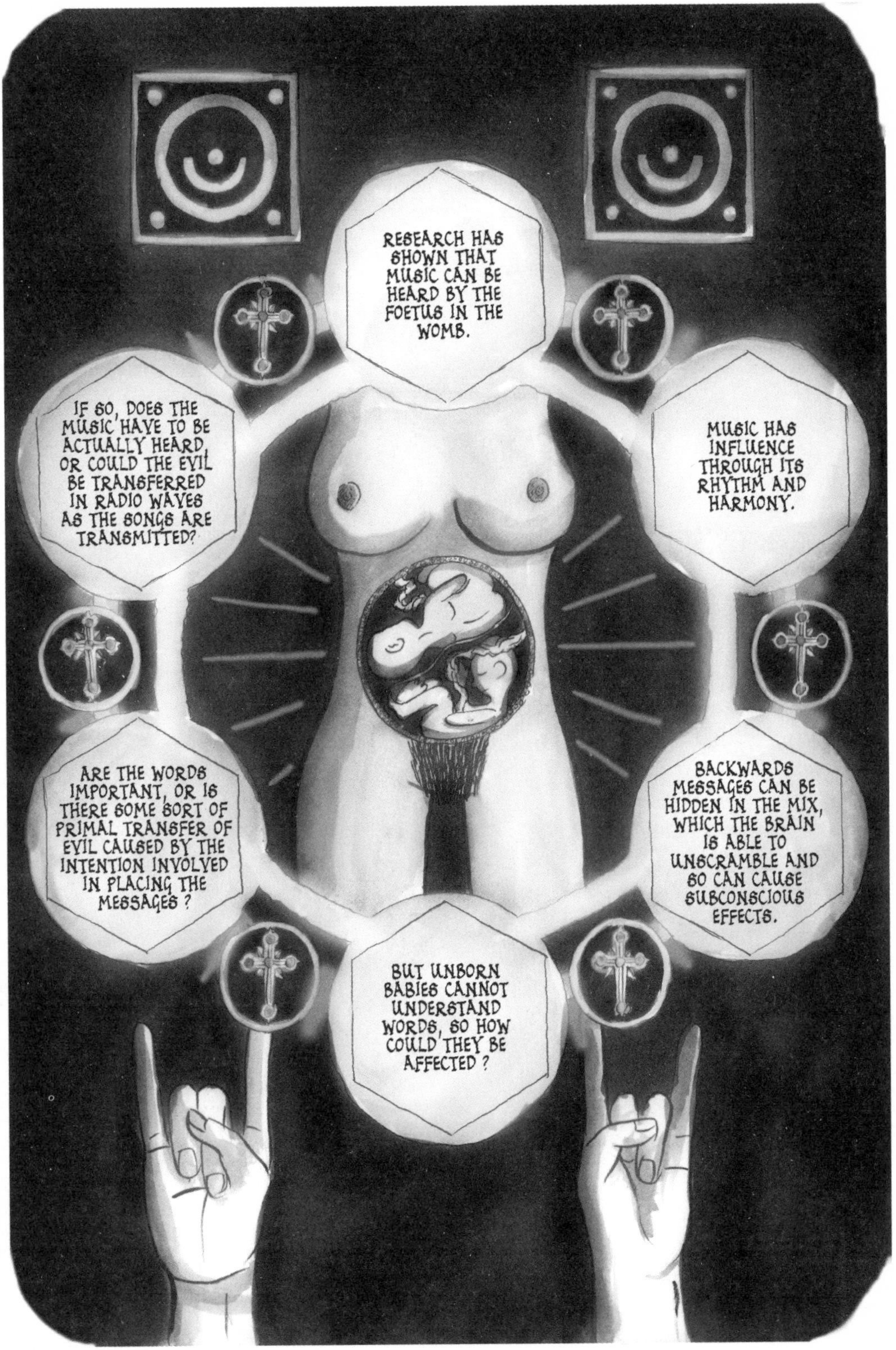
RESEARCH HAS SHOWN THAT MUSIC CAN BE HEARD BY THE FOETUS IN THE WOMB.
MUSIC HAS INFLUENCE THROUGH ITS RHYTHM AND HARMONY.
BACKWARDS MESSAGES CAN BE HIDDEN IN THE MIX, WHICH THE BRAIN IS ABLE TO UNSCRAMBLE AND SO CAN CAUSE SUBCONSCIOUS EFFECTS.
BUT UNBORN BABIES CANNOT UNDERSTAND WORDS, SO HOW COULD THEY BE AFFECTED ?
ARE THE WORDS IMPORTANT, OR IS THERE SOME SORT OF PRIMAL TRANSFER OF EVIL CAUSED BY THE INTENTION INVOLVED IN PLACING THE MESSAGES ?
IF SO, DOES THE MUSIC HAVE TO BE ACTUALLY HEARD, OR COULD THE EVIL BE TRANSFERRED IN RADIO WAVES AS THE SONGS ARE TRANSMITTED?

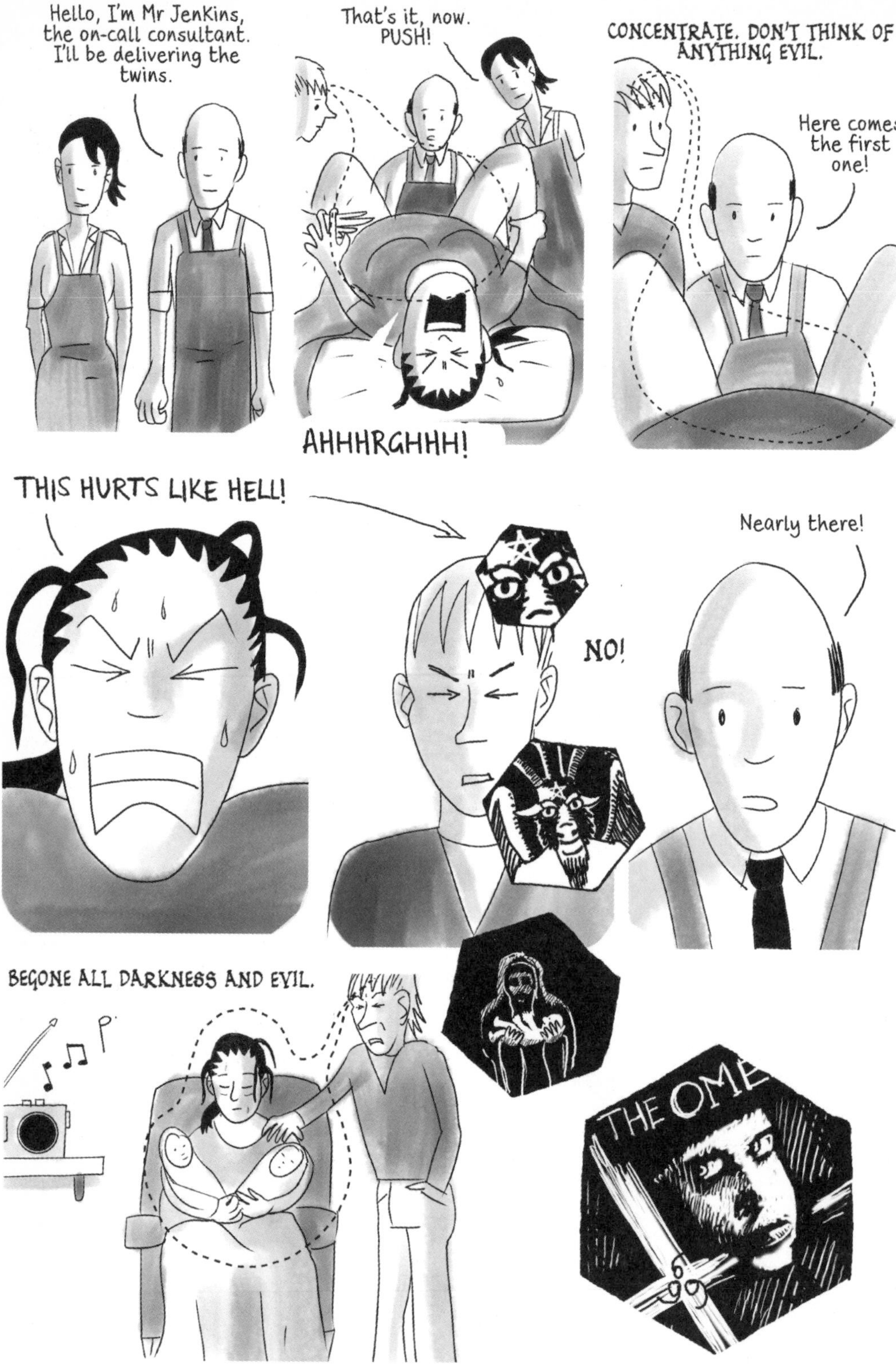

Hello, I'm Mr Jenkins, the on-call consultant. I'll be delivering the twins.
That's it, now. PUSH!
AHHHRGHHH!
CONCENTRATE. DON'T THINK OF ANYTHING EVIL.
Here comes the first one!
THIS HURTS LIKE HELL!
NO!
Nearly there!
BEGONE ALL DARKNESS AND EVIL.
THE OME

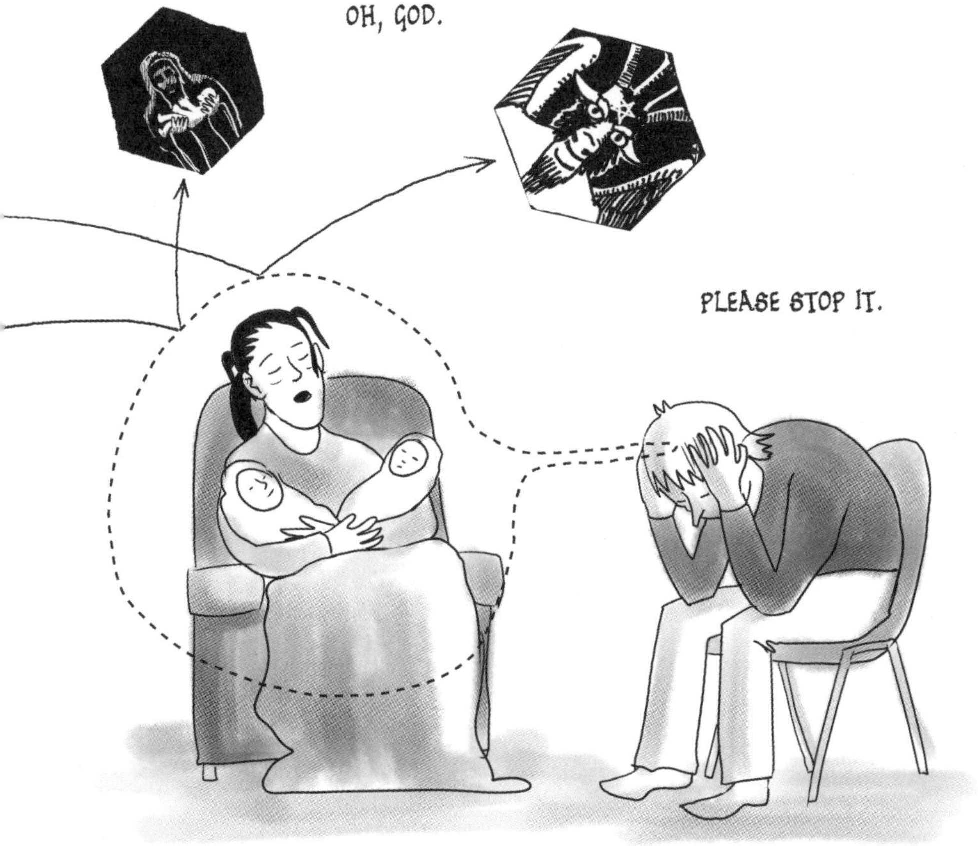
OH, GOD.
PLEASE STOP IT.

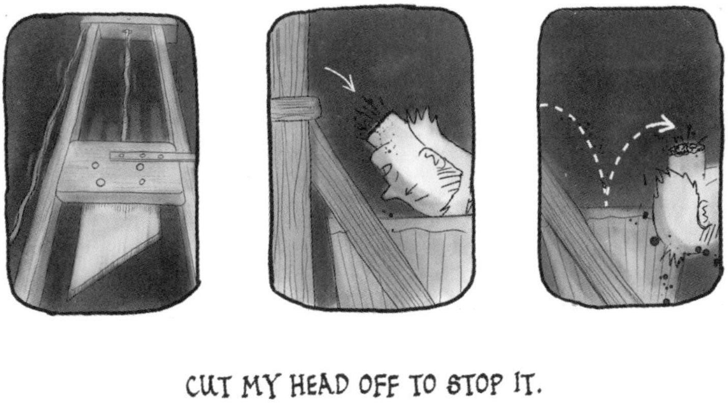
CUT MY HEAD OFF TO STOP IT.

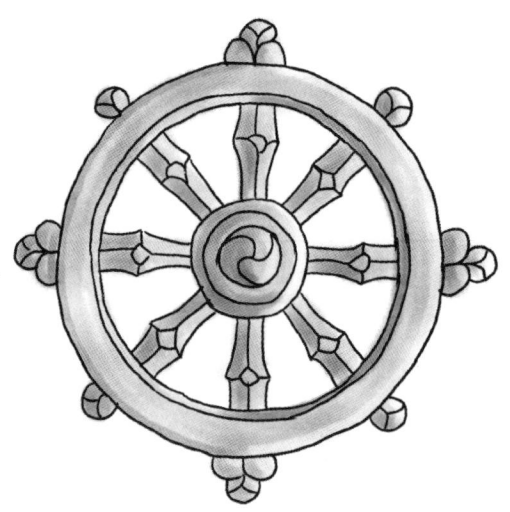

Hello, Doctor.
Hi, Mr Pryce, what can I do for you?
Sore throat.
We'd better have a look.
OKay. Open wide.
AHHHHHH
ULP!
Sorry, Doctor.

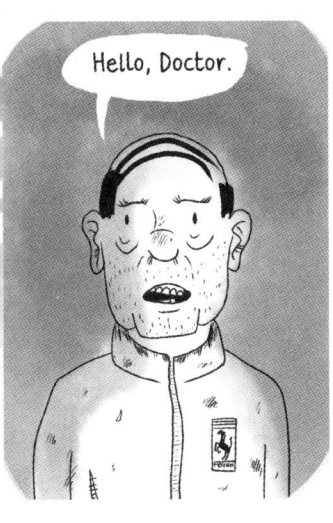

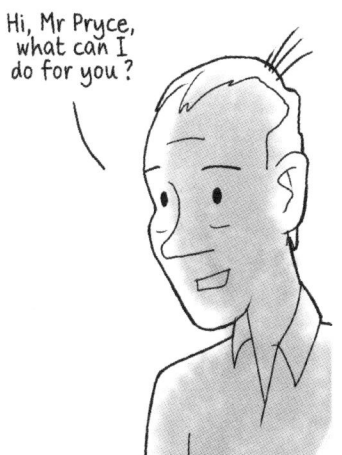

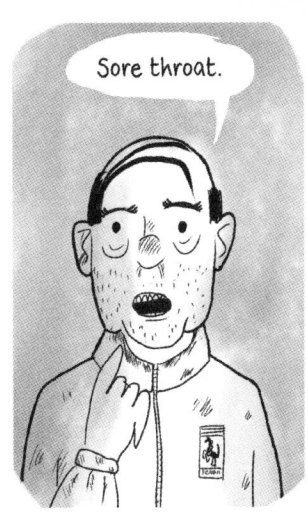

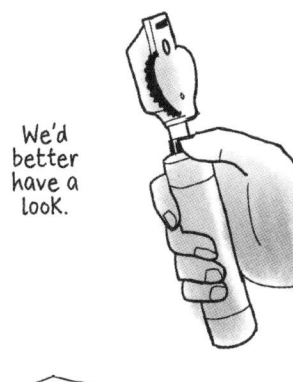

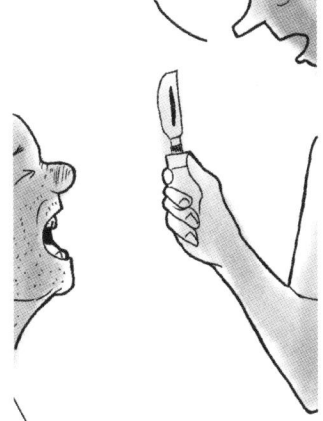

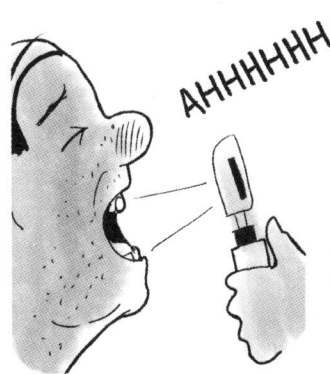

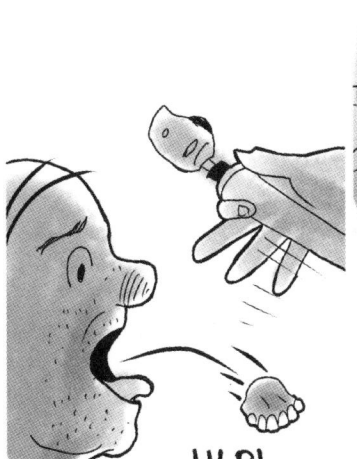

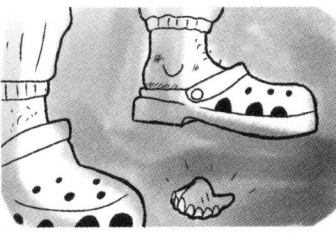

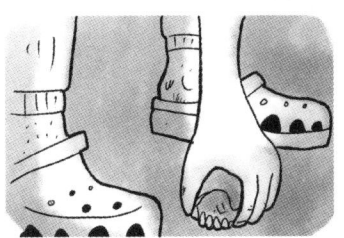

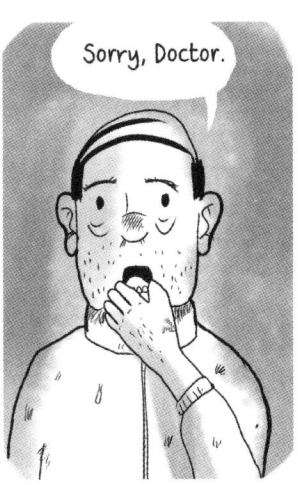

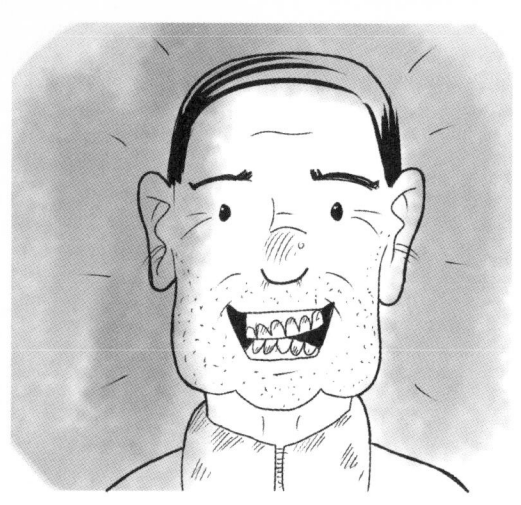
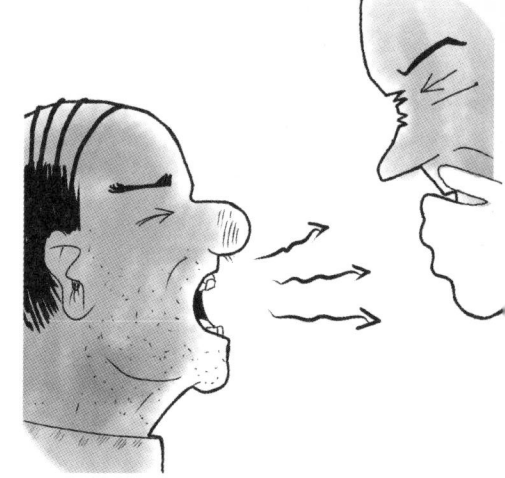

Your teeth don't seem to fit your mouth properly.

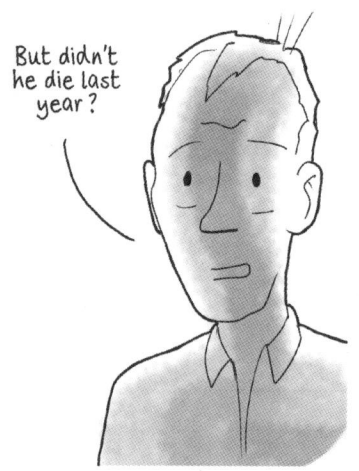

No, they're not my teeth.

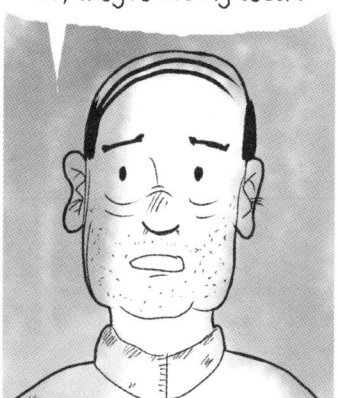

They're my brother's.

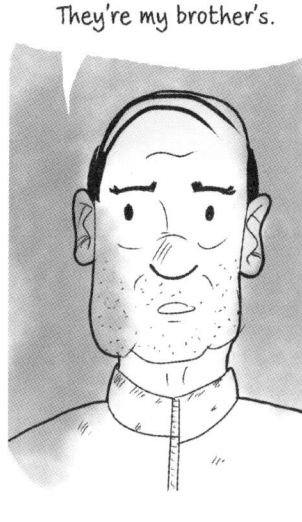

But didn't he die last year?

That's right, Doctor.

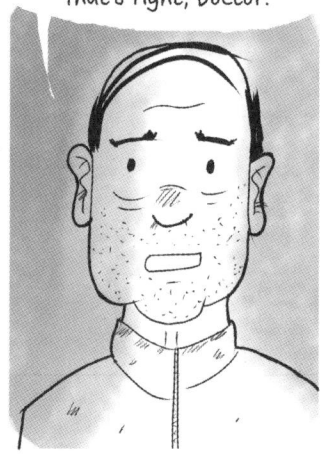
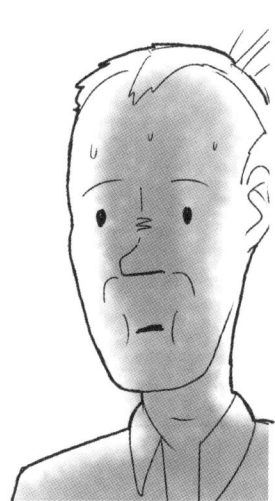

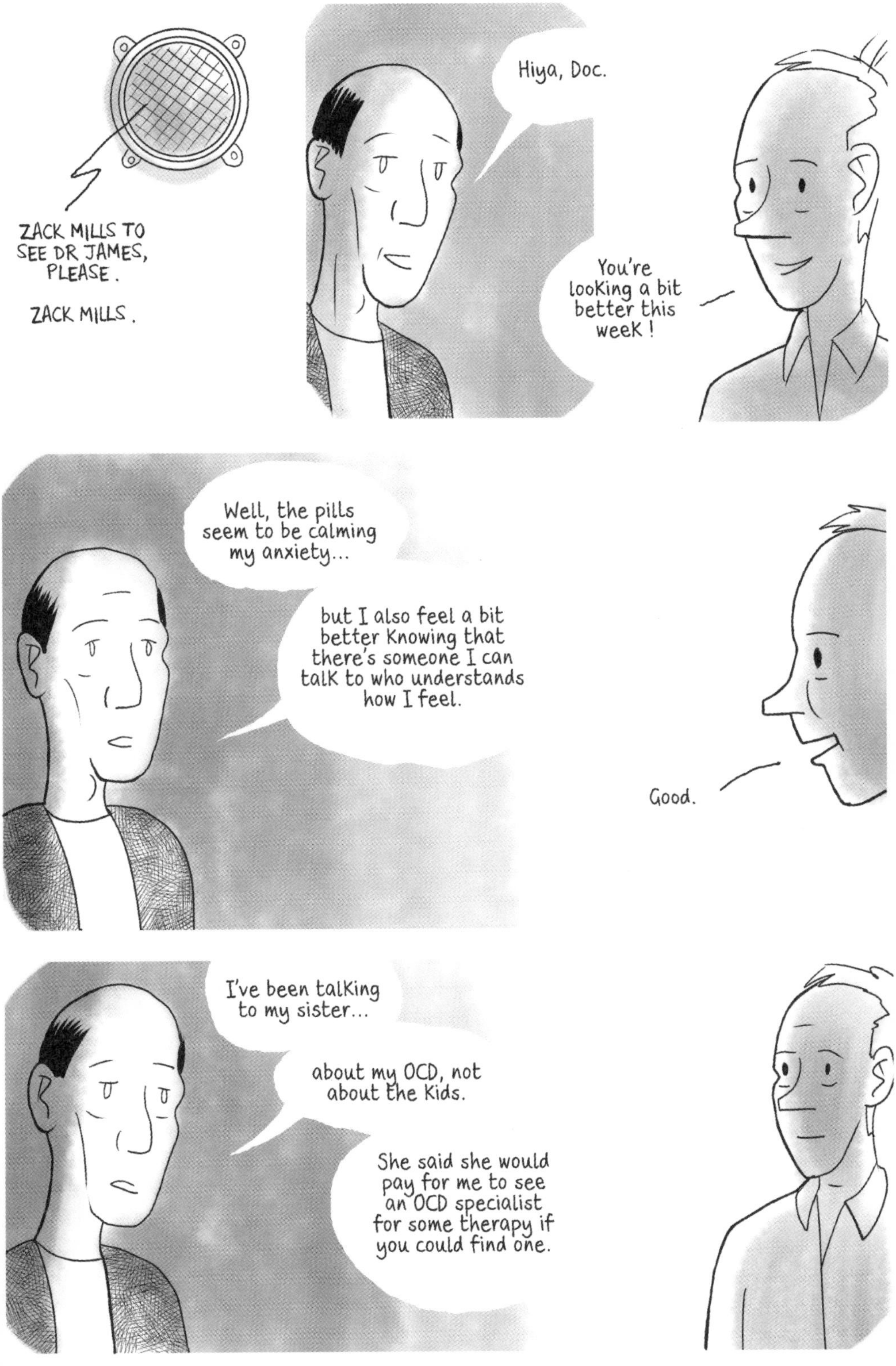
ZACK MILLS TO SEE DR JAMES, PLEASE.
ZACK MILLS.
Hiya, Doc.
You're looking a bit better this week!
Well, the pills seem to be calming my anxiety...
but I also feel a bit better knowing that there's someone I can talk to who understands how I feel.
Good.
I've been talking to my sister...
about my OCD, not about the kids.
She said she would pay for me to see an OCD specialist for some therapy if you could find one.

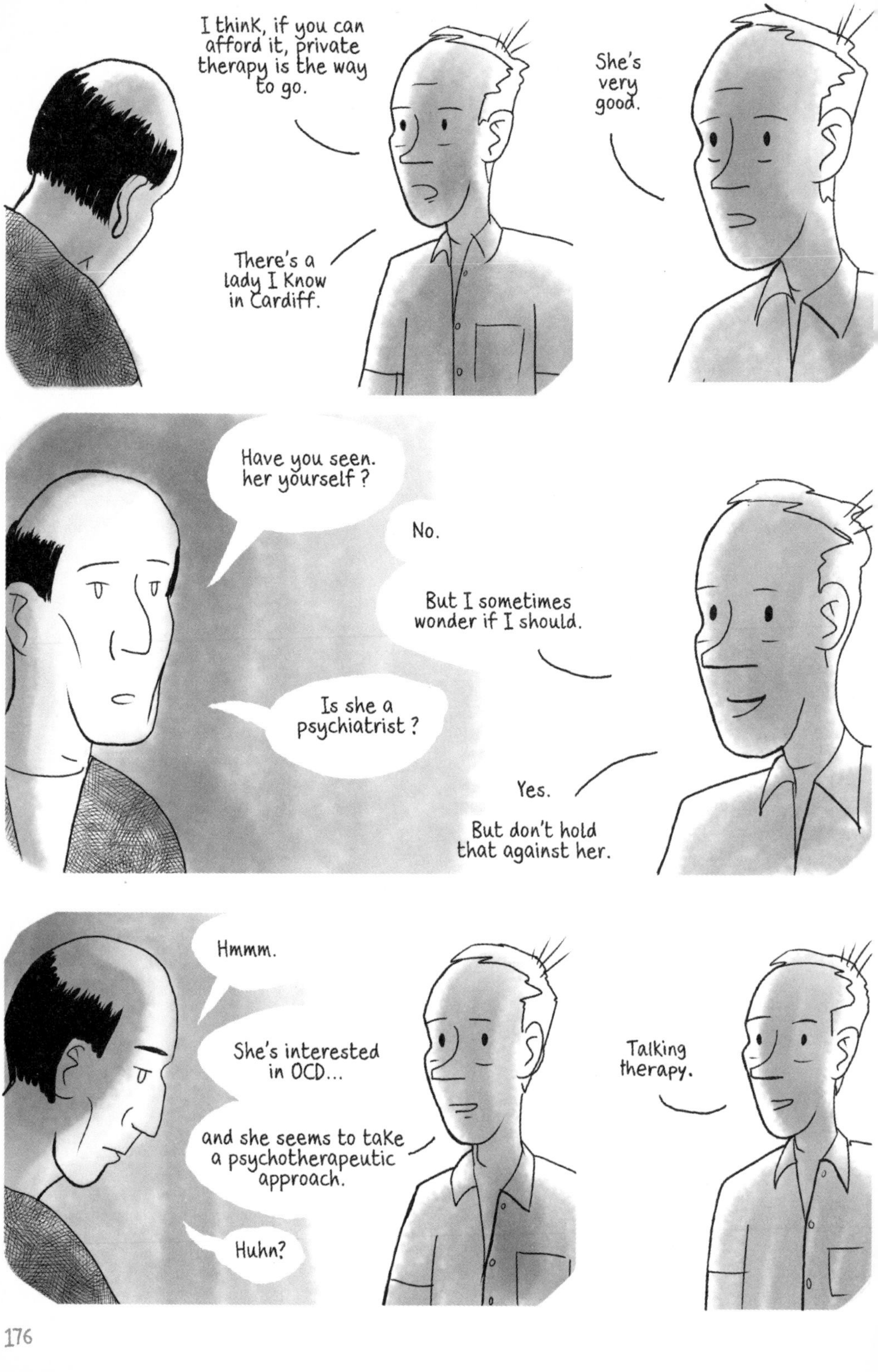
I think, if you can afford it, private therapy is the way to go.
There's a lady I know in Cardiff.
She's very good.
Have you seen. her yourself?
No.
But I sometimes wonder if I should.
Is she a psychiatrist?
Yes.
But don't hold that against her.
Hmmm.
She's interested in OCD...
and she seems to take a psychotherapeutic approach.
Huhn?
Talking therapy.

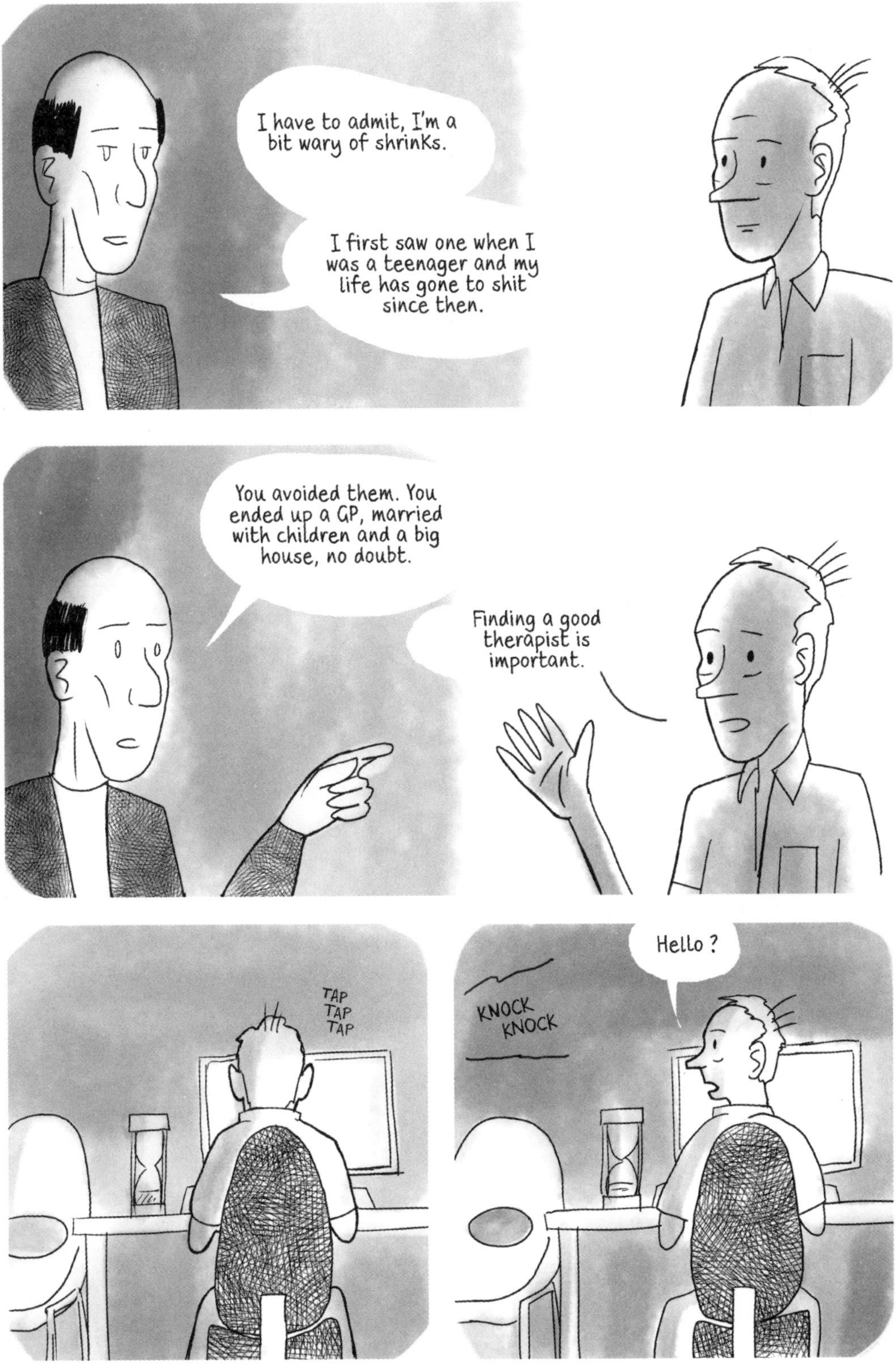
I have to admit, I'm a bit wary of shrinks.
I first saw one when I was a teenager and my life has gone to shit since then.
You avoided them. You ended up a GP, married with children and a big house, no doubt.
Finding a good therapist is important.
TAP TAP TAP
KNOCK KNOCK
Hello ?

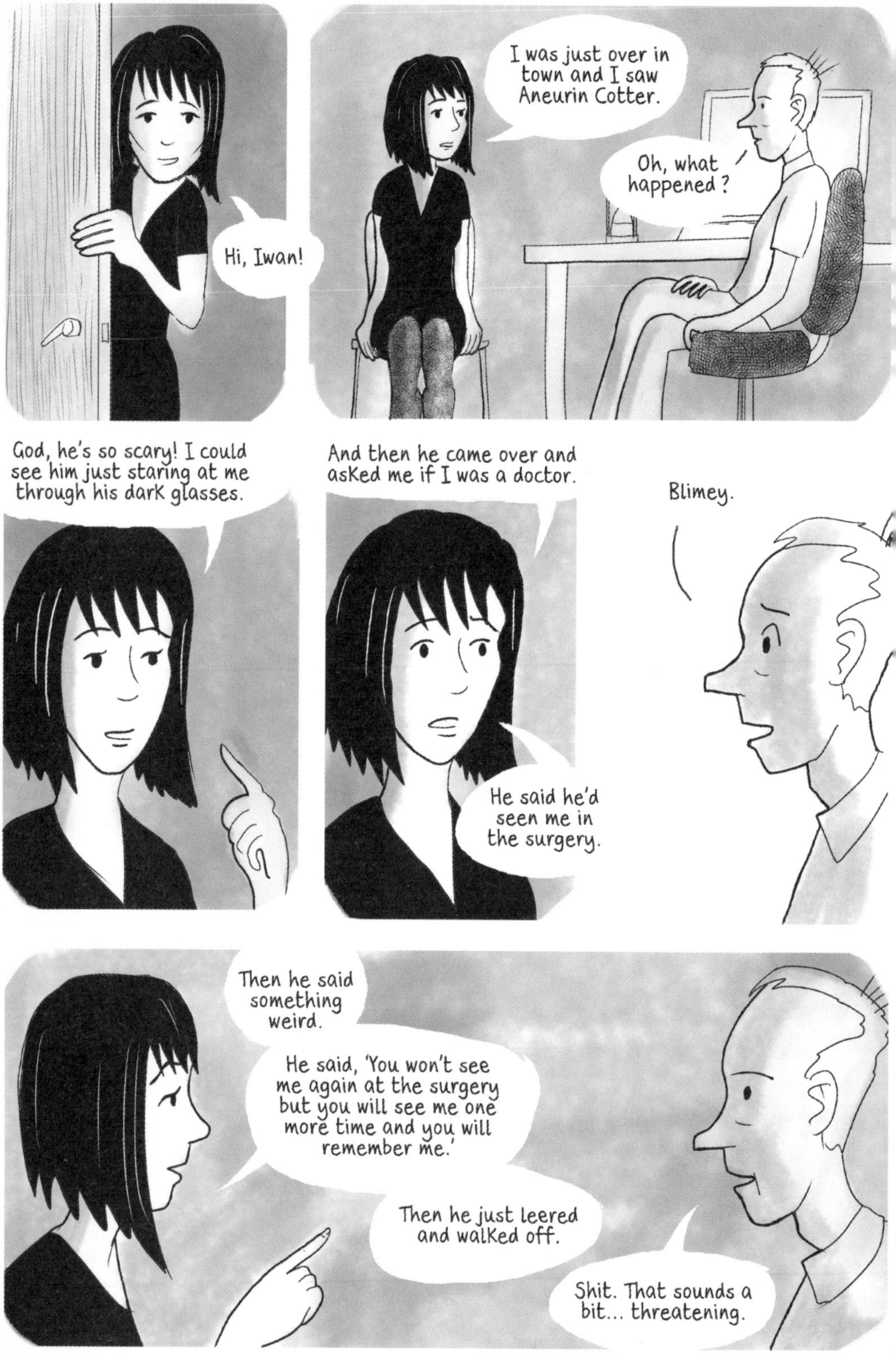
Hi, Iwan!
I was just over in town and I saw Aneurin Cotter.
Oh, what happened?
God, he's so scary! I could see him just staring at me through his dark glasses.
And then he came over and asked me if I was a doctor.
He said he'd seen me in the surgery.
Blimey.
Then he said something weird.
He said, 'You won't see me again at the surgery but you will see me one more time and you will remember me.'
Then he just leered and walked off.
Shit. That sounds a bit... threatening.

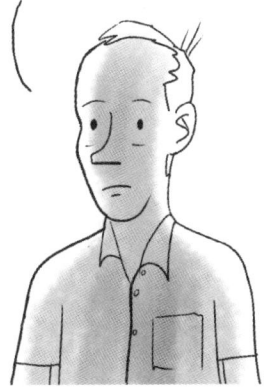

What do you think he meant?

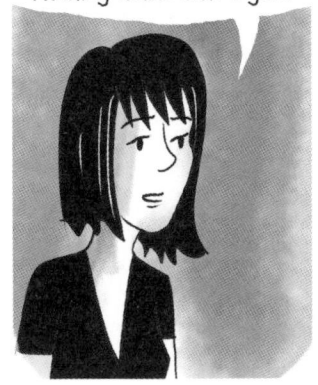

I don't Know. He's so scary, I could imagine him running amoK with a gun!

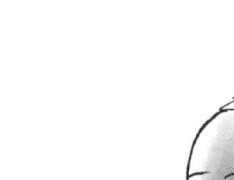

God! He was pretty unpleasant last time he was here.

Do you think we should do anything about it?

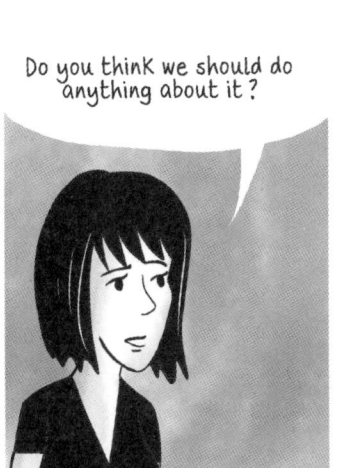

Like what? He hasn't made any specific threats.

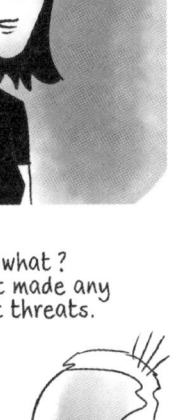

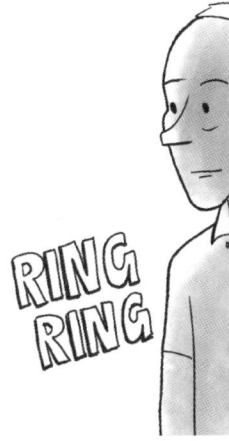

RING RING

RING RING

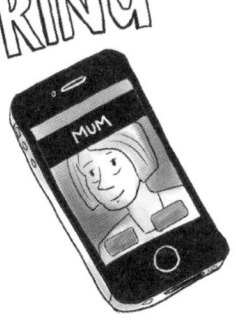

MUM

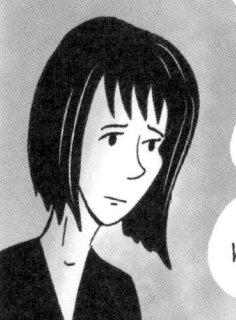

Hello... Mum? What's up?

Shit!

He's in hospital?

What happened?

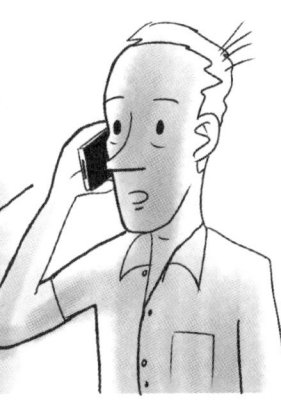

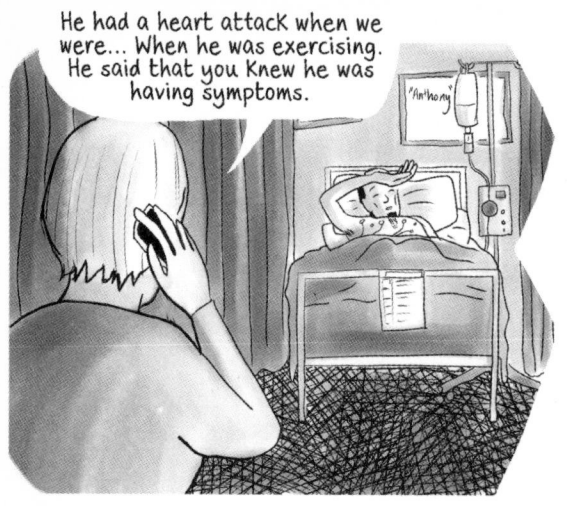

He had a heart attack when we were... When he was exercising. He said that you knew he was having symptoms.

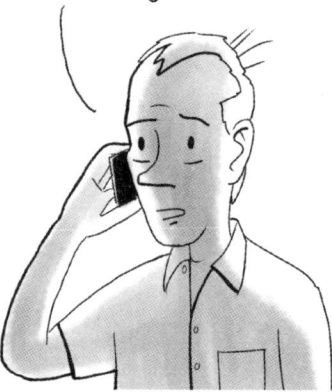

Yes, he told me. But Dr Jones has been treating him and sending him for investigations.

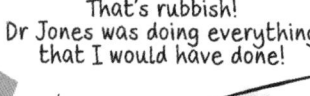

He's not taking it too well... He says he feels he's been let down by the 'Sons of Hippocrates'.

That's rubbish! Dr Jones was doing everything that I would have done!

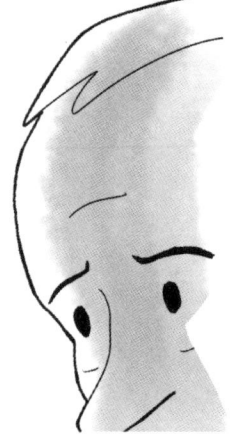

He's a bit annoyed. He says that Dr Jones is an old fart but he expected better advice from you...

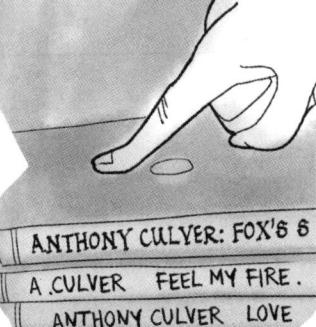

ANTHONY CULVER: FOX'S 8
A .CULVER   FEEL MY FIRE .
ANTHONY CULVER   LOVE

BUT I'M NOT HIS SODDING DOCTOR!

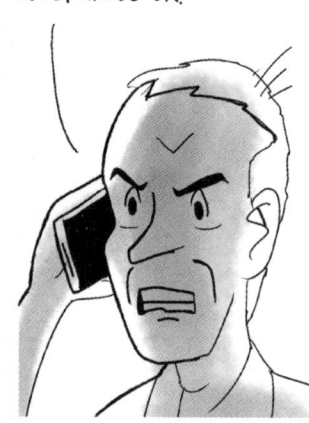

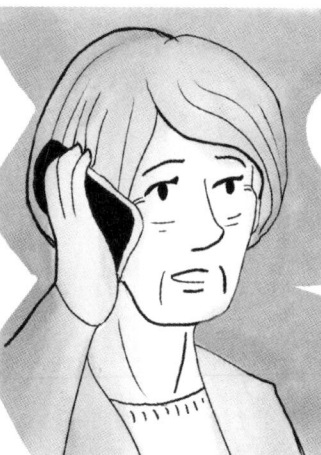

Luckily, the cardiologist is a poetry fan! He's into William Carlos Williams.

Anthony has given him signed copies of each of his collections.

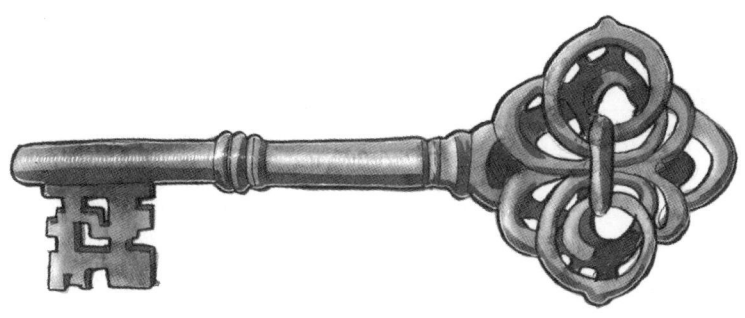

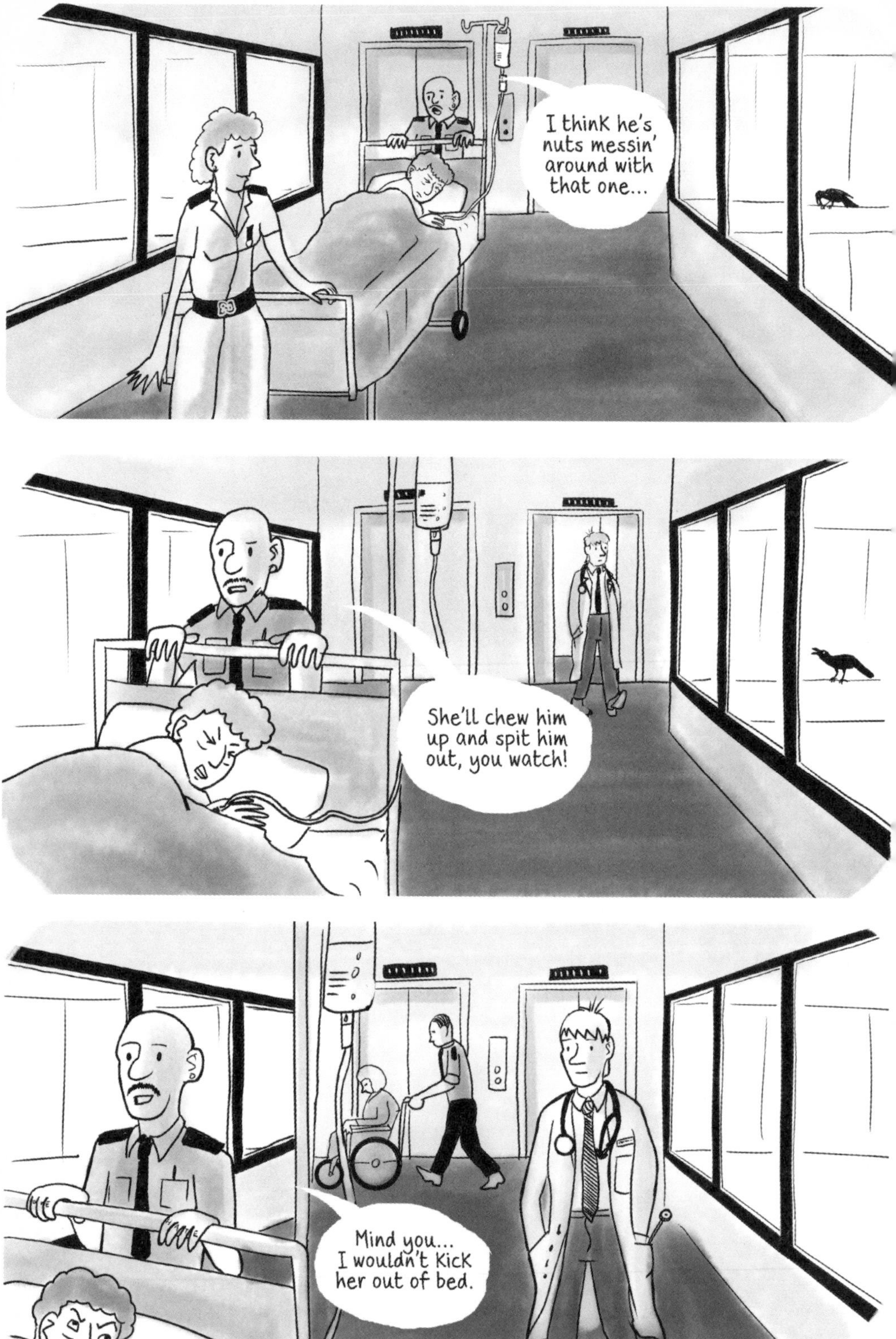
I think he's nuts messin' around with that one...
She'll chew him up and spit him out, you watch!
Mind you... I wouldn't kick her out of bed.

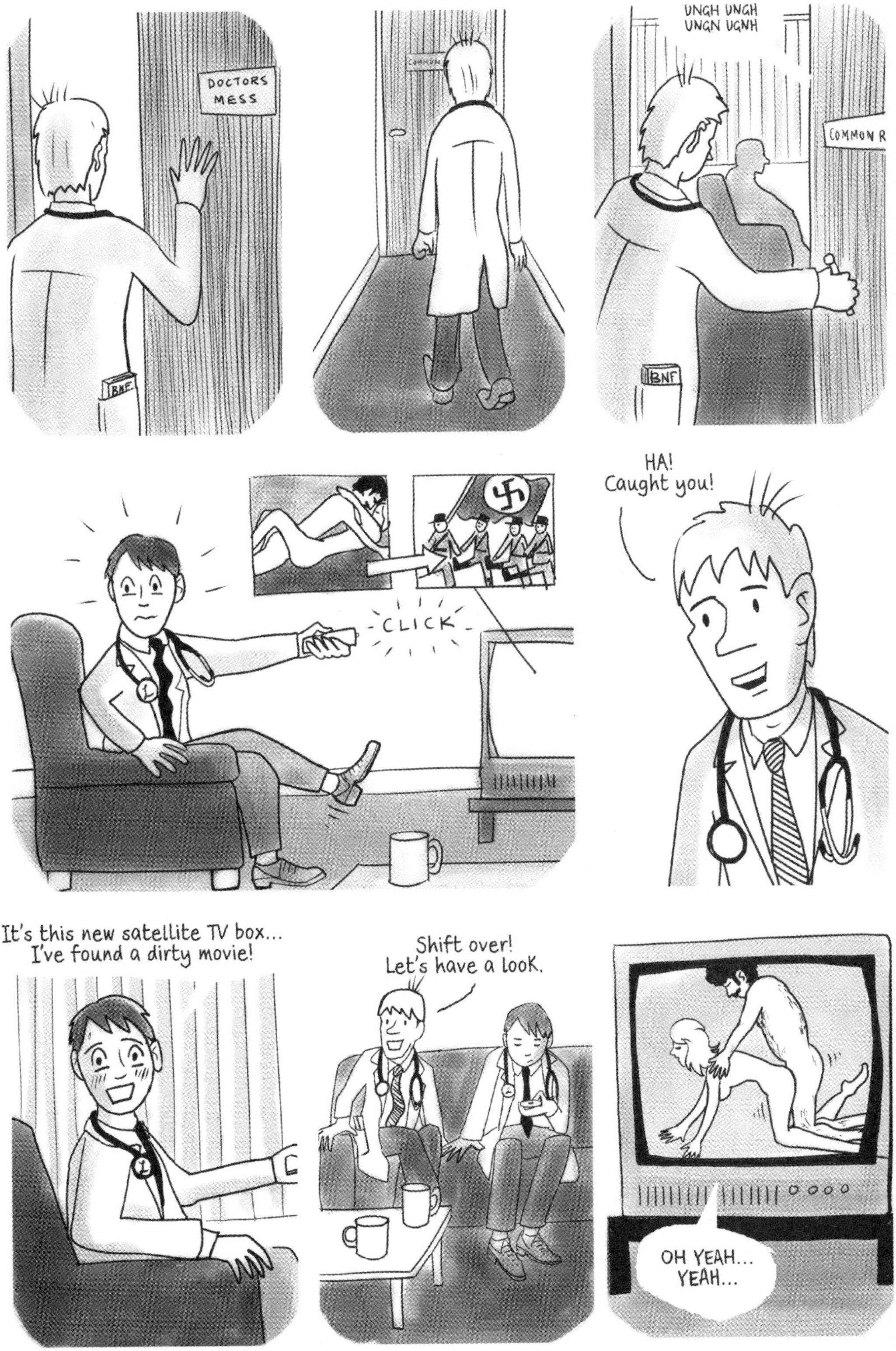
DOCTORS MESS
BNF
COMMON
UNGH UNGH UNGN UGNH
COMMON R
BNF
CLICK
HA! Caught you!
It's this new satellite TV box... I've found a dirty movie!
Shift over! Let's have a look.
OH YEAH... YEAH...

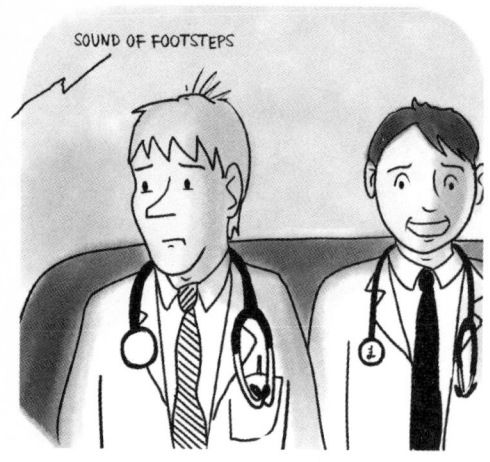

SOUND OF FOOTSTEPS

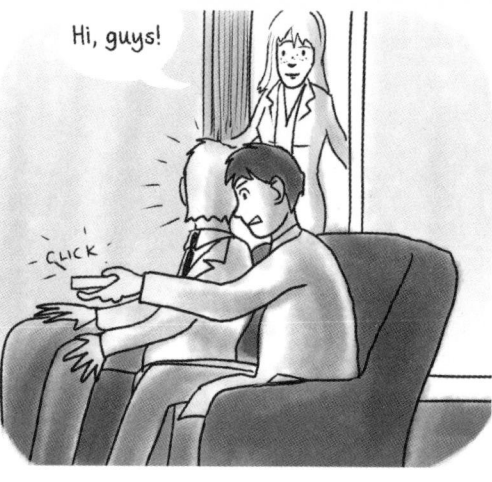

Hi, guys!

CLICK

What are you watching?

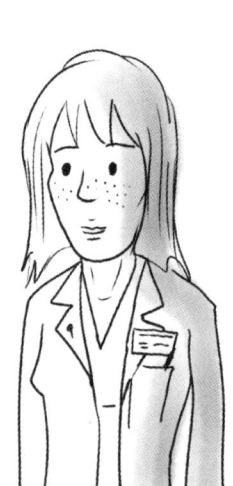

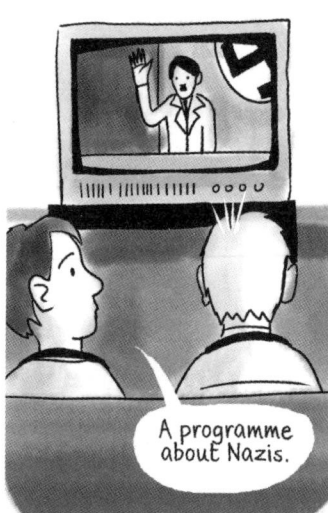

A programme about Nazis.

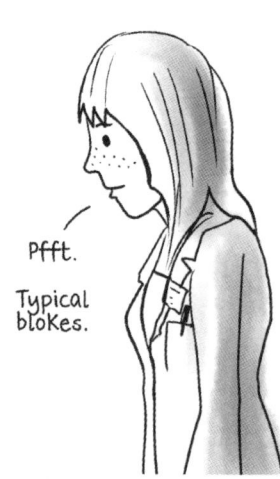

Pfft.

Typical blokes.

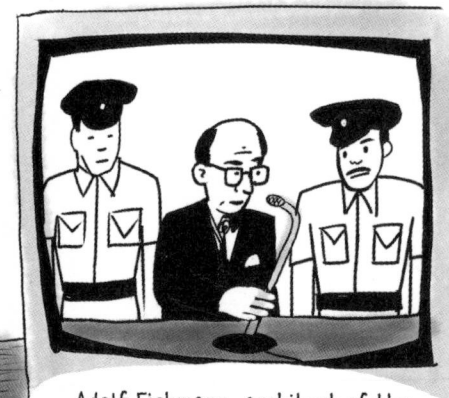

Adolf Eichmann, architect of the Holocaust, at his trial in Jerusalem.

He had been kidnapped in Argentina by Mossad agents and smuggled back to Israel to face trial.

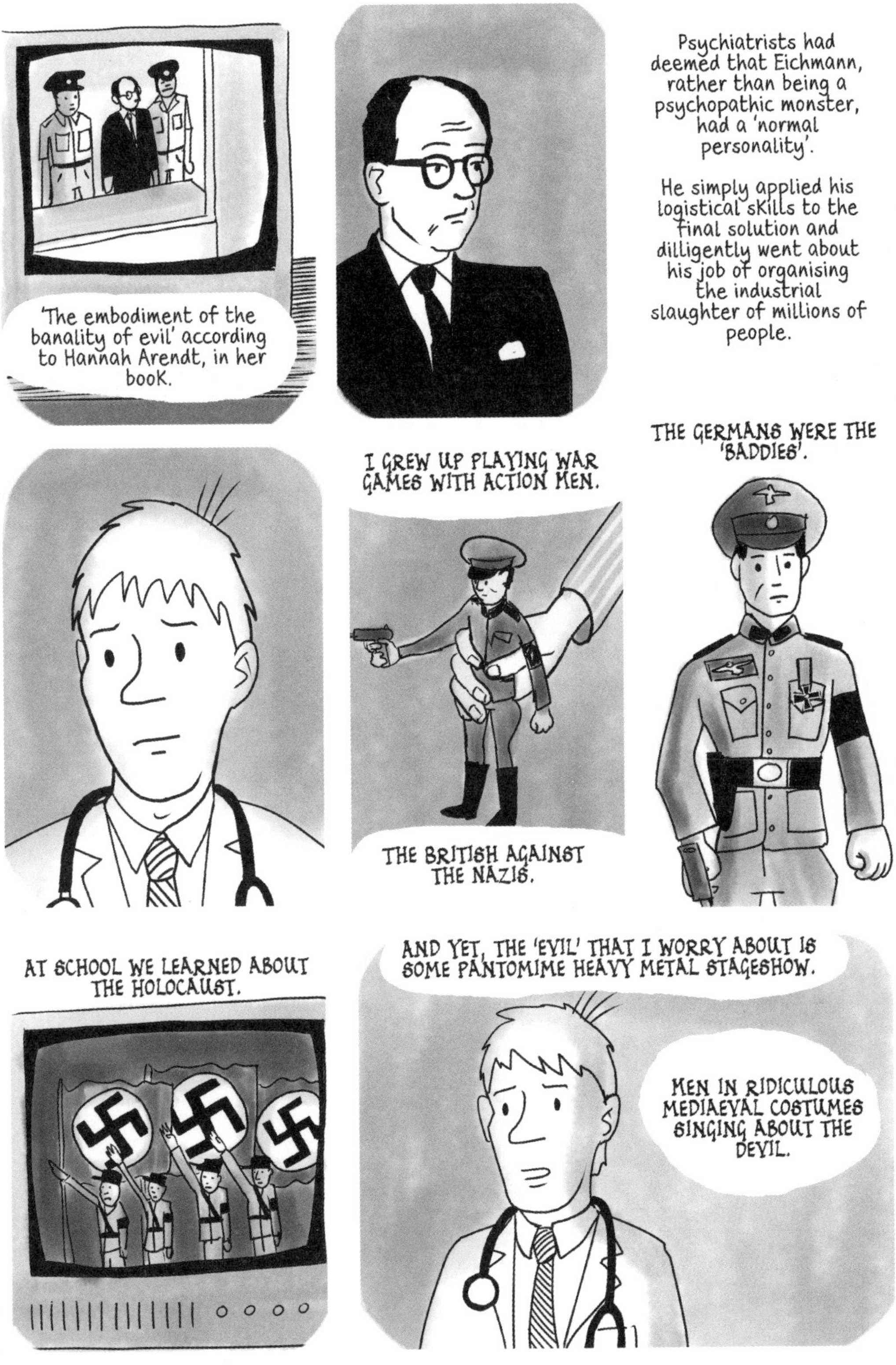
'The embodiment of the banality of evil' according to Hannah Arendt, in her book.
Psychiatrists had deemed that Eichmann, rather than being a psychopathic monster, had a 'normal personality'.
He simply applied his logistical skills to the final solution and dilligently went about his job of organising the industrial slaughter of millions of people.
I GREW UP PLAYING WAR GAMES WITH ACTION MEN.
THE BRITISH AGAINST THE NAZIS.
THE GERMANS WERE THE 'BADDIES'.
AT SCHOOL WE LEARNED ABOUT THE HOLOCAUST.
AND YET, THE 'EVIL' THAT I WORRY ABOUT IS SOME PANTOMIME HEAVY METAL STAGESHOW.
MEN IN RIDICULOUS MEDIAEVAL COSTUMES SINGING ABOUT THE DEVIL.

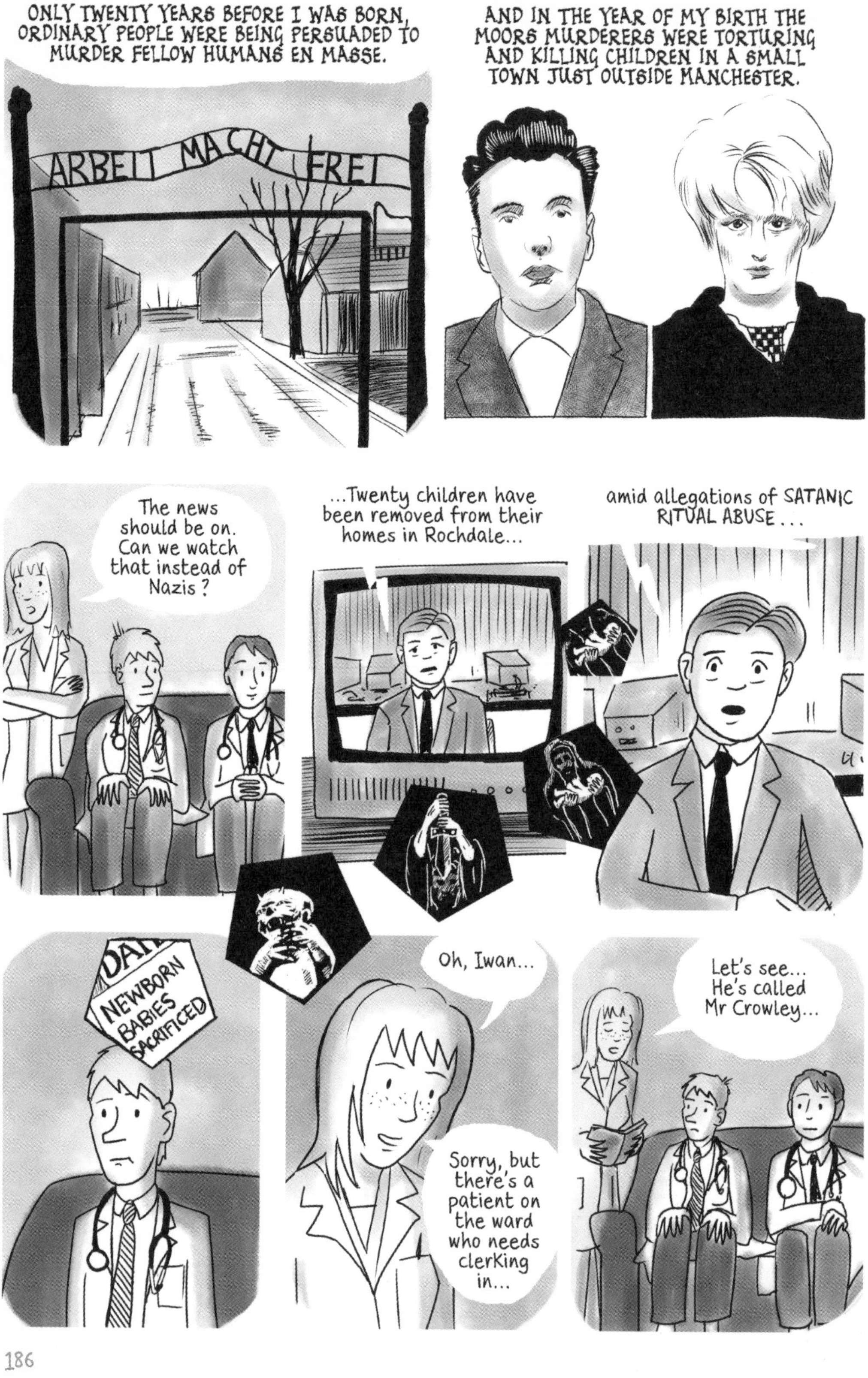

ONLY TWENTY YEARS BEFORE I WAS BORN, ORDINARY PEOPLE WERE BEING PERSUADED TO MURDER FELLOW HUMANS EN MASSE.
ARBEIT MACHT FREI
AND IN THE YEAR OF MY BIRTH THE MOORS MURDERERS WERE TORTURING AND KILLING CHILDREN IN A SMALL TOWN JUST OUTSIDE MANCHESTER.
The news should be on. Can we watch that instead of Nazis ?
...Twenty children have been removed from their homes in Rochdale...
amid allegations of SATANIC RITUAL ABUSE...
NEWBORN BABIES SACRIFICED
Oh, Iwan...
Sorry, but there's a patient on the ward who needs clerKing in...
Let's see... He's called Mr Crowley...

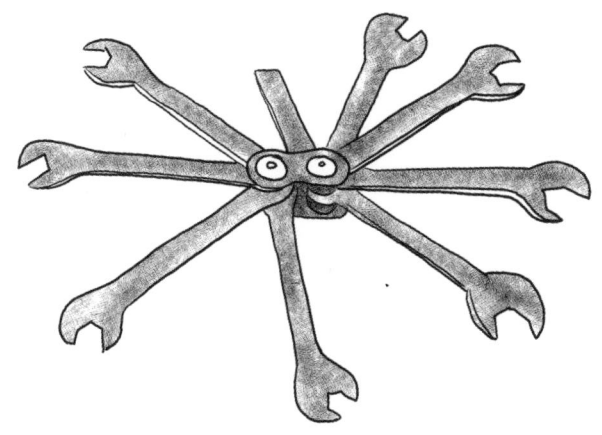

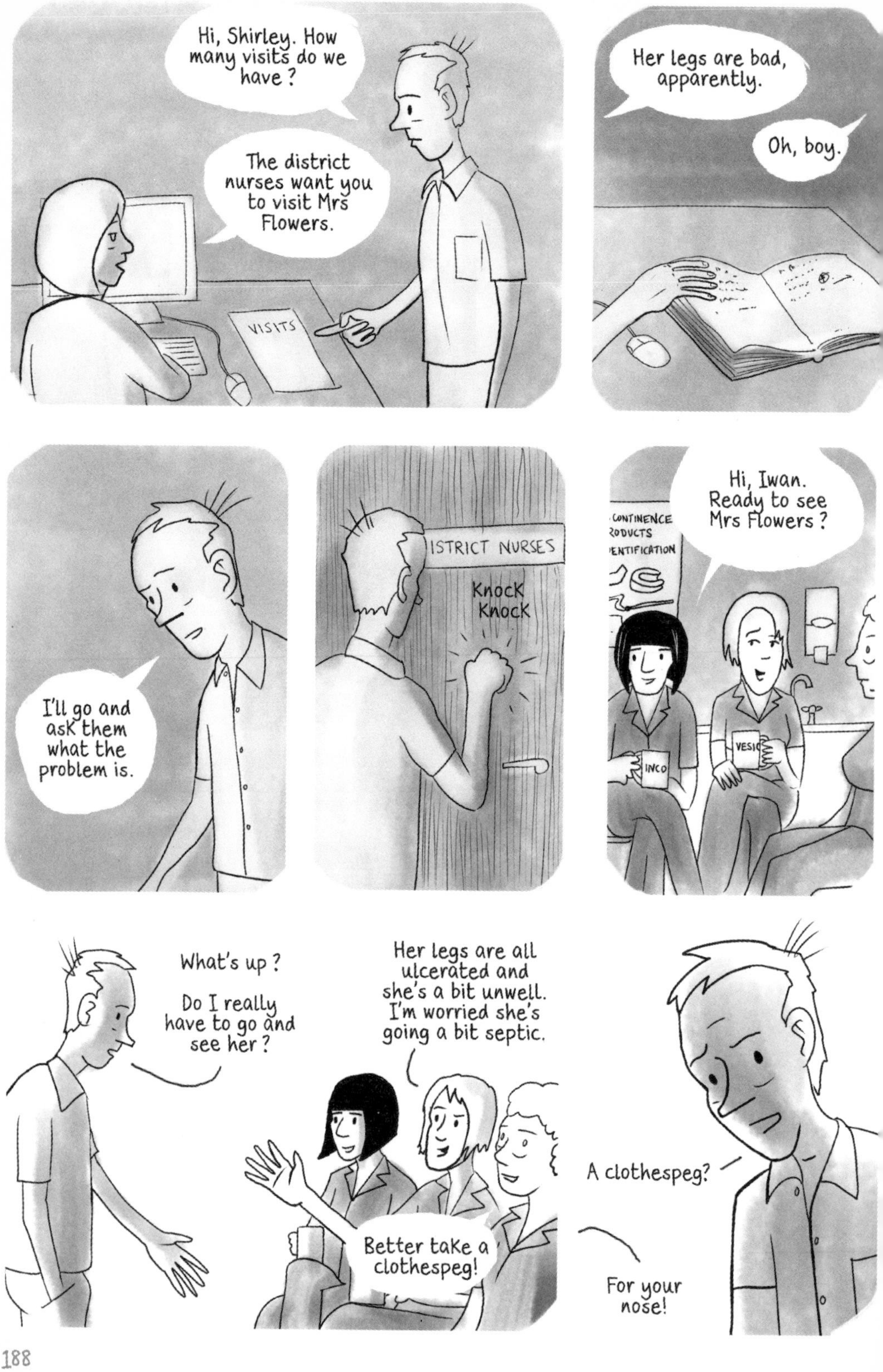
Hi, Shirley. How many visits do we have?
The district nurses want you to visit Mrs Flowers.
VISITS
Her legs are bad, apparently.
Oh, boy.
I'll go and ask them what the problem is.
ISTRICT NURSES
Knock Knock
CONTINENCE
RODUCTS
ENTIFICATION
Hi, Iwan. Ready to see Mrs Flowers?
INCO
VESIC
What's up?
Do I really have to go and see her?
Her legs are all ulcerated and she's a bit unwell. I'm worried she's going a bit septic.
Better take a clothespeg!
A clothespeg?
For your nose!

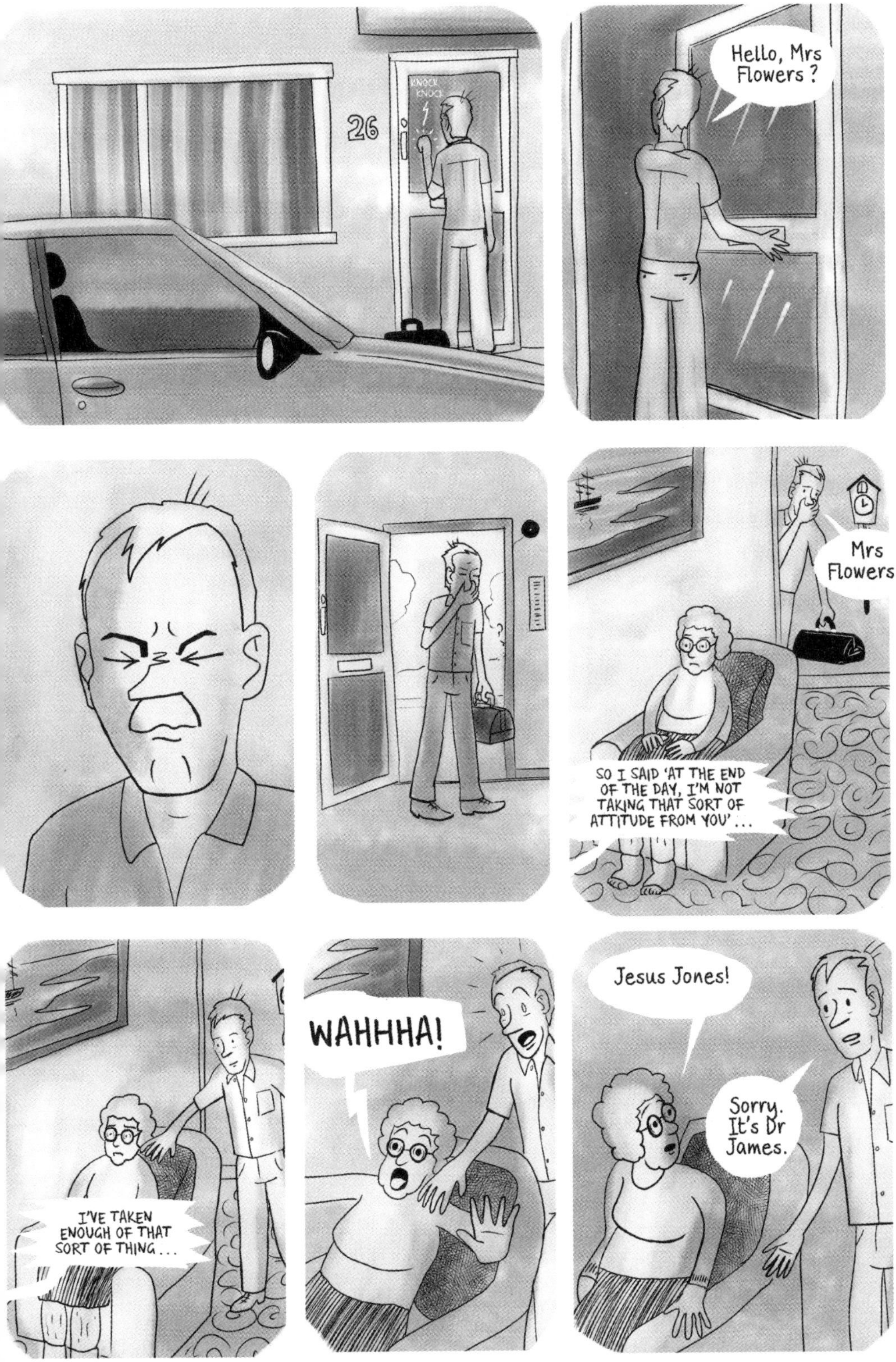
KNOCK KNOCK
26
Hello, Mrs Flowers?
Mrs Flowers?
SO I SAID 'AT THE END OF THE DAY, I'M NOT TAKING THAT SORT OF ATTITUDE FROM YOU'...
I'VE TAKEN ENOUGH OF THAT SORT OF THING...
WAHHHA!
Jesus Jones!
Sorry. It's Dr James.

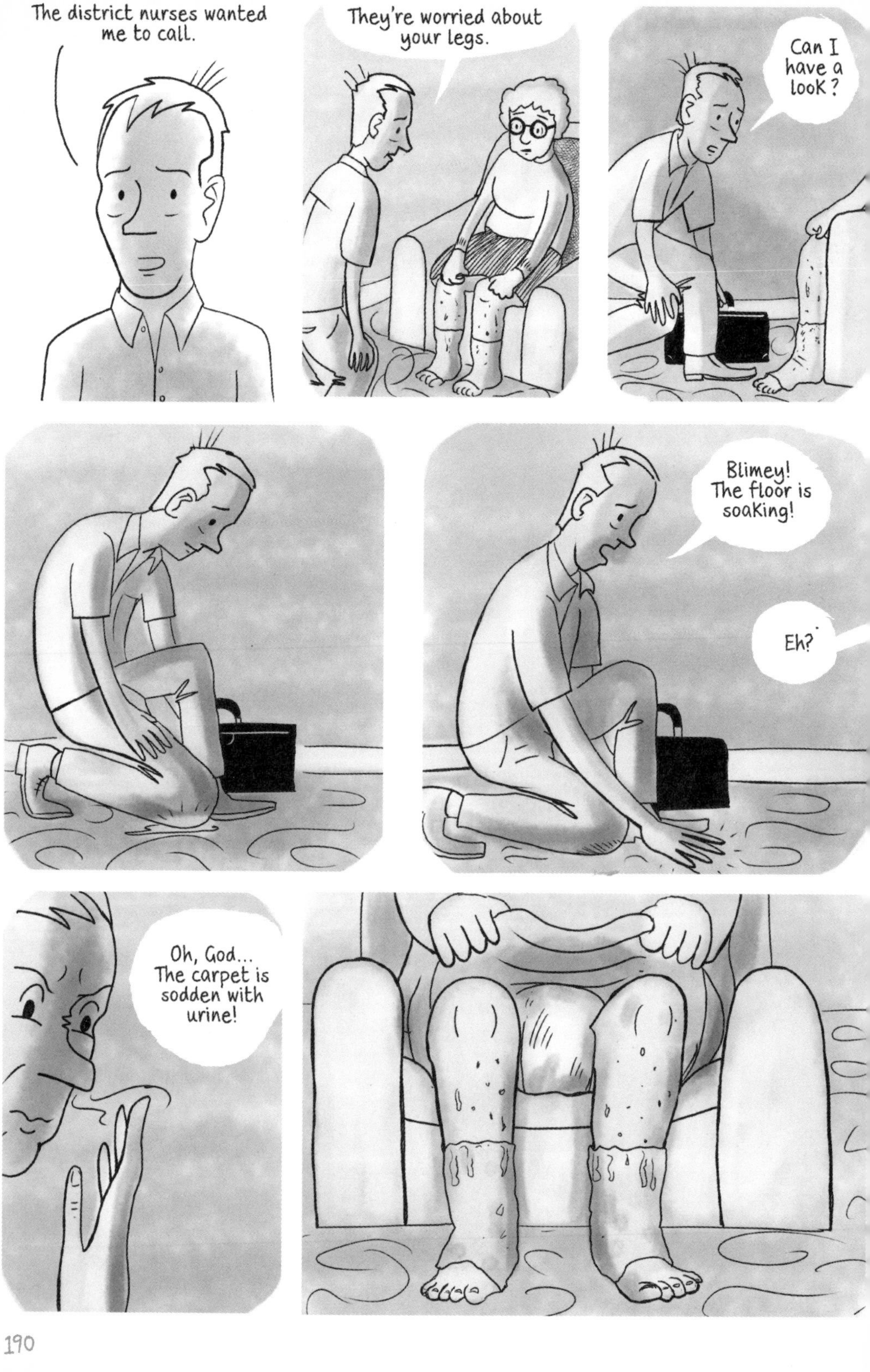
The district nurses wanted me to call.
They're worried about your legs.
Can I have a look?
Blimey! The floor is soaking!
Eh?
Oh, God... The carpet is sodden with urine!

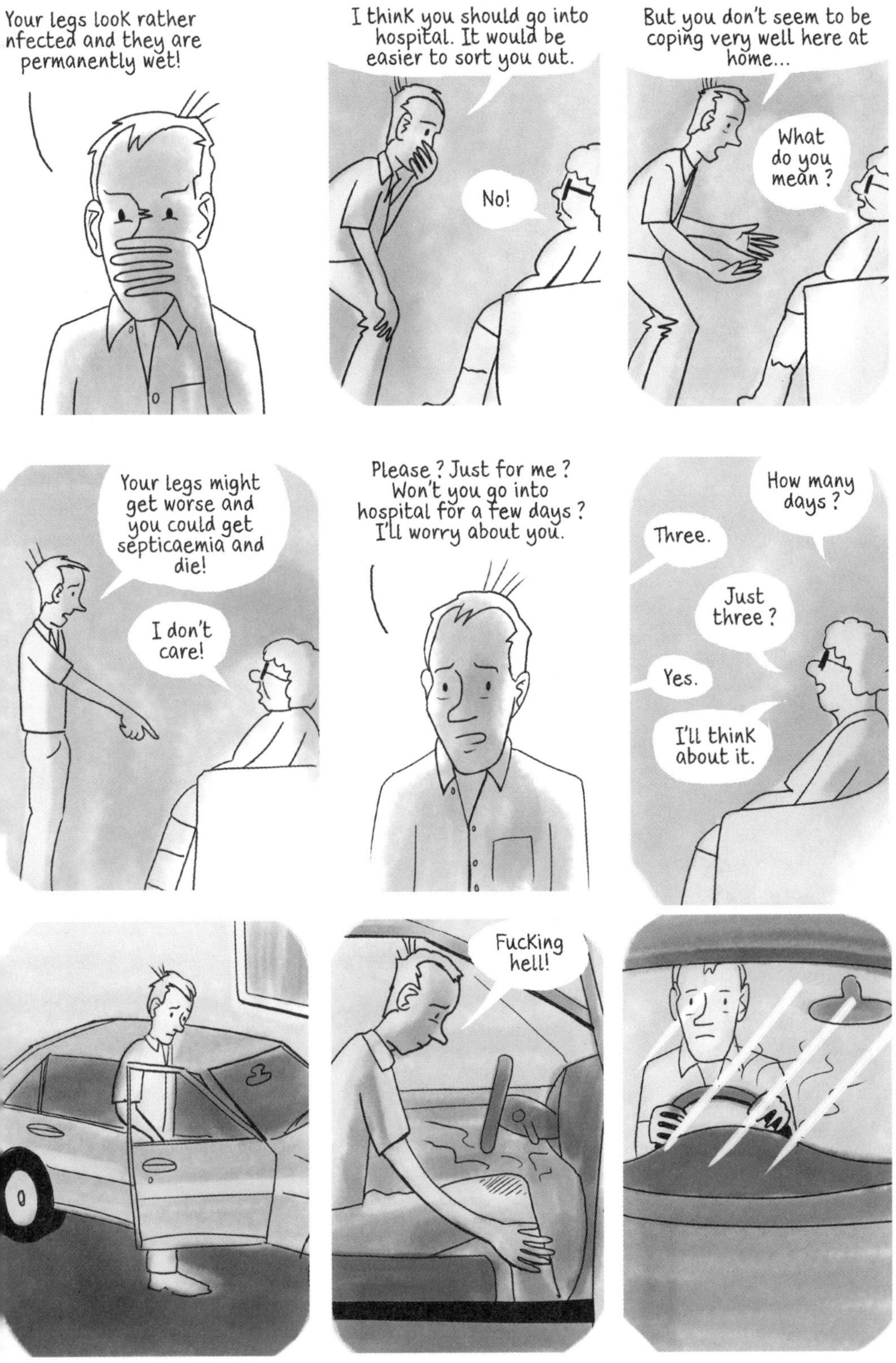
Your legs look rather nfected and they are permanently wet!
I think you should go into hospital. It would be easier to sort you out.
No!
But you don't seem to be coping very well here at home...
What do you mean ?
Your legs might get worse and you could get septicaemia and die!
I don't care!
Please ? Just for me ? Won't you go into hospital for a few days ? I'll worry about you.
How many days ?
Three.
Just three ?
Yes.
I'll think about it.
Fucking hell!

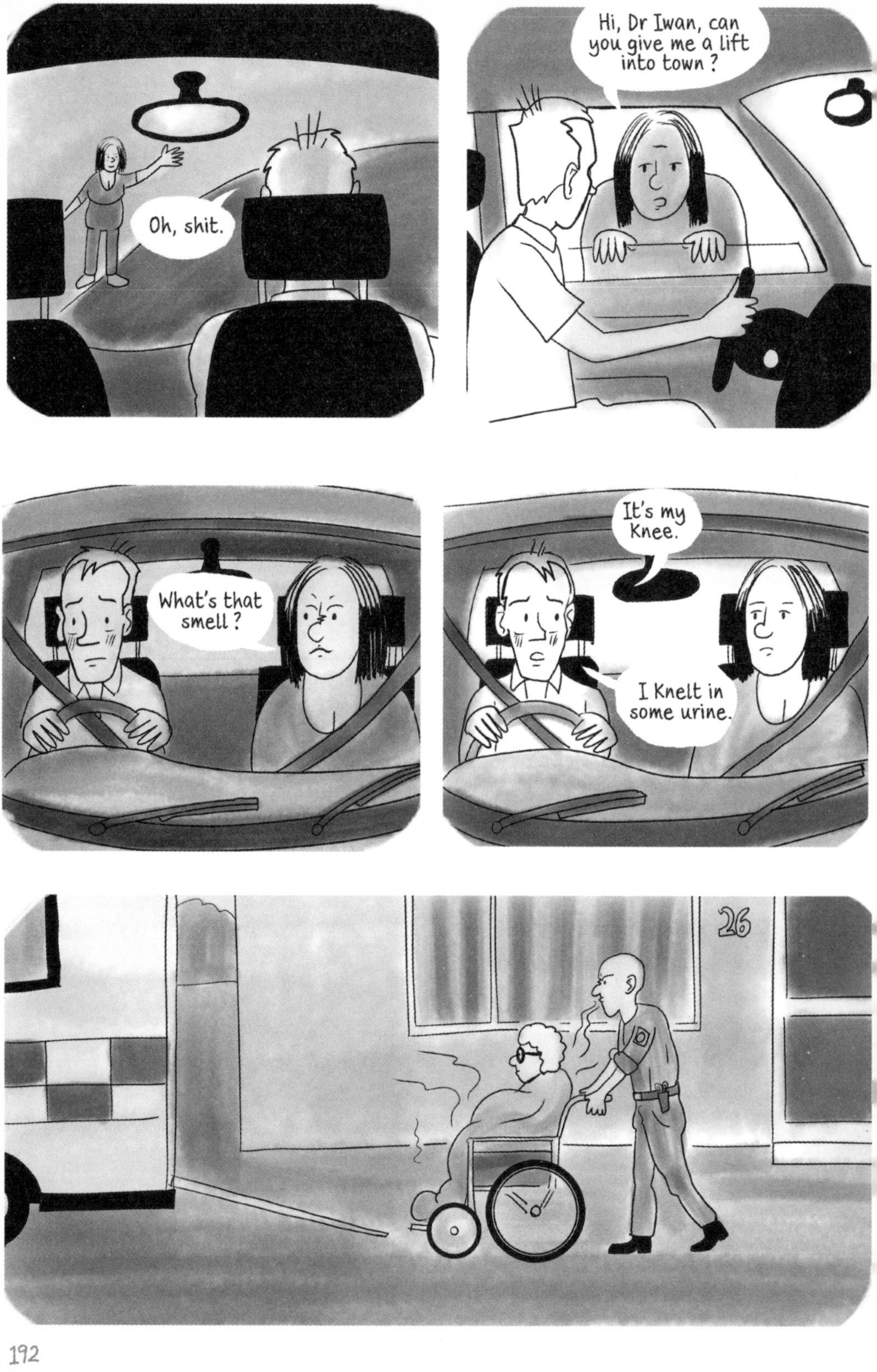
Oh, shit.
Hi, Dr Iwan, can you give me a lift into town?
What's that smell?
It's my Knee.
I Knelt in some urine.
26

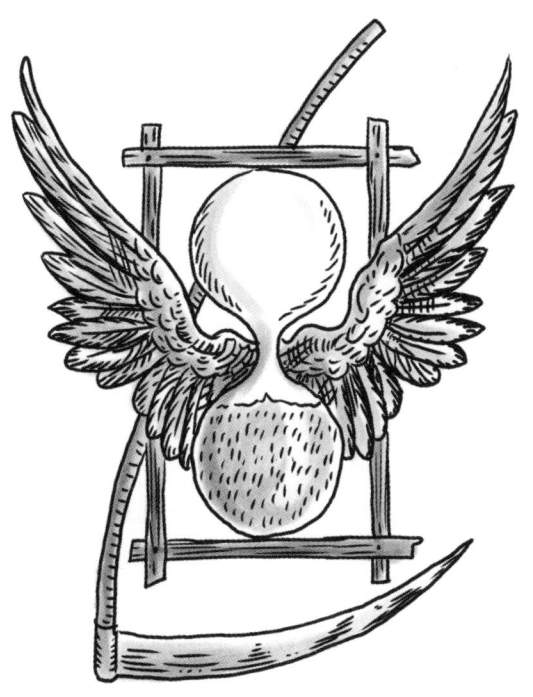

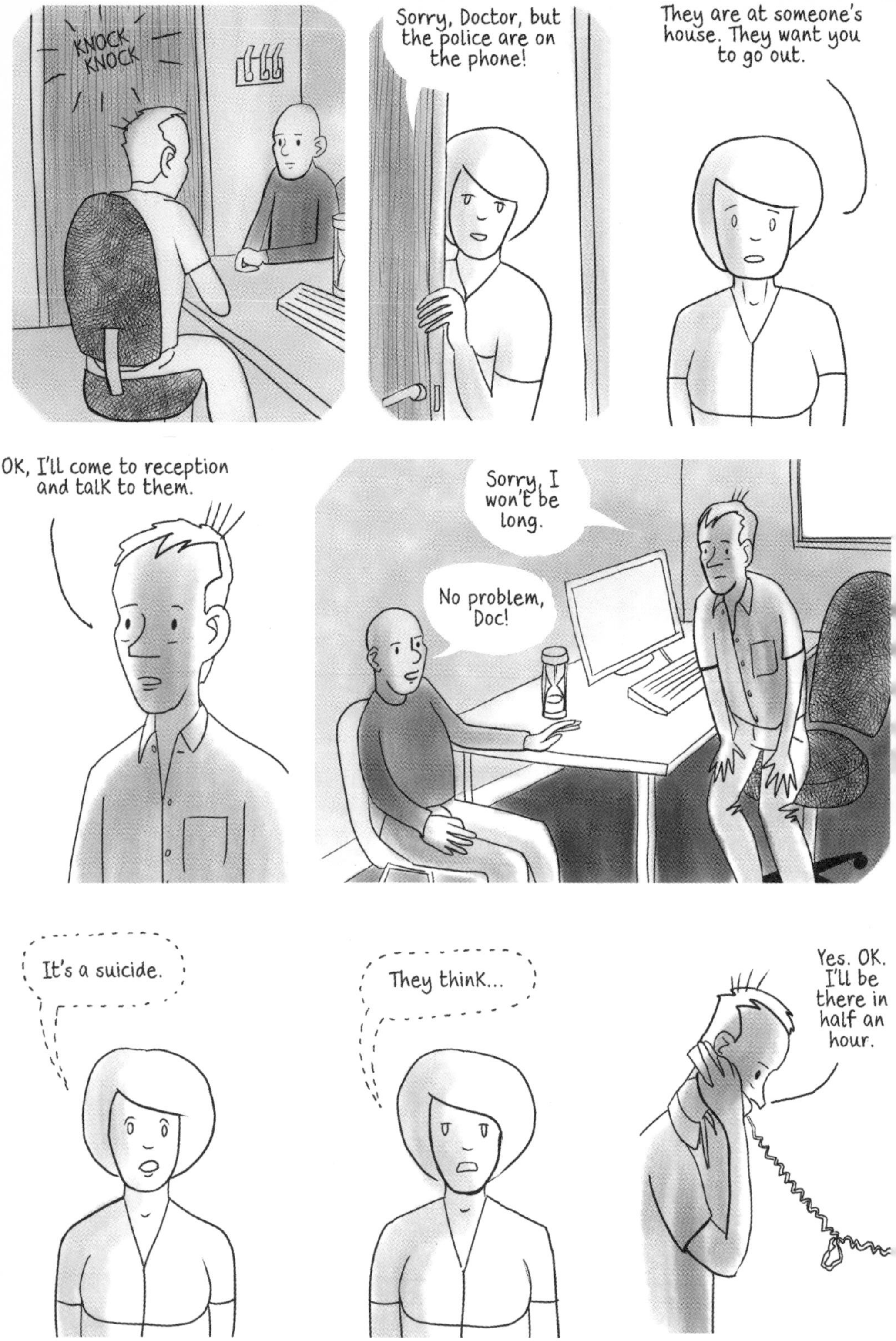
KNOCK KNOCK
Sorry, Doctor, but the police are on the phone!
They are at someone's house. They want you to go out.
OK, I'll come to reception and talk to them.
Sorry, I won't be long.
No problem, Doc!
It's a suicide.
They think...
Yes. OK. I'll be there in half an hour.

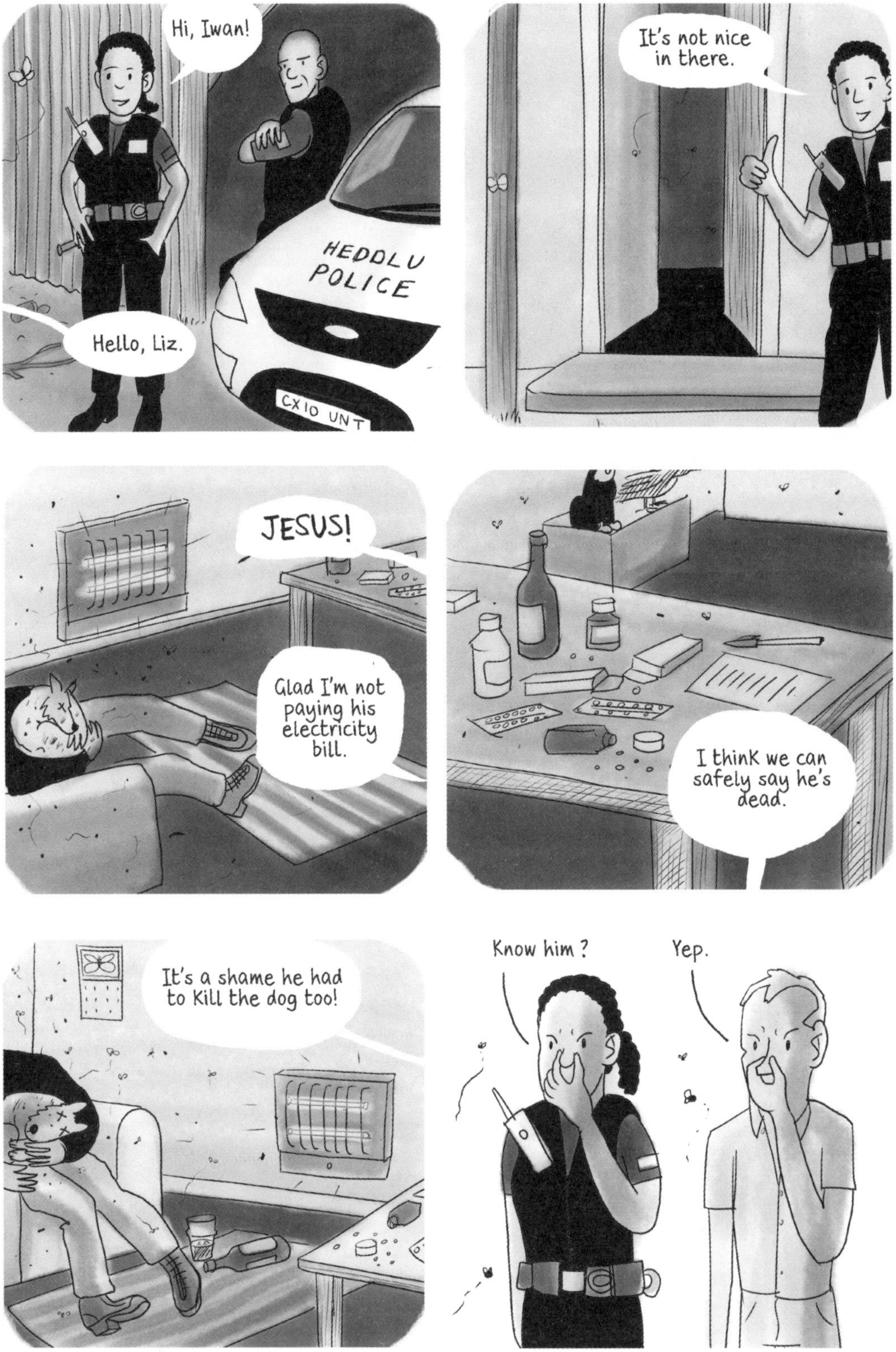
Hi, Iwan!
Hello, Liz.
HEDDLU
POLICE
CX10 UNT
It's not nice in there.
JESUS!
Glad I'm not paying his electricity bill.
I think we can safely say he's dead.
It's a shame he had to Kill the dog too!
Know him ?
Yep.

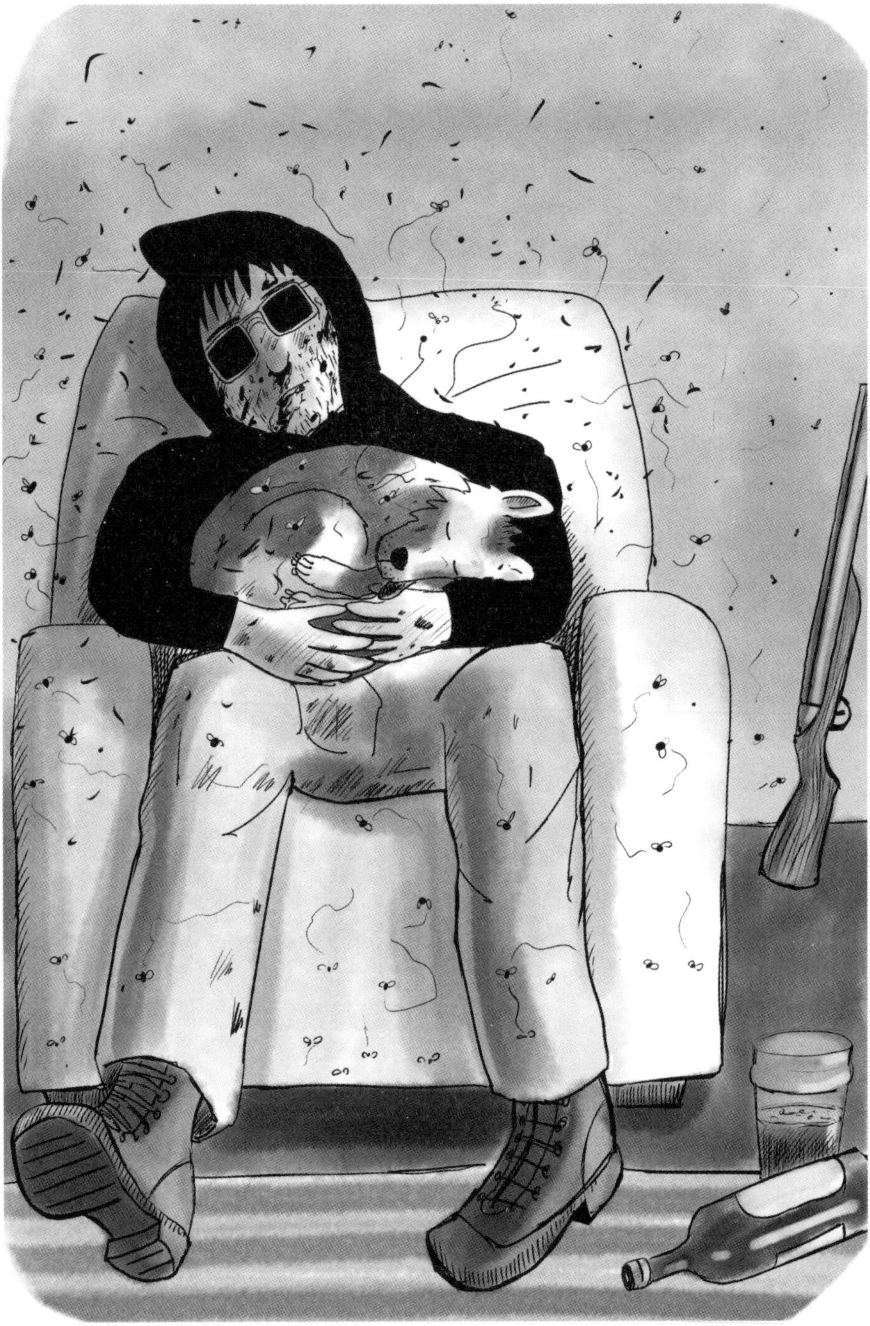

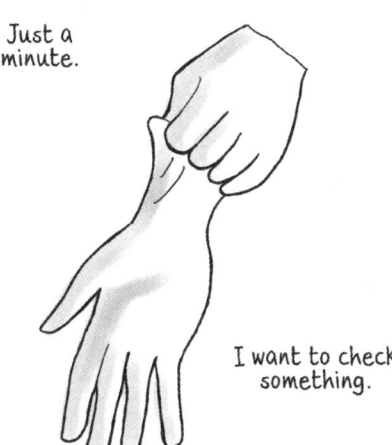

Just a minute.

I want to check something.

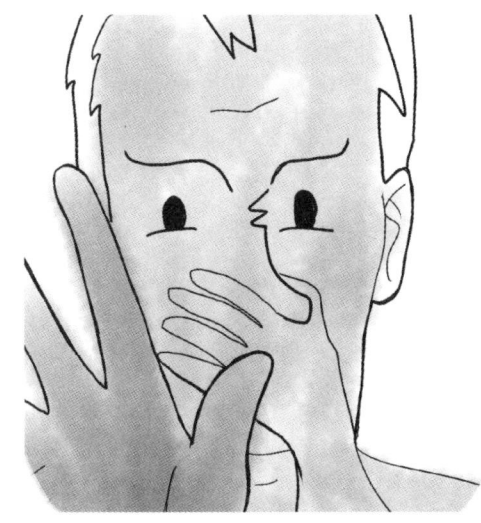

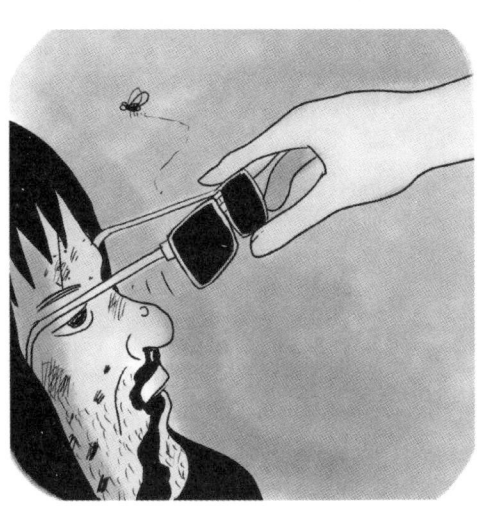

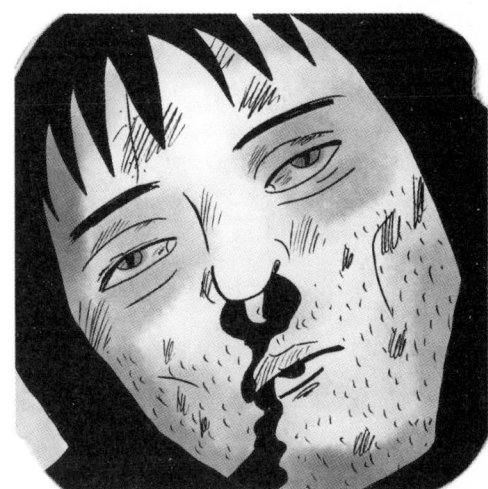

He's got bilateral colobomas... defects of the iris. That's where the 'goat eye' rumour came from.

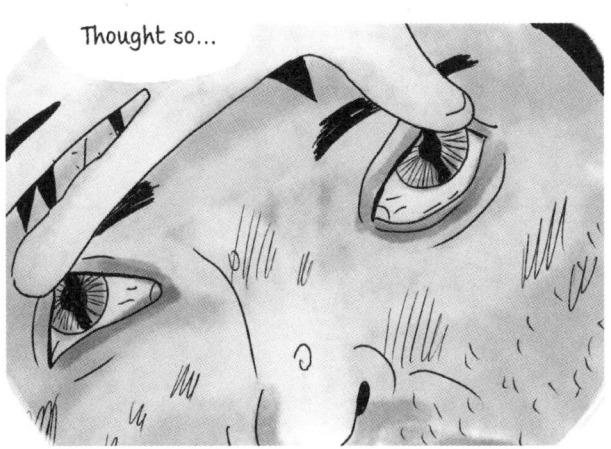

Thought so...

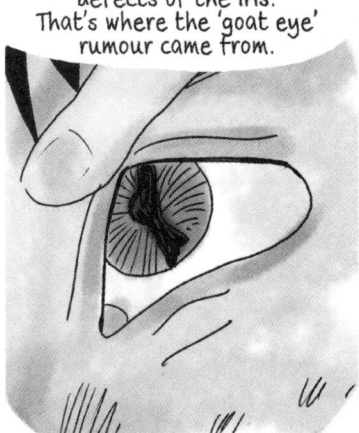

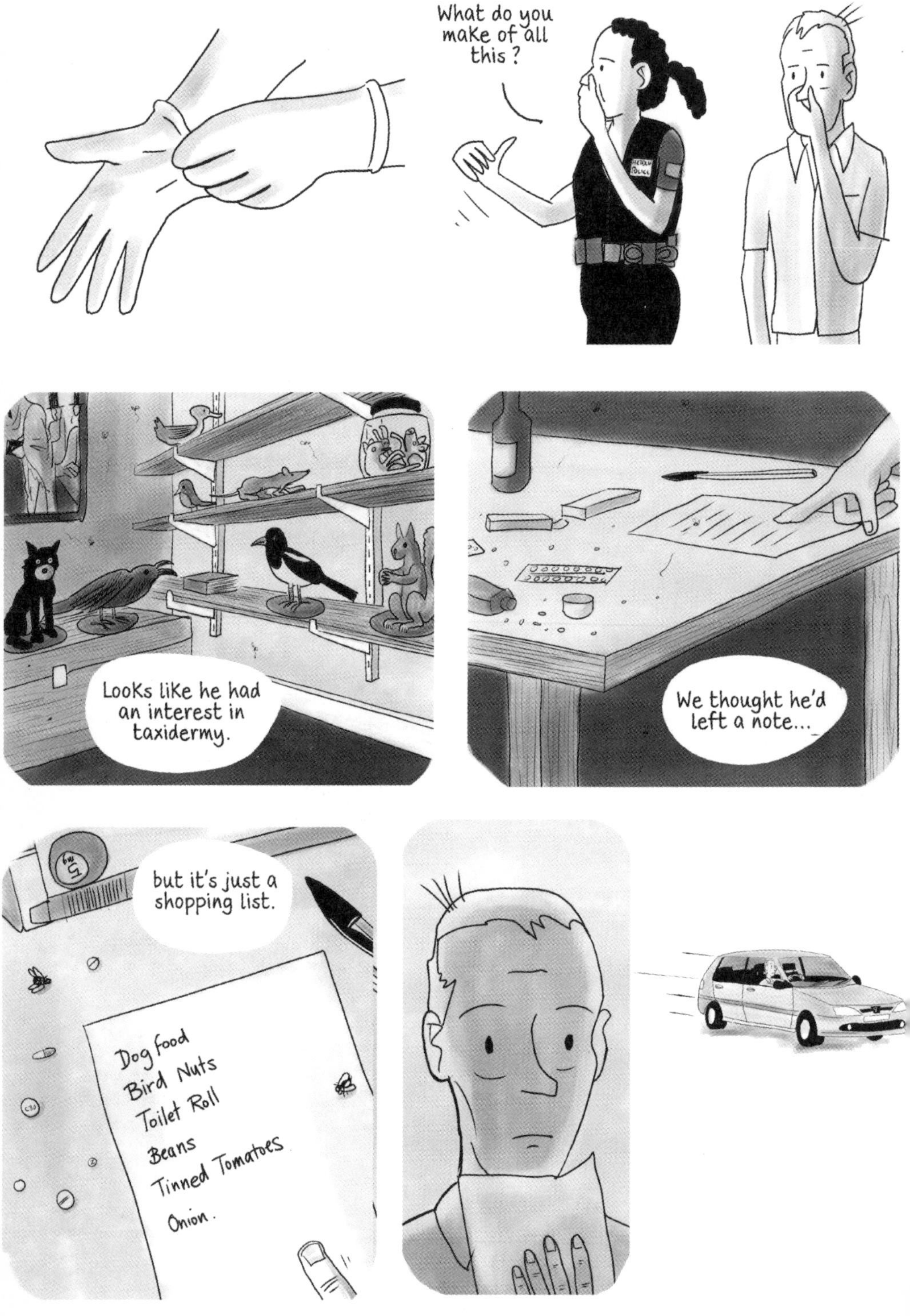

What do you make of all this ?
Looks like he had an interest in taxidermy.
We thought he'd left a note...
but it's just a shopping list.
Dog food
Bird Nuts
Toilet Roll
Beans
Tinned Tomatoes
Onion.

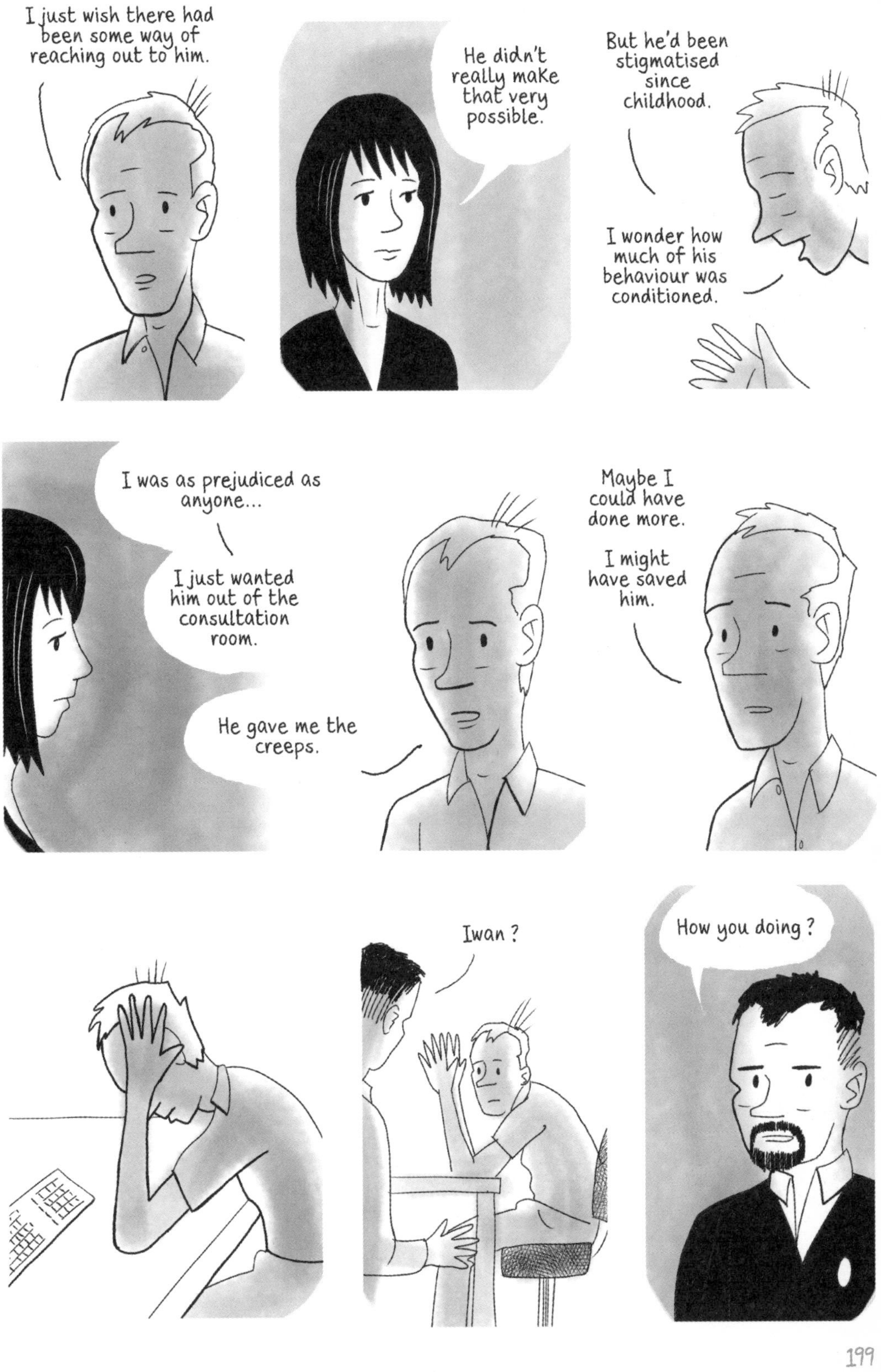

I just wish there had been some way of reaching out to him.
He didn't really make that very possible.
But he'd been stigmatised since childhood.
I wonder how much of his behaviour was conditioned.
I was as prejudiced as anyone...
I just wanted him out of the consultation room.
He gave me the creeps.
Maybe I could have done more.
I might have saved him.
Iwan ?
How you doing ?

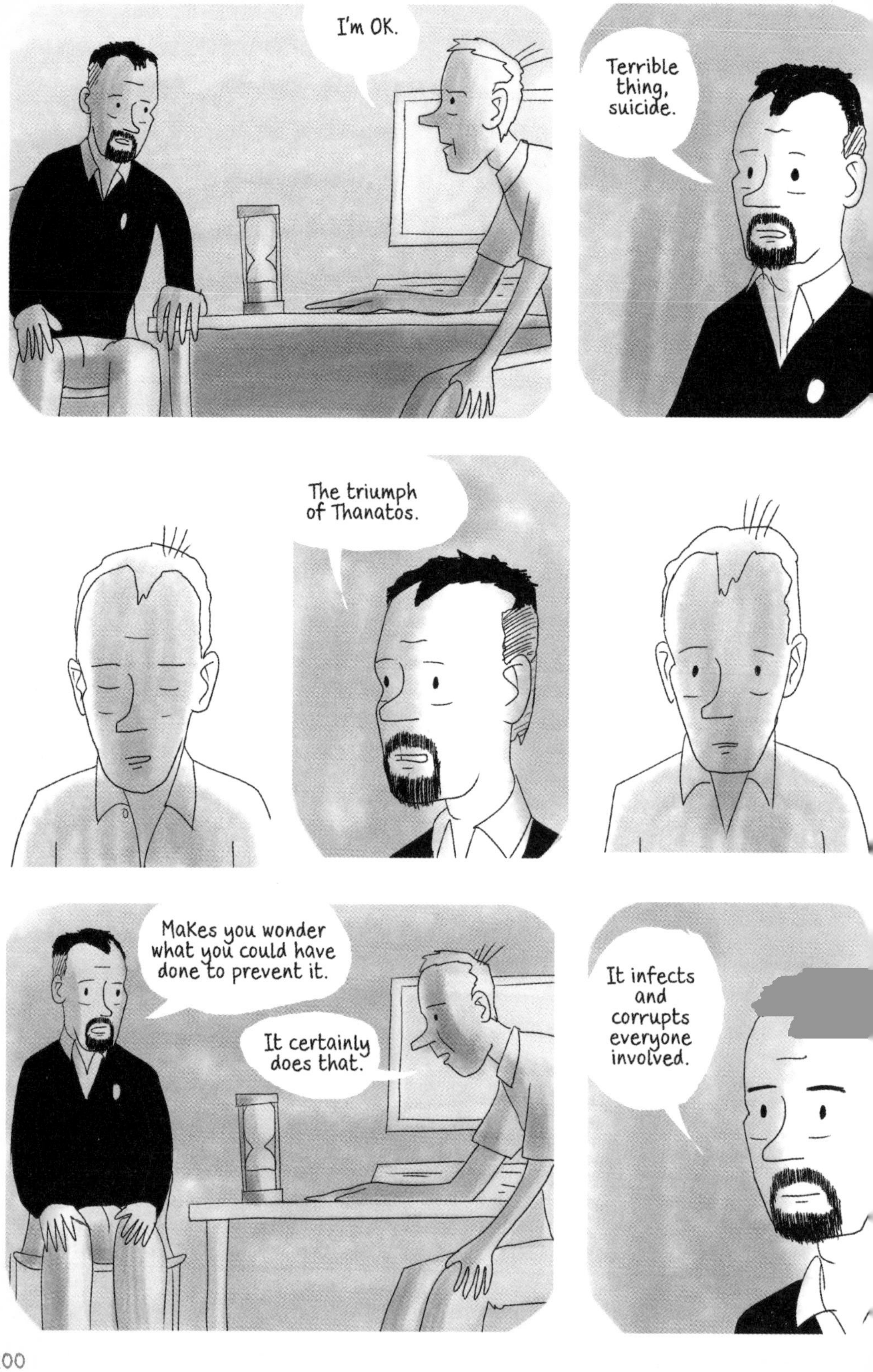
I'm OK.
Terrible thing, suicide.
The triumph of Thanatos.
Makes you wonder what you could have done to prevent it.
It certainly does that.
It infects and corrupts everyone involved.

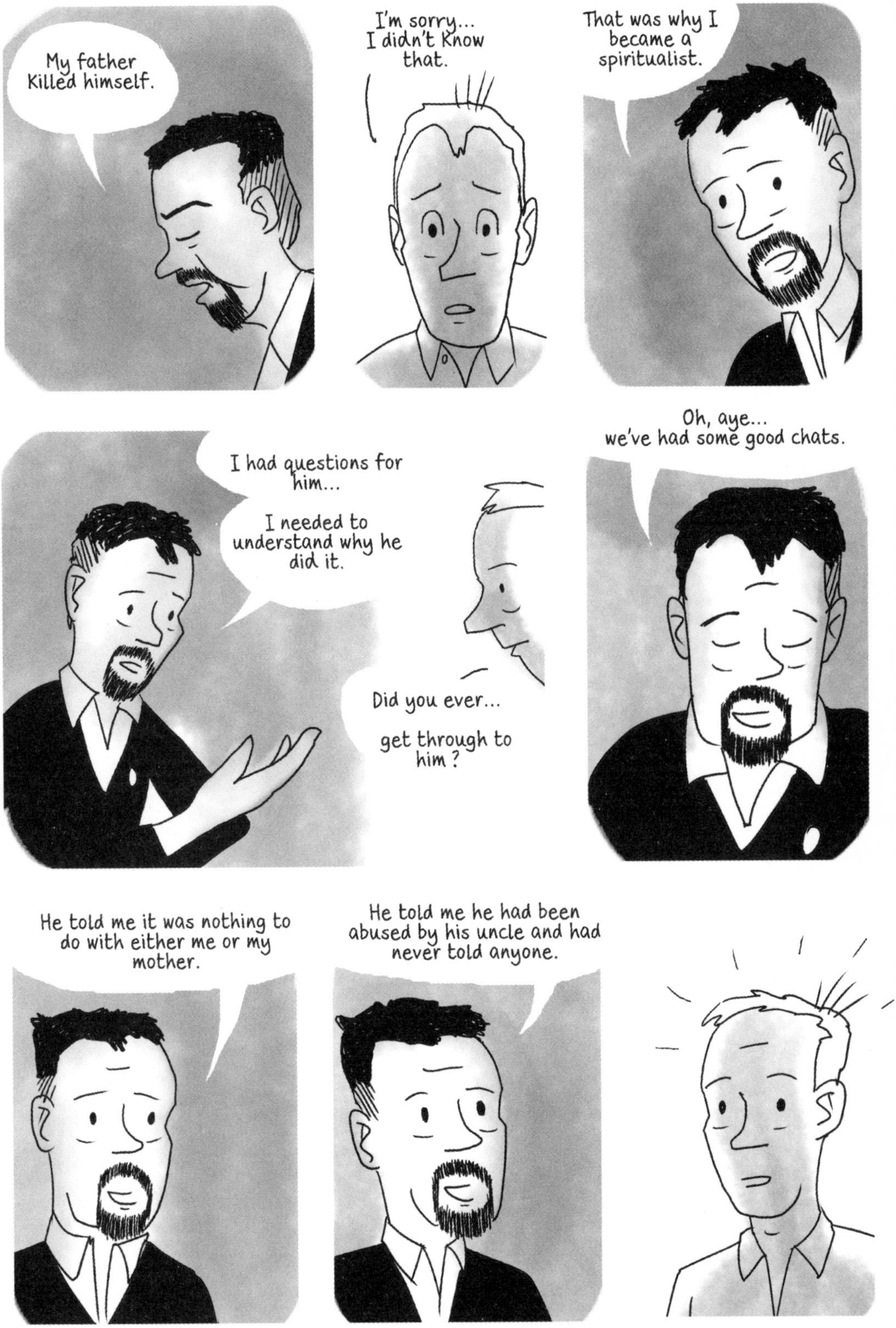
My father Killed himself.
I'm sorry... I didn't Know that.
That was why I became a spiritualist.
I had questions for him...
I needed to understand why he did it.
Did you ever...
get through to him?
Oh, aye... we've had some good chats.
He told me it was nothing to do with either me or my mother.
He told me he had been abused by his uncle and had never told anyone.

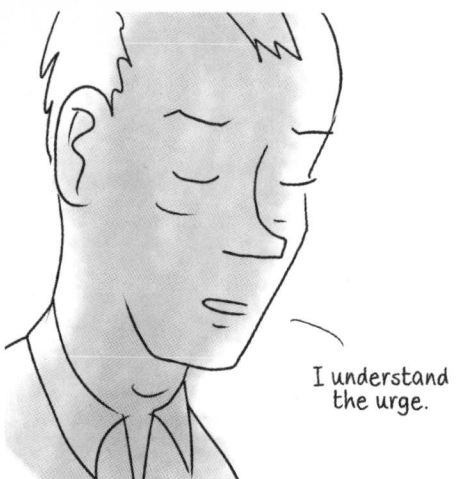

I understand the urge.

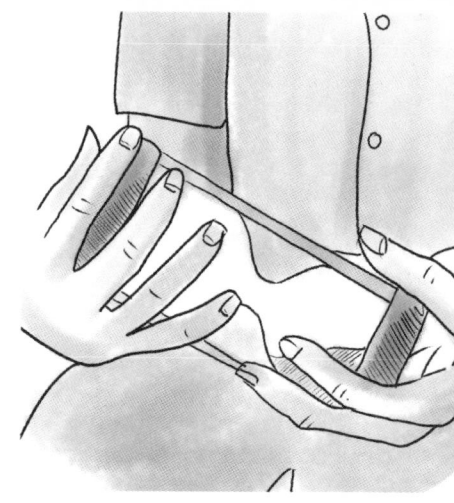

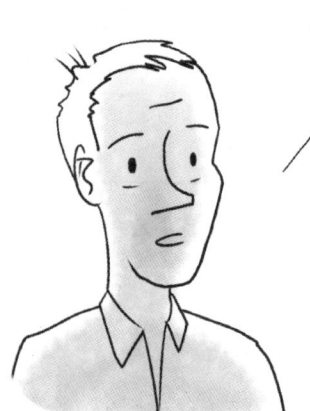

Have done since I was a teenager.

What the hell are you talking about?

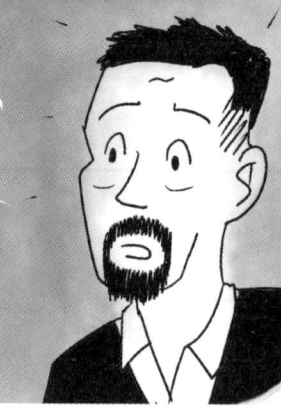

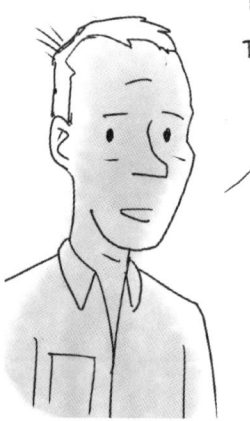

Thanatos.

The death drive.

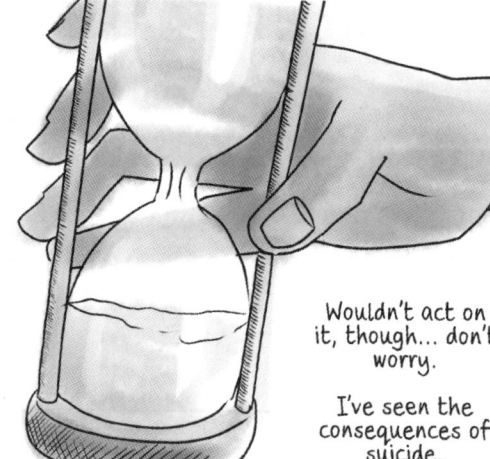

Wouldn't act on it, though... don't worry.

I've seen the consequences of suicide.

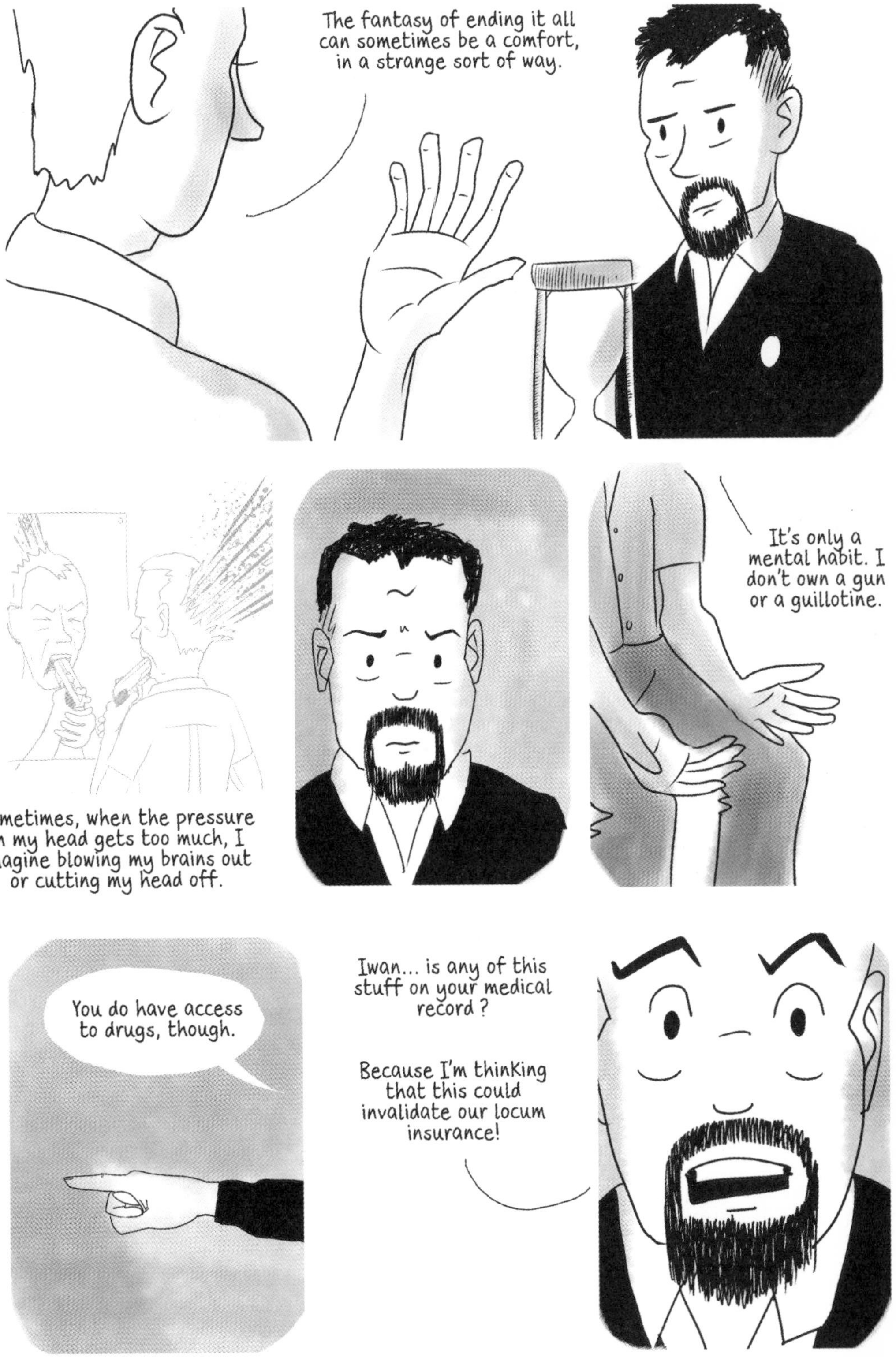
The fantasy of ending it all can sometimes be a comfort, in a strange sort of way.
ometimes, when the pressure n my head gets too much, I nagine blowing my brains out or cutting my head off.
It's only a mental habit. I don't own a gun or a guillotine.
You do have access to drugs, though.
Iwan... is any of this stuff on your medical record?
Because I'm thinking that this could invalidate our locum insurance!

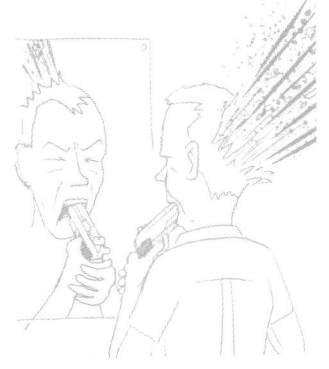

N
OCTOBER
SEPTEMBER
AUGUST
Y
JUNE

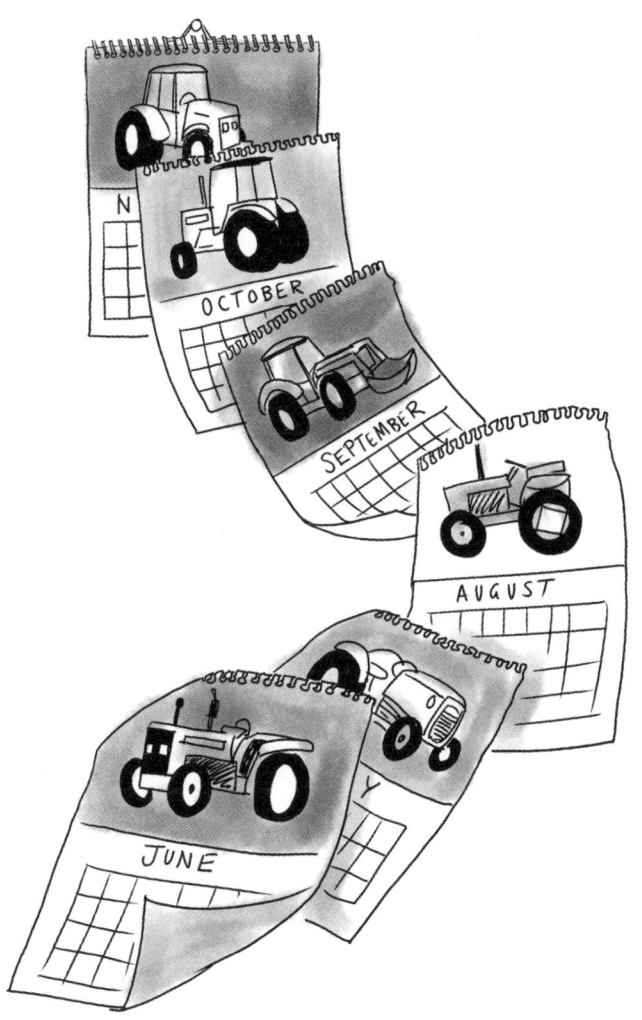

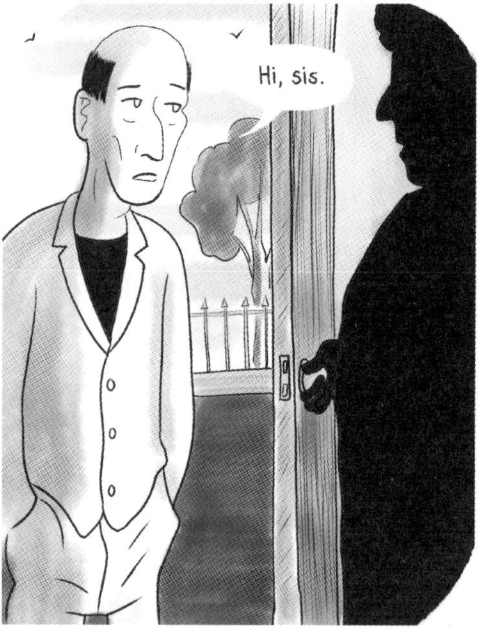
Hi, sis.

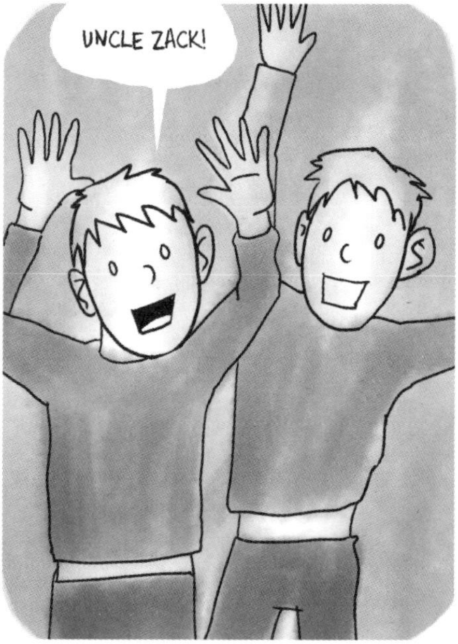
UNCLE ZACK!

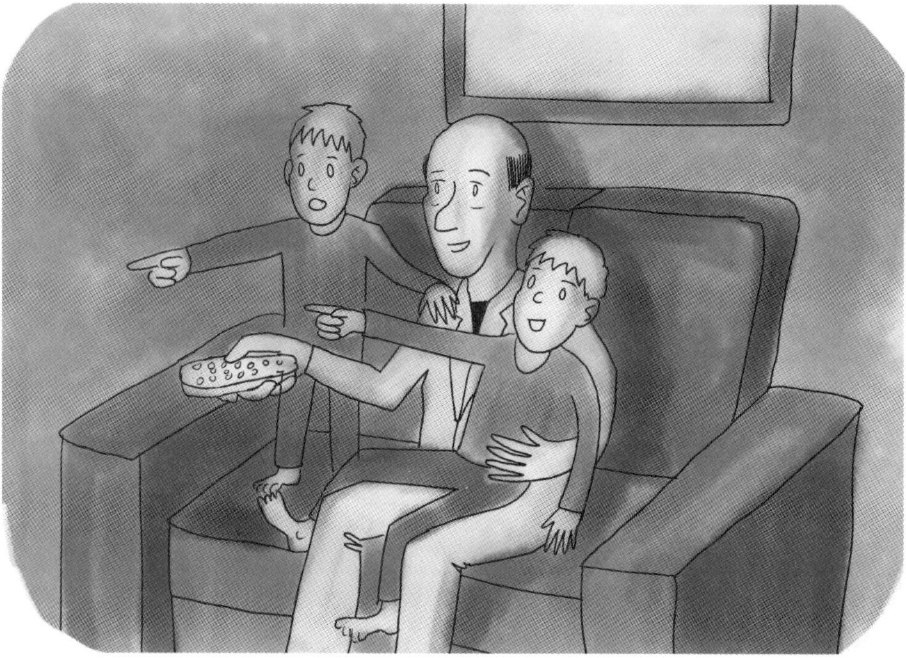

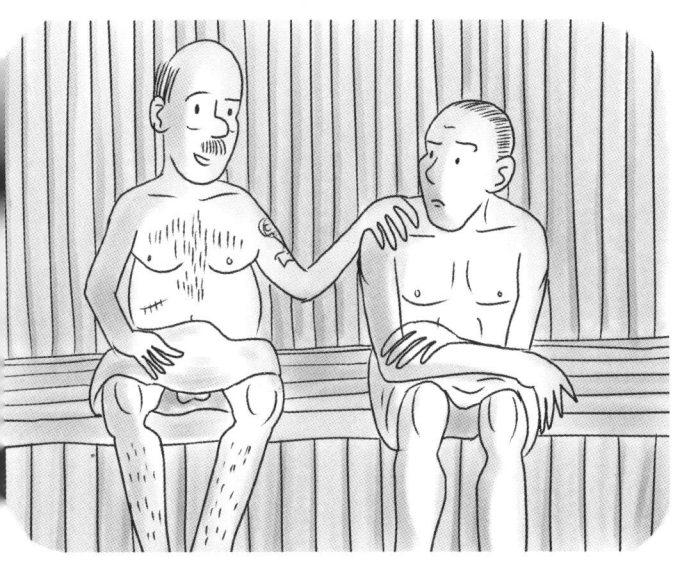

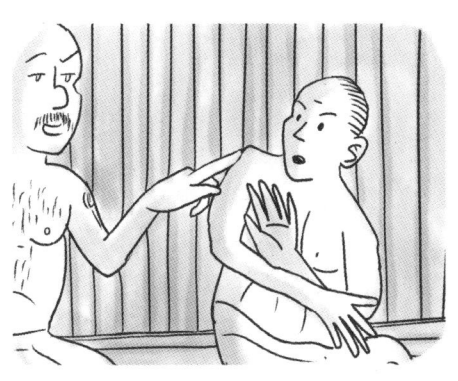

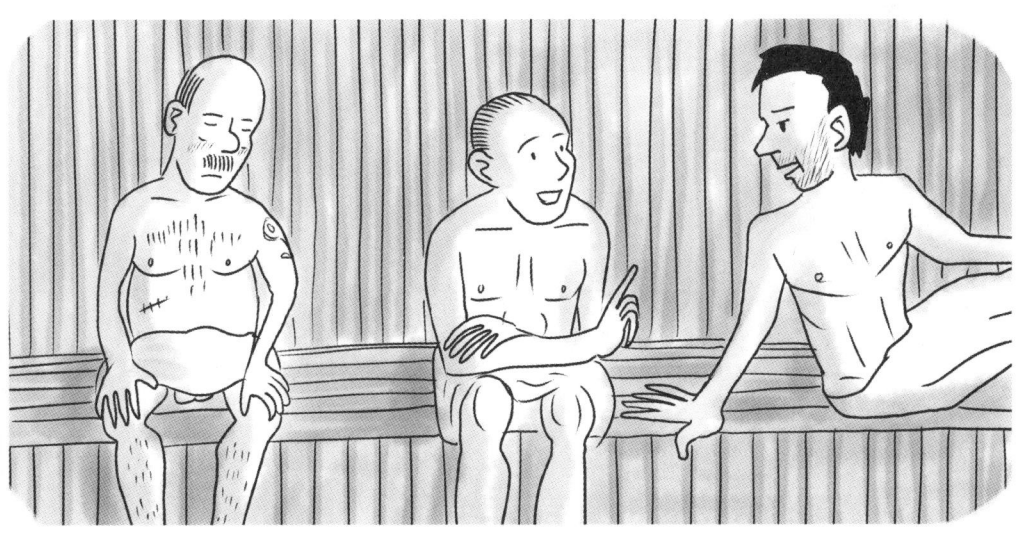

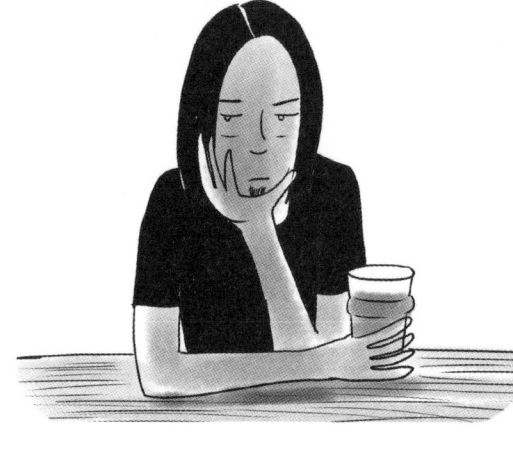

So, Lois... what happened with Dave?

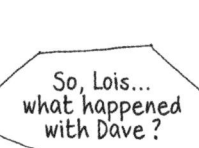

I thought that things were going great...

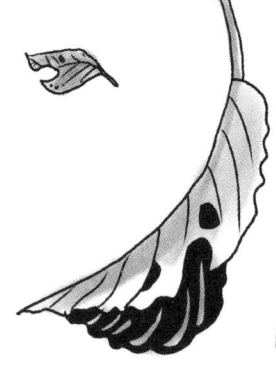

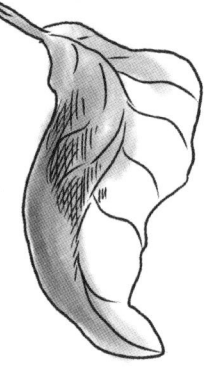

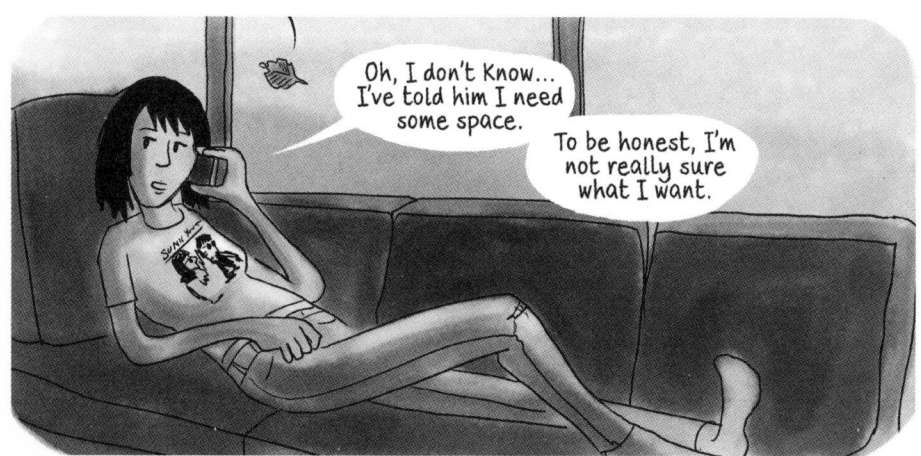

Oh, I don't know... I've told him I need some space.

To be honest, I'm not really sure what I want.

ANTHONY CULVER
1950 – 2012
POET

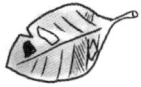

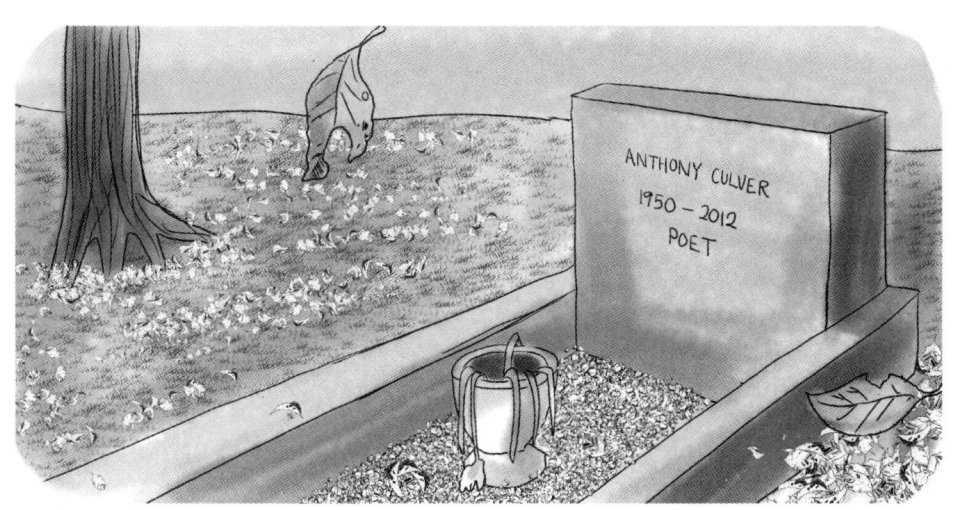

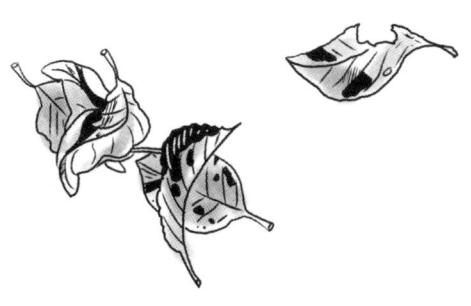

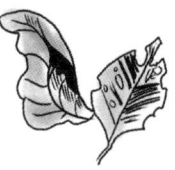

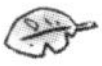

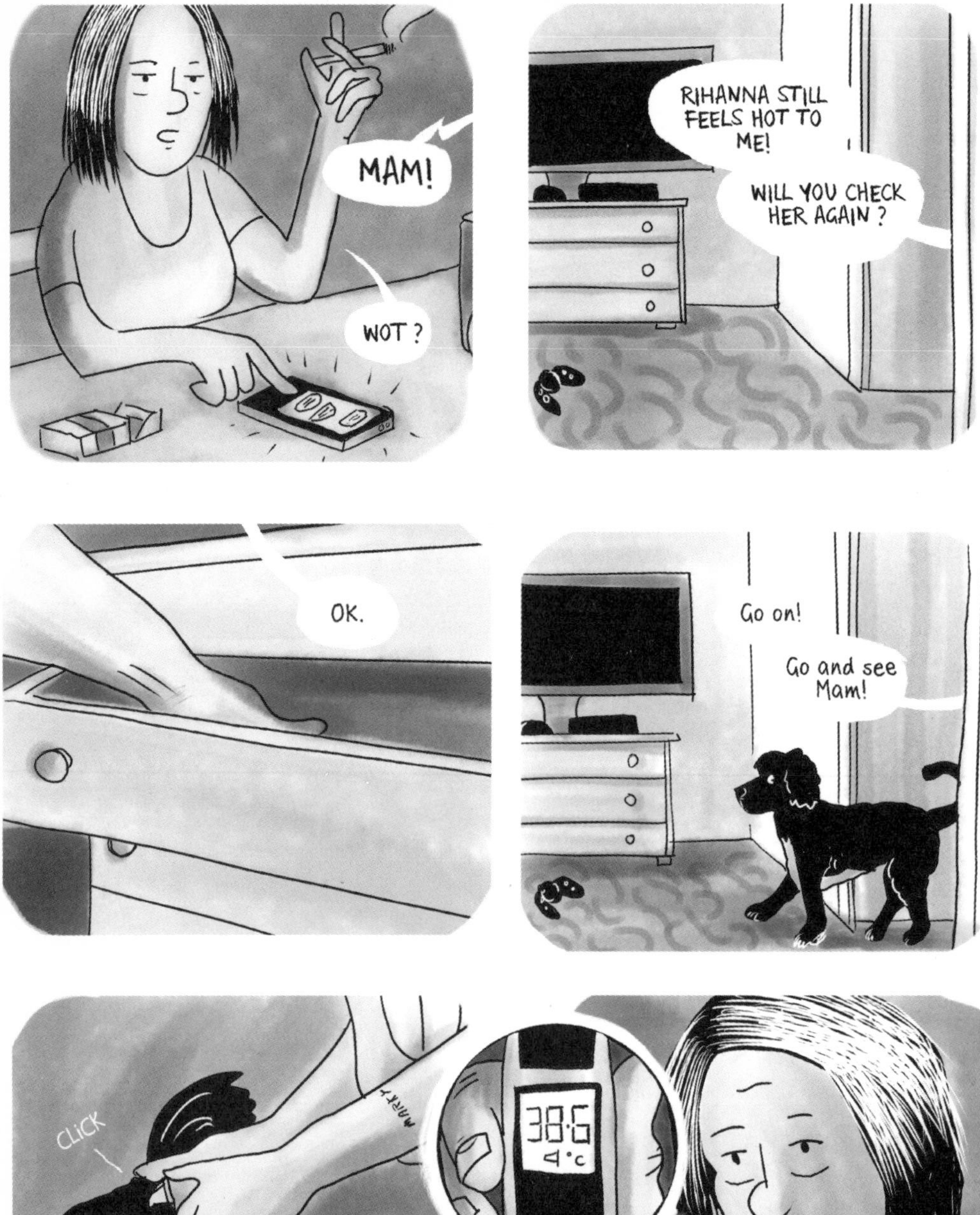
MAM!
WOT ?
RIHANNA STILL FEELS HOT TO ME!
WILL YOU CHECK HER AGAIN ?
OK.
Go on!
Go and see Mam!
CLICK
38.6 °c
YELP!
She's fine.

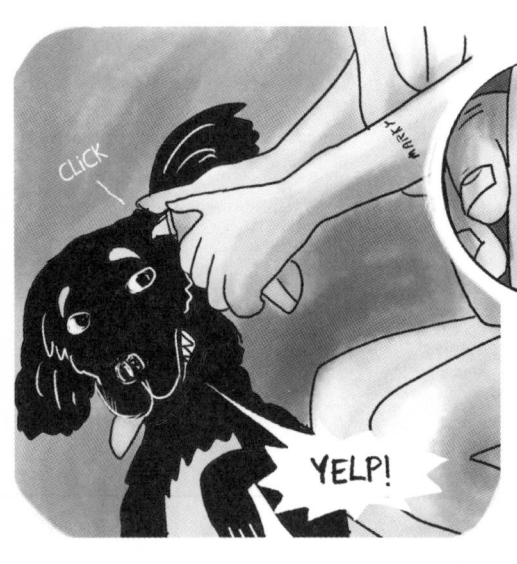

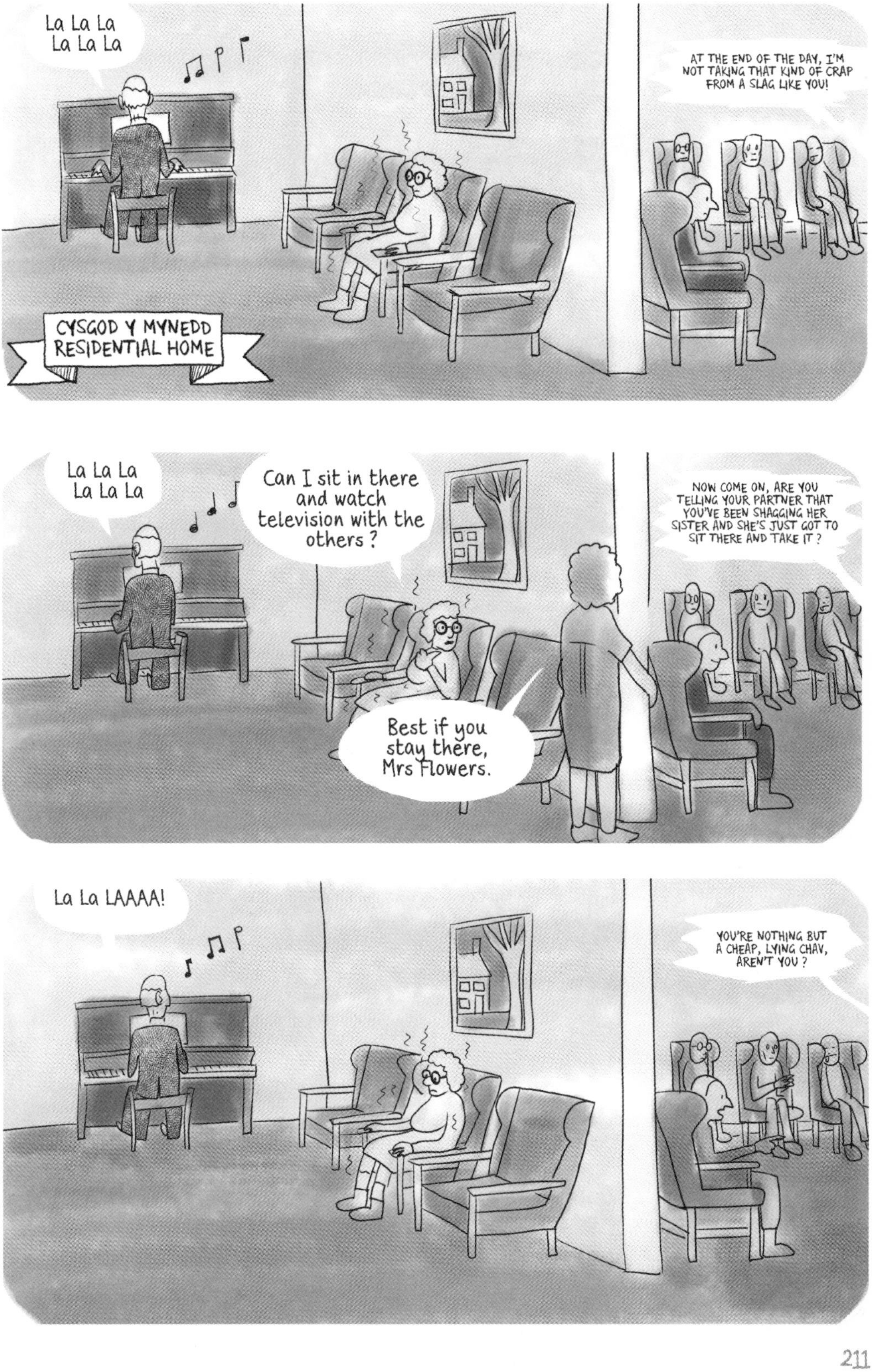

La La La La La La
AT THE END OF THE DAY, I'M NOT TAKING THAT KIND OF CRAP FROM A SLAG LIKE YOU!
CYSGOD Y MYNEDD RESIDENTIAL HOME
La La La La La La
Can I sit in there and watch television with the others ?
NOW COME ON, ARE YOU TELLING YOUR PARTNER THAT YOU'VE BEEN SHAGGING HER SISTER AND SHE'S JUST GOT TO SIT THERE AND TAKE IT ?
Best if you stay there, Mrs Flowers.
La La LAAAA!
YOU'RE NOTHING BUT A CHEAP, LYING CHAV, AREN'T YOU ?

X
T
A
R
O
WHEEL of FORTUNE

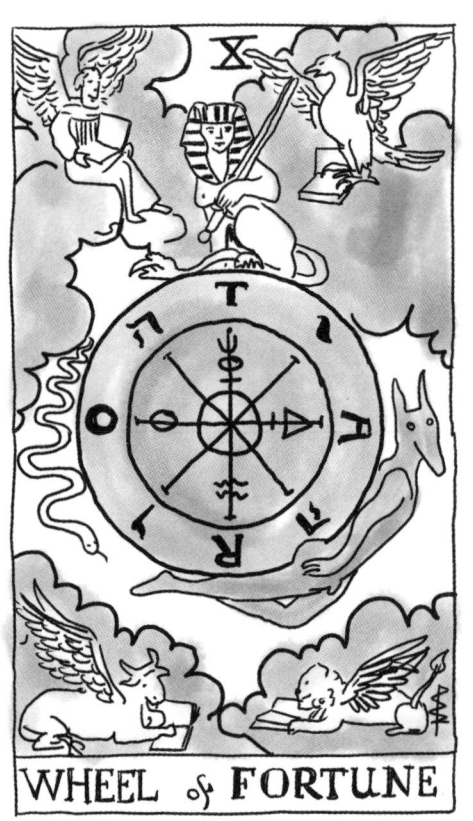

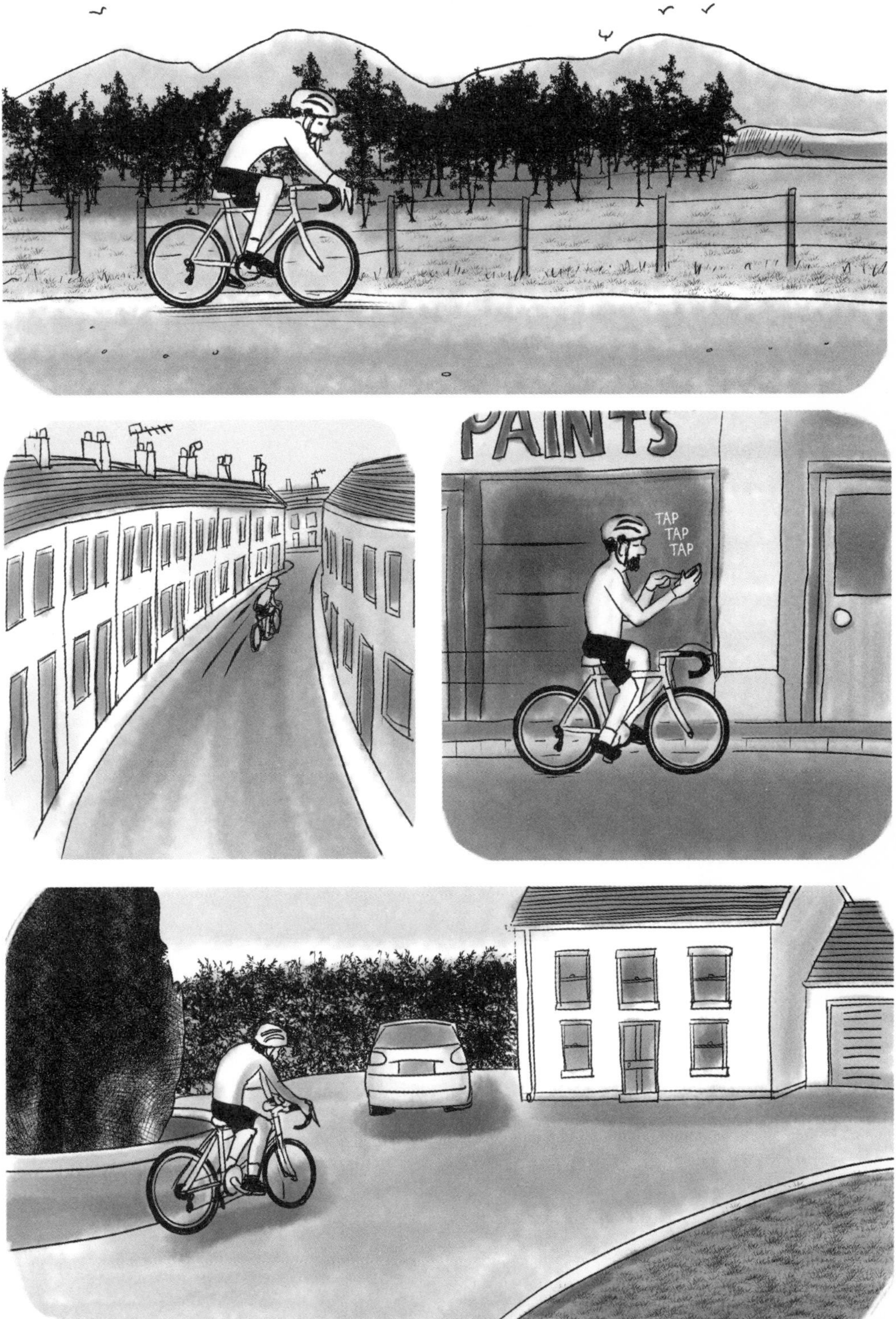
PAINTS
TAP
TAP
TAP

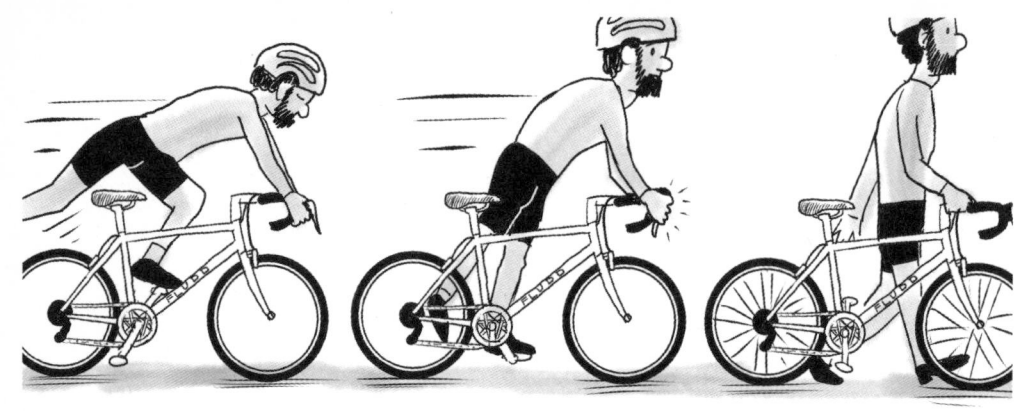

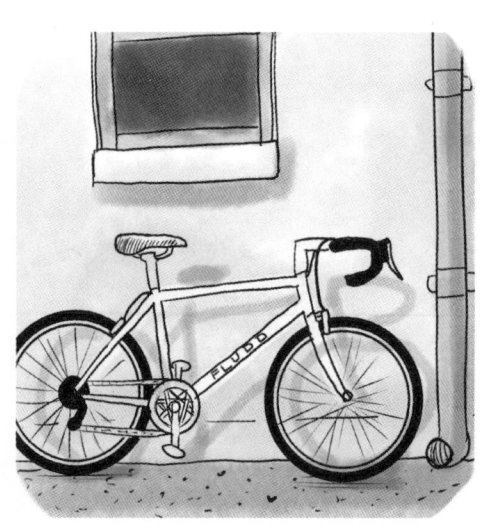

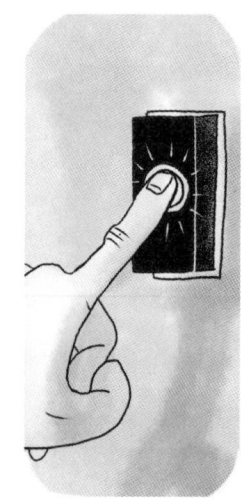

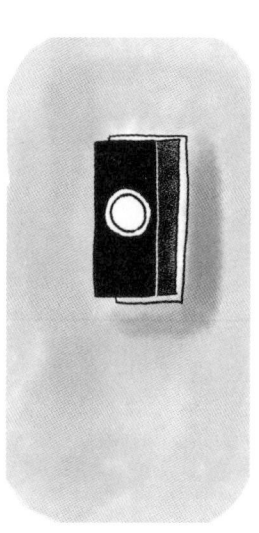

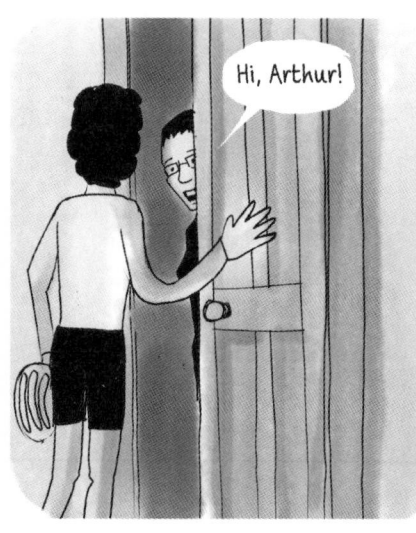

Hi, Arthur!

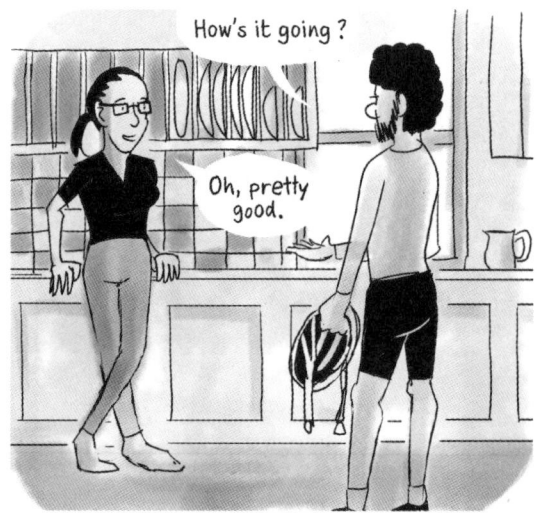

How's it going?

Oh, pretty good.

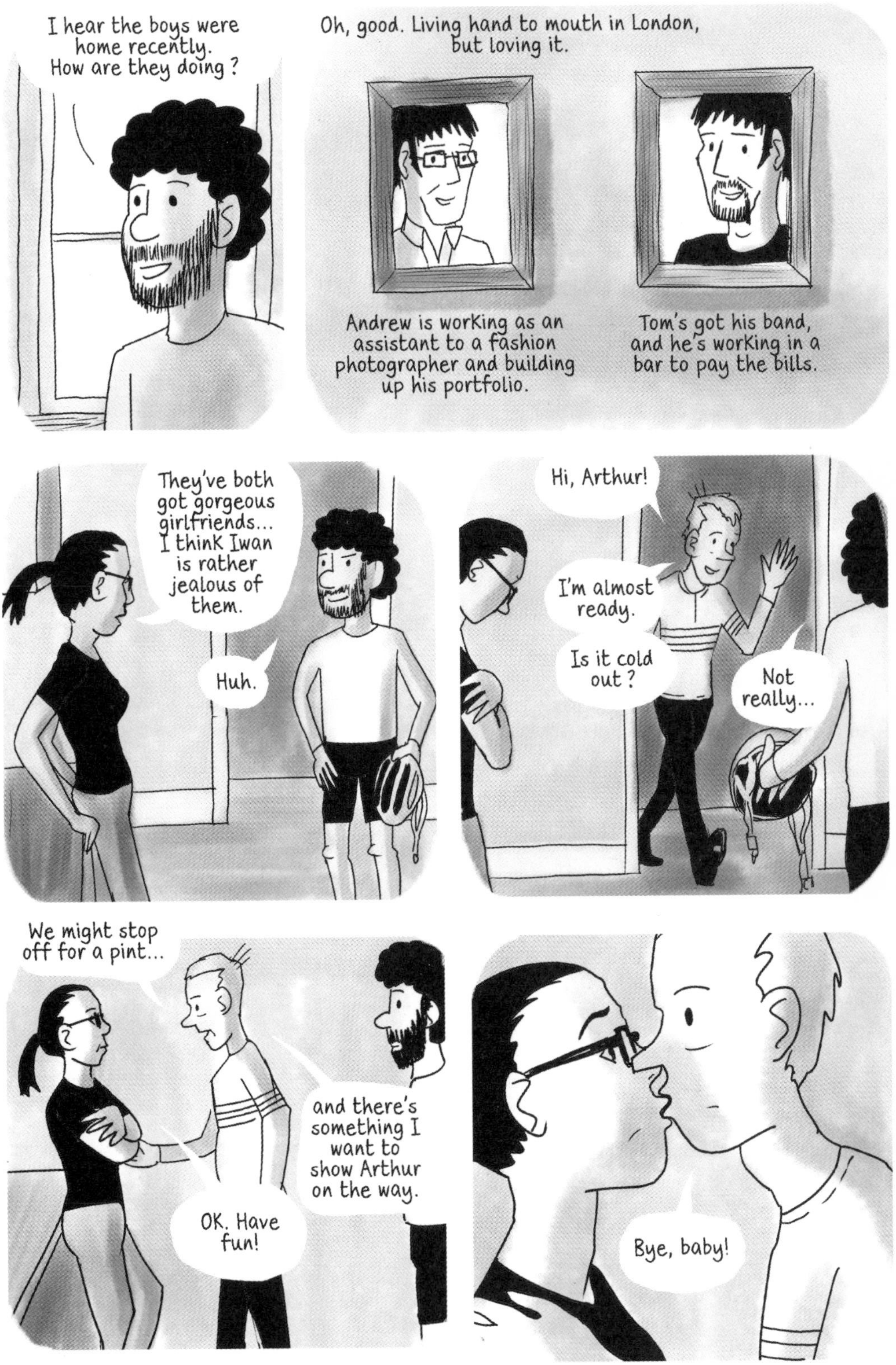
I hear the boys were home recently. How are they doing ?
Oh, good. Living hand to mouth in London, but loving it.
Andrew is working as an assistant to a fashion photographer and building up his portfolio.
Tom's got his band, and he's working in a bar to pay the bills.
They've both got gorgeous girlfriends... I think Iwan is rather jealous of them.
Huh.
Hi, Arthur!
I'm almost ready.
Is it cold out ?
Not really...
We might stop off for a pint...
and there's something I want to show Arthur on the way.
OK. Have fun!
Bye, baby!

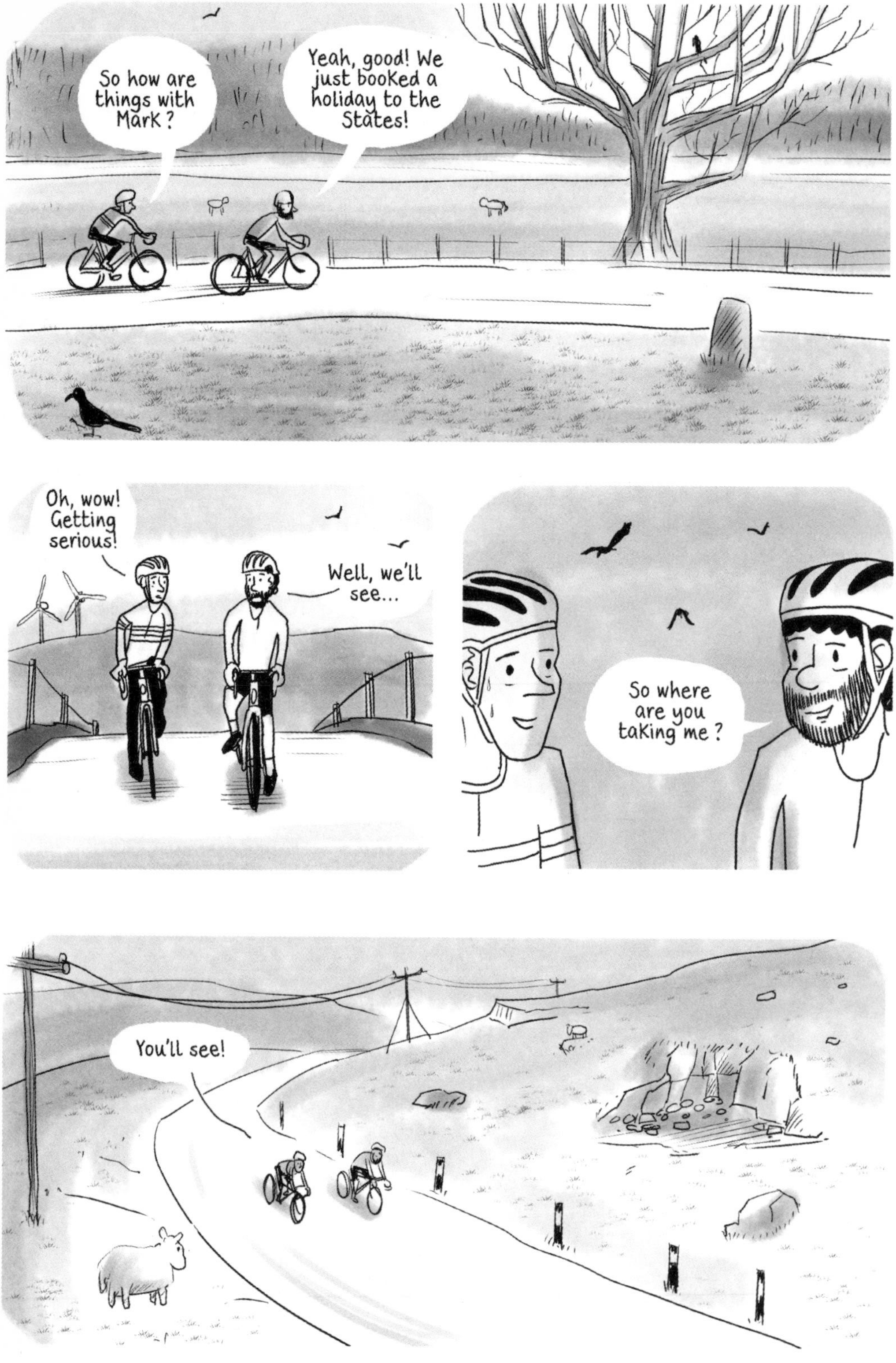
So how are things with Mark?
Yeah, good! We just booked a holiday to the States!
Oh, wow! Getting serious!
Well, we'll see...
So where are you taking me?
You'll see!

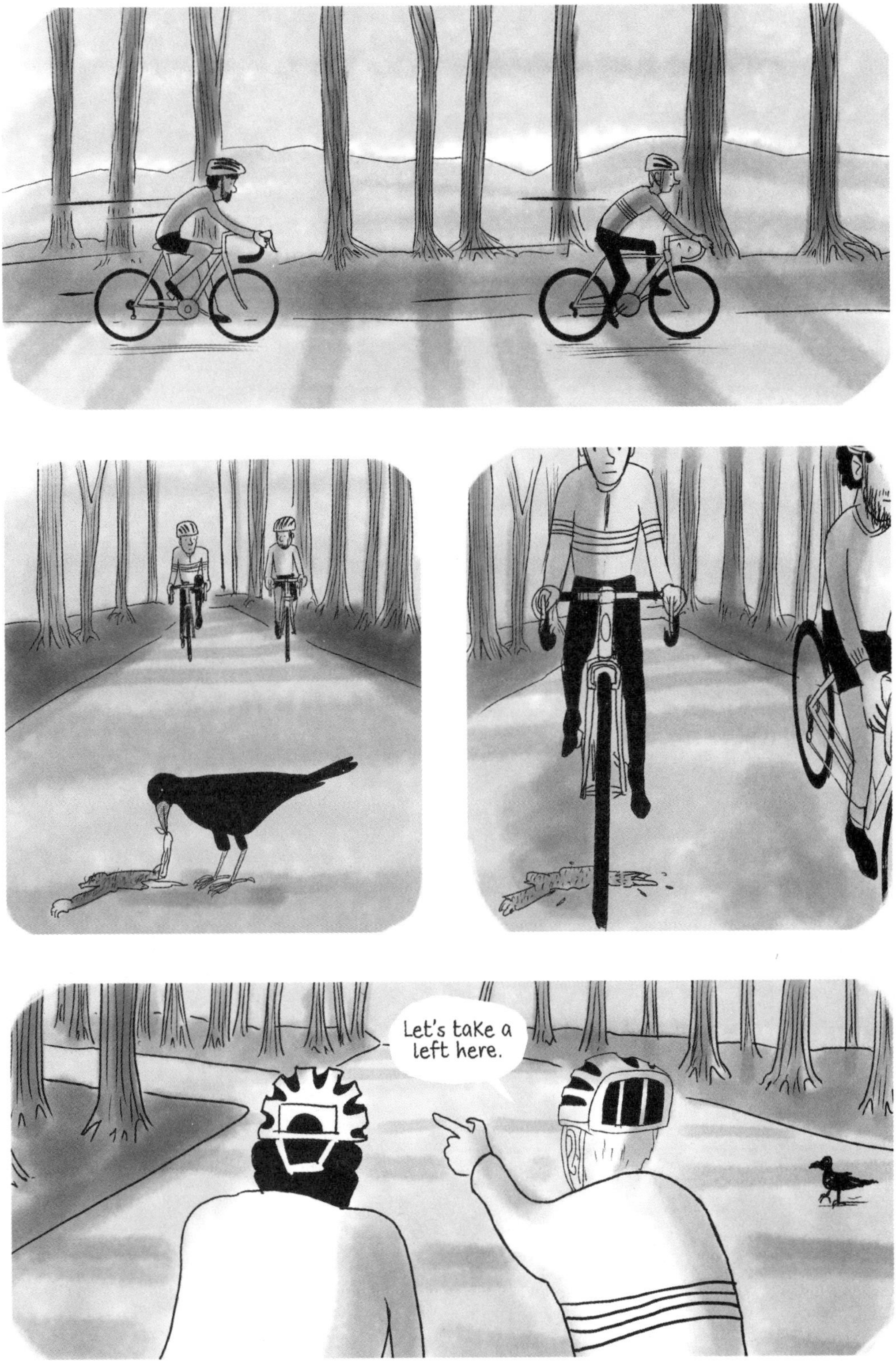
Let's take a left here.

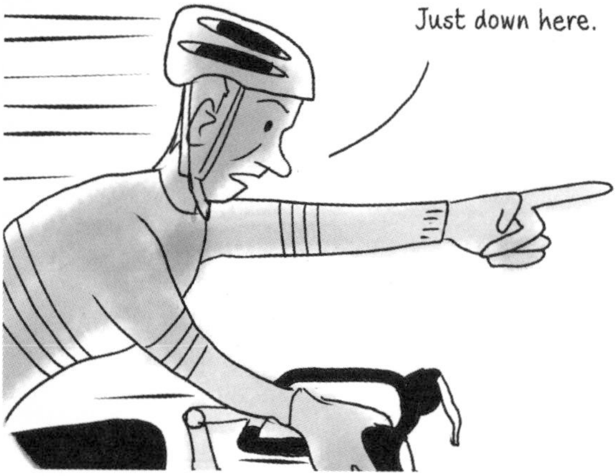
Just down here.

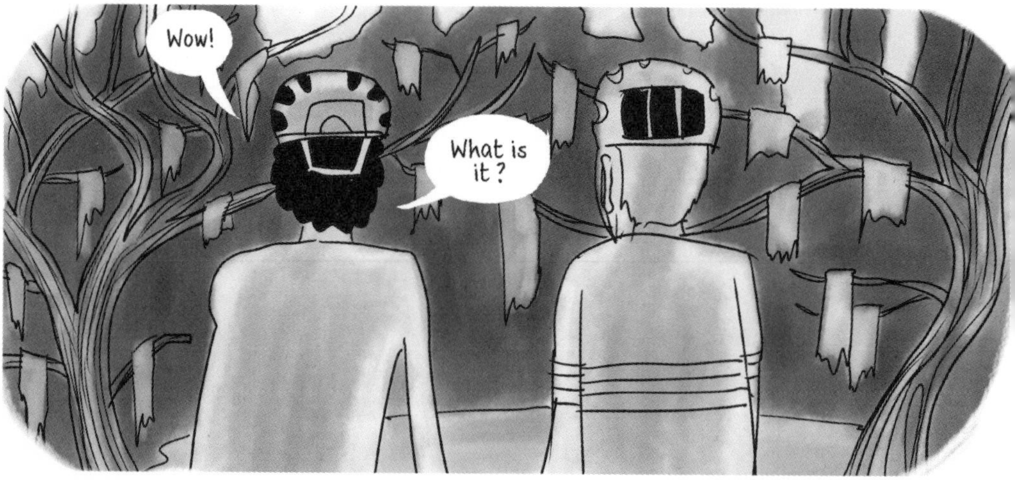
Wow!
What is it?

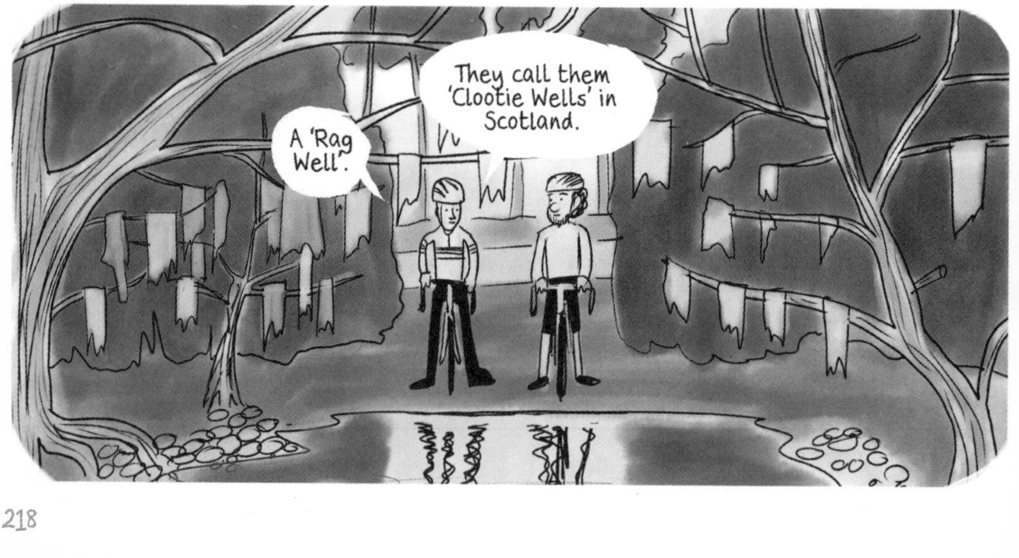
A 'Rag Well'.
They call them 'Clootie Wells' in Scotland.

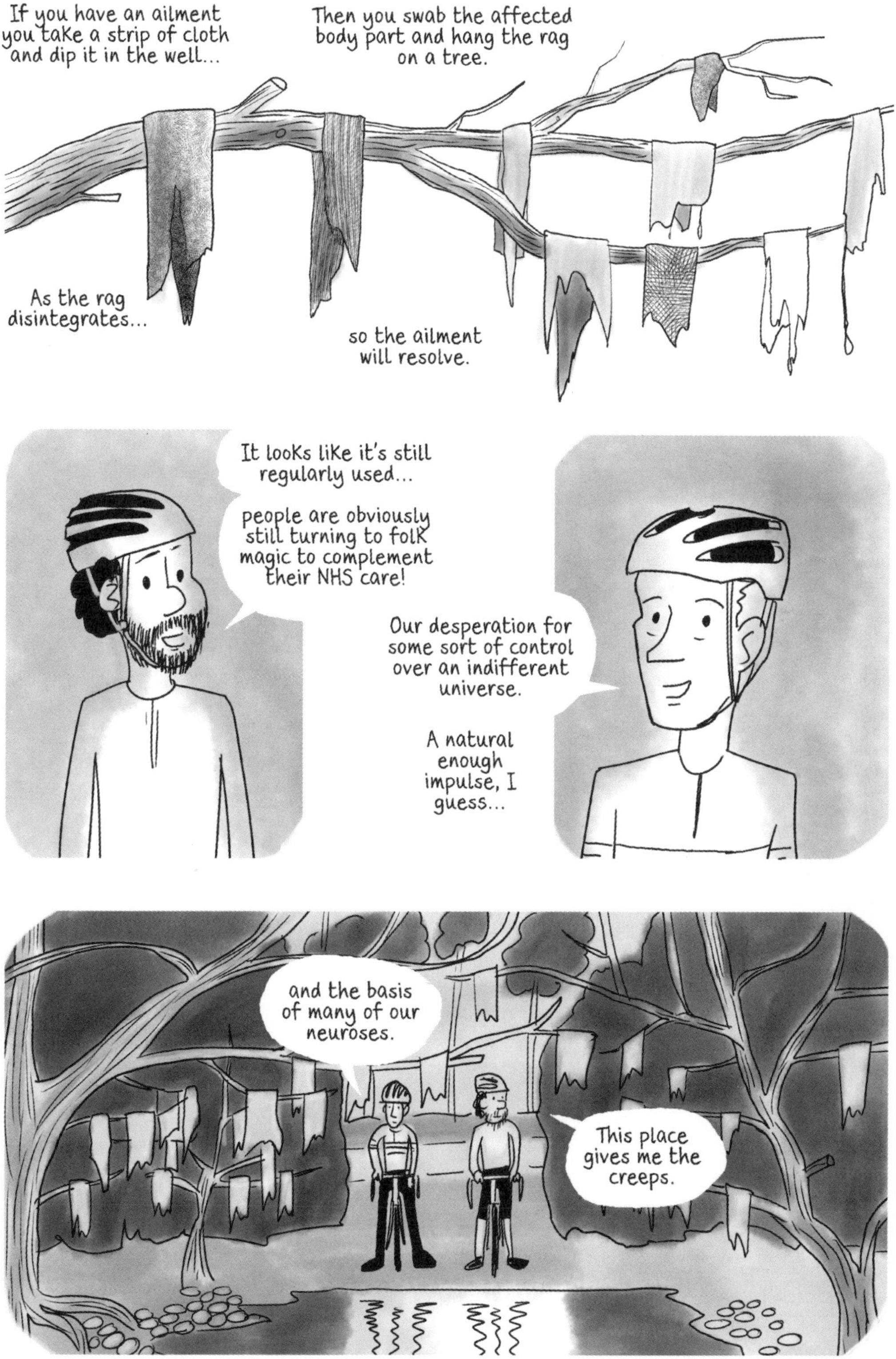
If you have an ailment you take a strip of cloth and dip it in the well...
Then you swab the affected body part and hang the rag on a tree.
As the rag disintegrates...
so the ailment will resolve.
It looks like it's still regularly used...
people are obviously still turning to folk magic to complement their NHS care!
Our desperation for some sort of control over an indifferent universe.
A natural enough impulse, I guess...
and the basis of many of our neuroses.
This place gives me the creeps.

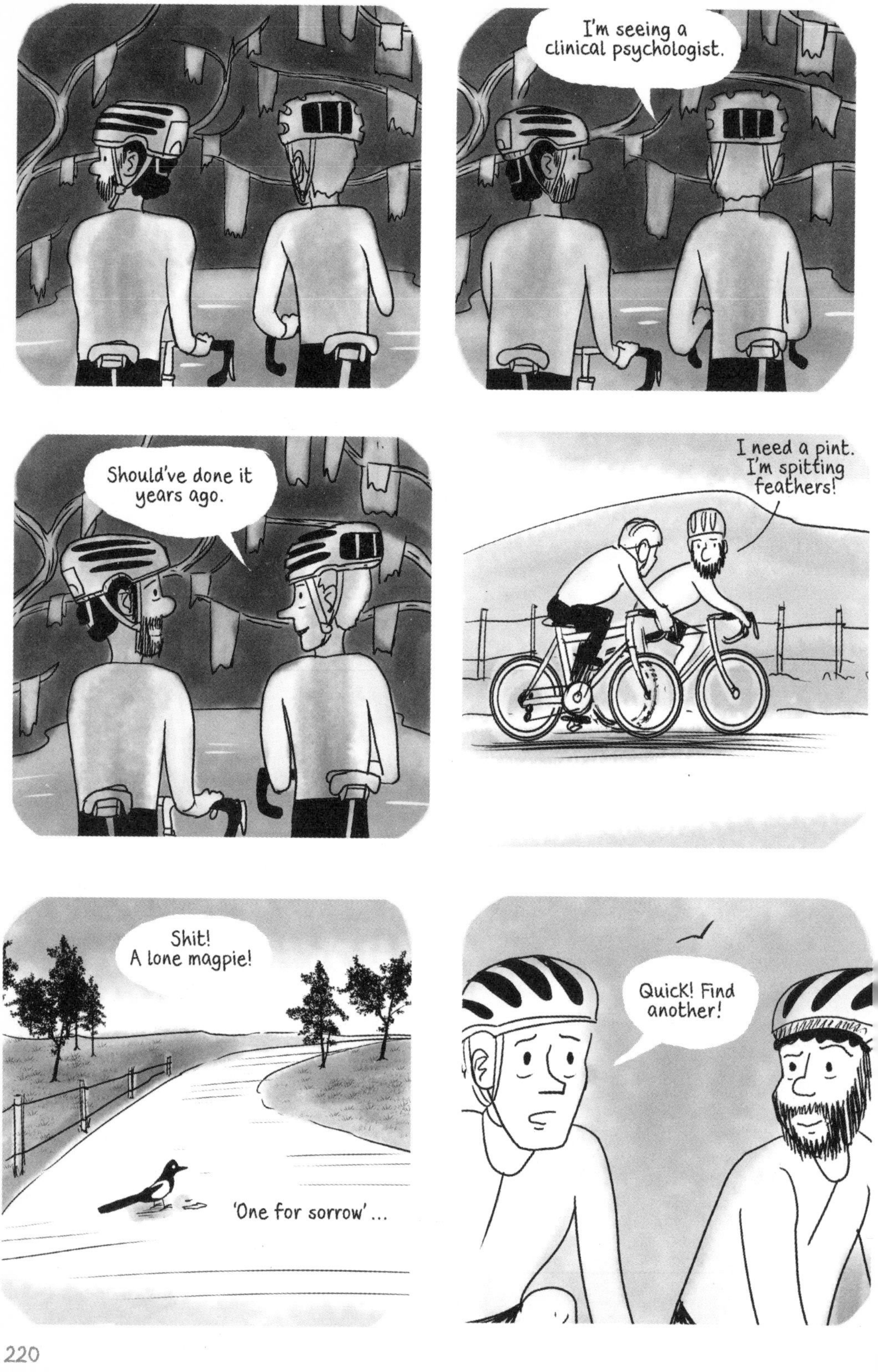
I'm seeing a clinical psychologist.
Should've done it years ago.
I need a pint. I'm spitting feathers!
Shit! A lone magpie!
'One for sorrow'...
Quick! Find another!

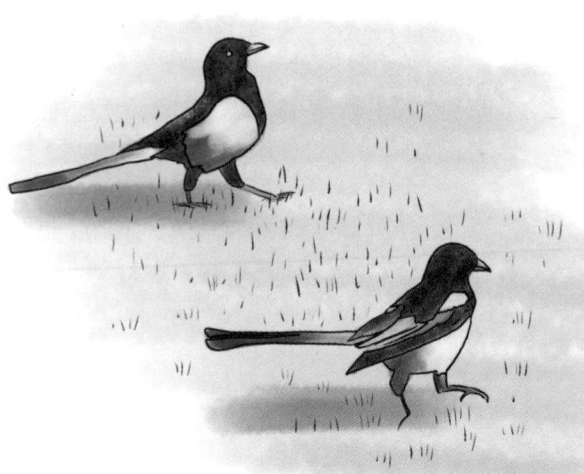

ACKNOWLEDGEMENTS:

I would like to thank Corinne Pearlman and Candida Lacey of Myriad Editions for having faith in me and for sound guidance throughout the production of this book.

I would like to thank the following people (in alphabetical order) for love, support, advice or encouragement during the various stages of this project:

Hannah Berry, Darryl Cunningham, MK Czerwiec, Megan Donnolly, Lizzie Enfield, Jamie Evans, Becky Farrington, Paul Gravett, Justin Green, Matt Green, Cindy Homan, Laura Jones, Paula Knight, Sarah Lightman, Mita Mahato, Linda McQueen, John Miers, Simon Moreton, Philippa Perry, Columba Quigley, David Small, Nicola Streeten, Ravi Thornton, Victoria Tischler, Emma Jane Unsworth, Maria Vaccarella and my parents.

I would also like to thank the Arts Council of Wales.

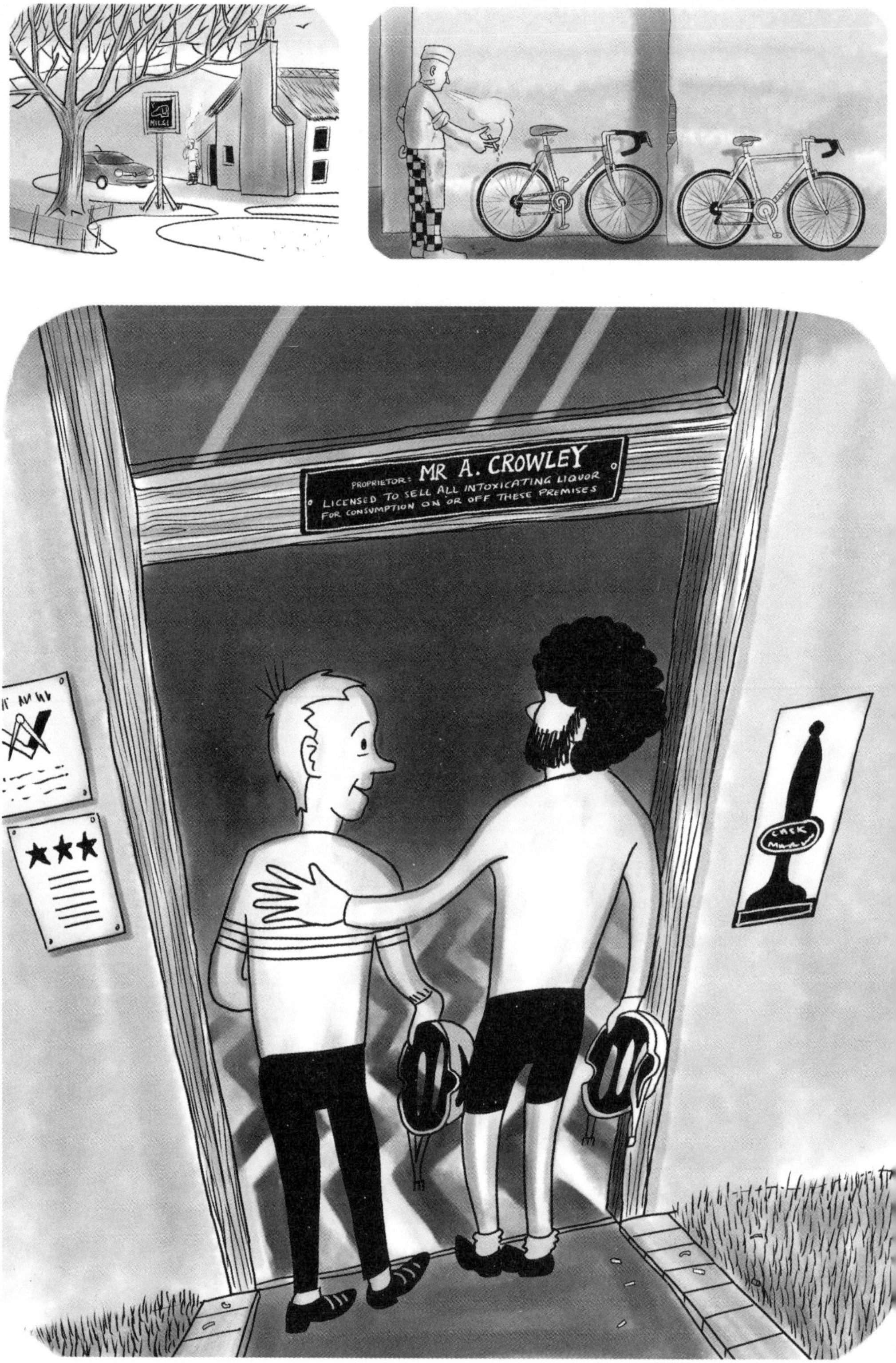
PROPRIETOR: MR A. CROWLEY
LICENSED TO SELL ALL INTOXICATING LIQUOR
FOR CONSUMPTION ON OR OFF THESE PREMISES